Hepatitis C: Infection and Disease

Hepatitis C: Infection and Disease

Edited by Terry May

AMERICAN
MEDICAL PUBLISHERS
www.americanmedicalpublishers.com

American Medical Publishers,
41 Flatbush Avenue,
1st Floor, New York,
NY 11217, USA

Visit us on the World Wide Web at:
www.americanmedicalpublishers.com

ISBN: 978-1-63927-190-0

Cataloging-in-Publication Data

Hepatitis C : infection and disease / edited by Terry May.
p. cm.
Includes bibliographical references and index.
ISBN 978-1-63927-190-0
1. Hepatitis C. 2. Hepatitis C--Infections. 3. Hepatitis C virus. I. May, Terry.
RC848.H425 H46 2022
616.362 3--dc23

Table of Contents

Preface

This book aims to highlight the current researches and provides a platform to further the scope of innovations in this area. This book is a product of the combined efforts of many researchers and scientists, after going through thorough studies and analysis from different parts of the world. The objective of this book is to provide the readers with the latest information of the field.

Hepatitis C is an infectious disease that is caused by the hepatitis C virus (HCV). It primarily affects the liver. It causes symptoms such as decreased appetite, fatigue and nausea in case of an acute infection. In case of chronic infections, it causes fatigue and mild cognitive problems. The chronic infection often leads to liver cirrhosis which can cause liver failure. It can also result in liver cancer or dilated blood vessels in the esophagus and stomach. Hepatitis C is a transmissible disease. It is often transmitted from drug use, sexual intercourse, blood transfusion and body modification such as tattooing. The diagnostic tests of hepatitis C include HCV antibody enzyme immunoassay, recombinant immunoblot assay and quantitative HCV RNA polymerase chain reaction. This book contains some path-breaking studies associated with hepatitis C. It brings forth some of the most innovative concepts and elucidates the unexplored aspects of diagnosis and treatment of hepatitis C. This book will serve as a valuable source of reference for graduate and postgraduate students.

I would like to express my sincere thanks to the authors for their dedicated efforts in the completion of this book. I acknowledge the efforts of the publisher for providing constant support. Lastly, I would like to thank my family for their support in all academic endeavors.

Editor

A population-based study of chronic hepatitis C in immigrants and non-immigrants in Quebec, Canada

Christina Greenaway[1,2*], Laurent Azoulay[2,3], Robert Allard[3,4], Joseph Cox[5], Viet Anh Tran[2], Claire Nour Abou Chakra[2], Russ Steele[2,6] and Marina Klein[7]

Abstract

Background: Immigrants originating from intermediate and high HCV prevalence countries may be at increased risk of exposure to hepatitis C infection (HCV) in their countries of origin, however they are not routinely screened after arrival in most low HCV prevalence host countries. We aimed to describe the epidemiology of HCV in immigrants compared to the Canadian born population.

Methods: Using the reportable infectious disease database linked to the landed immigration database and several provincial administrative databases, we assembled a cohort of all reported cases of HCV in Quebec, Canada (1998–2008). Underlying co-morbidities were identified in the health services databases. Stratum specific rates of reported cases/100,000, rate ratios (RRs) and trends over the study period were estimated.

Results: A total of 20,862 patients with HCV were identified, among whom 1922 (9.2%) were immigrants. Immigrants were older and diagnosed a mean of 9.8 ± 7 years after arrival. The Canadian born population was more likely to have behavior co-morbidities (problematic alcohol or drug use) and HIV co-infection. Immigrants from Sub-Saharan Africa, Asia and Eastern Europe had the highest HCV reported rates with RRs compared to non-immigrants ranging from 1.5 to 1.7. The age and sex adjusted rates decreased by 4.9% per year in non-immigrants but remained unchanged in immigrants. The proportion of HCV occurring in immigrants doubled over the study period from 5 to 11%.

Conclusions: Immigrants from intermediate and high HCV prevalence countries are at increased risk for HCV and had a mean delay in diagnosis of almost 10 years after arrival suggesting that they may benefit from targeted HCV screening and earlier linkage to care.

Keywords: Hepatitis C, Immigrant, Incidence, Rates, Viral hepatitis

Background

Health care utilization, costs and mortality due to hepatitis C infection are increasing in many low HCV prevalence countries in North America and Europe resulting in an enormous burden on society and health care systems [1–8]. Undetected chronic infections remain asymptomatic for decades until they progress to chronic liver disease and liver cancer [9]. HCV is now the leading infectious cause of death and the primary indication for liver transplants in Canada and the US [2, 3, 10, 11]. These sequelae are preventable through early screening and providing highly effective therapy that cures infection, stops the progression to liver disease and decreases all-cause mortality [12, 13]. Despite the benefits of curative therapy and recommendations for risk factor based screening almost half of all HCV infected persons in these low HCV prevalence countries remain undiagnosed [9, 14, 15]. Risk factor based programs recommend screening for those at increased risk for HCV exposure such as current or past intravenous drug use, those who have received blood products prior to routine HCV

* Correspondence: ca.greenaway@mcgill.ca
[1]Division of Infectious Diseases, Jewish General Hospital, McGill University, 3755 Côte St. Catherine Road, Room E-0057, Montreal PQ H3T 1E2, Canada
[2]Centre for Clinical Epidemiology, Lady Davis Research Institute for Medical Research, Jewish General Hospital, McGill University, Montreal, Canada
Full list of author information is available at the end of the article

screening of the blood supply, hemodialysis, and incarceration [16–18]. Identifying all HCV infected individuals and successfully linking them to care is therefore an urgent priority to reverse the escalating burden of HCV.

Immigrants living in low HCV prevalence countries are a large underappreciated group that are disproportionately affected by HCV infection. Many were born in intermediate and high HCV prevalence countries and thus at increased risk to have been exposed to HCV in their countries of origin [19, 20]. In intermediate and high HCV prevalence countries HCV infection are acquired primarily iatrogenically through contaminated needles, medical procedures, or due to the receipt of unscreened contaminated blood products whereas in low HCV prevalence countries, the primary mode of transmission is through intravenous drug use (IDU) [16–18, 21]. Many immigrants from intermediate/high HCV prevalence countries will therefore be missed in current risk factor based screening programs. In certain low HCV prevalence countries such as Japan and Italy, the HCV epidemiology is more complex and reflects changing temporal patterns of HCV transmission with high HCV rates in older cohorts that were remotely infected through iatrogenic transmission (eg. blood transfusions and unsafe medical procedures), whereas recent infections are occurring in those with percutaneous exposure such as intravenous drug users, and/or among incarcerated individuals [9, 22, 23]. Recent estimates suggest that the foreign-born population has a higher HCV seroprevalence (~2%) compared to host populations and account for a substantial proportion of HCV cases (35–50% or more) in Canada and many European countries, even though immigrants make up less than 20% of the population [15, 19, 24]. Despite this, immigrants are not routinely screened for viral hepatitis before or after arrival in most host countries. In a population-based cohort, we aimed to determine the rates of newly reported HCV cases, the trend over time, and behavioral risk factors for exposure to HCV in immigrants as compared to the Canadian born population. The objective of this study was to identify immigrant groups who would benefit most from targeted HCV screening and early linkage to care. These data may ultimately be used to inform policy making and health care planning.

Methods

We conducted a population-based retrospective study of all reported cases of hepatitis C and their associated health services in Quebec, Canada between January 1, 1998 and June 30, 2008 by linking three Quebec provincial administrative databases.

Data sources

The Quebec public health mandatory reportable (notifiable) infectious disease (MADO) database in which all laboratory confirmed cases of HCV are reported using standard definitions since 1998 [25]. The majority of laboratories began reporting HCV in 1998 even though obligatory reporting of HCV came into effect in 2002. The *Régie de l'assurance maladie du Québec* (RAMQ), is the universal free health care plan in Quebec and covers over 99% of the Quebec born and landed immigrant population. RAMQ manages the following provincial administrative databases; 1) the Quebec hospital discharge database (MED-ECHO) in which discharge diagnoses are coded using the International Classification of Diseases, Ninth Revision (ICD-9) up until March 2006 and ICD-10 from April 2006 onward (ICD-10), 2) the physician reimbursement claims (RAMQ-PB) for inpatient and ambulatory medical services with visit diagnoses classified with ICD-9 codes and 3) the provincial prescription plan (RAMQ-Pharm) contains information on all dispensed medications and covers ~50% of the population. The Québec landed immigrant database (MIDI) contains demographic information on all immigrants and refugees (~1,258,000) who have arrived and were given permission to live in Quebec since 1985 [26].

Cohort assembly

All cases of chronic HCV present in the MADO database between Jan 1, 1998 and June 30, 2008, were deterministically linked to the RAMQ databases through a unique health card number. All immigrants present in the MIDI database from January 1, 1985 to June 30, 2008 were deterministically linked to the RAMQ demographic database thorough the presence of a unique immigration number and allowed for classification of cases as occurring in immigrants (who arrived between 1985 and 2008) or in non-immigrants.

Variables

All reported cases of chronic HCV present in the MADO database were included. Chronic HCV included those with either past or current (viremic) infection and were defined as the presence of HCV antibody (anti-HCV) detected by an enzyme immunoassay (EIA) confirmed by a second test (a different EIA, RIBA, INNO-LIA or PCR), or a very high level of anti-HCV antibodies not requiring a confirmatory test, or a positive HCV RNA by reverse transcriptase polymerase chain reaction (RT-PCR) [25]. Acute HCV cases were excluded. The MIDI database included information on country of origin, date of arrival, and immigrant class at time of landing. Countries of origin were grouped into regions of origin as classified by the World Bank (Additional file 1: Table A1) [27]. Immigration status at the time of acceptance as a permanent resident was classified as either a refugee or an immigrant. Hepatitis C behavioral risk factors including problematic drug use (both recreational and prescribed drugs) or underlying co-morbidities such as problematic alcohol use, alcohol-related liver disease, and HIV, occurring in the year prior to HCV diagnosis were identified in the MED-ECHO and RAMQ-PB databases through the presence of diagnoses classified by ICD-9/10 codes [28, 29]. Additional cases of drug use and HIV we identified through the use of methadone or HIV specific medications present in the RAMQ-Pharm database (Additional file 1: Table A2).

Statistical analyses

Standard descriptive statistics were used when appropriate (*t*-test, Chi-2, and Fisher's exact test). Rates of reported HCV cases/100,000 with 95% confidence intervals (CIs) for the entire study period and per year in immigrants and non-immigrants were estimated with a Poisson distribution. Stratum-specific rates by age, sex, region of origin, and immigration class for immigrants and by age and sex for non-immigrants were also estimated. Numerators were derived from the database produced in this study. The denominator was estimated using census data for the population of Quebec in 1996, 2001, and 2006, with linear interpolation for the intercensal years. Rate ratios (RRs) and 95% CI of overall and stratum specific rates of reported HCV cases in immigrants as compared to the Canadian-born population were calculated with Poisson regression. The age and sex adjusted trends of reported rates of HCV cases over the study period were modeled with Poisson regression in immigrants and non-immigrants, separately. To estimate the impact of unlinked cases [19.8% of all cases ($N = 5255$)] on the calculated rates and to determine if the linkage was differential for immigrants and non-immigrants, inverse probability weighting was used [30, 31]. Two separate models were constructed using age, sex, address, and year of diagnosis from complete cases as predictive variables for immigrant status. These variables were chosen as immigrants were older, less likely to be male and to live in different neighbourhoods compared to non-immigrants. Additional methods and results are shown in the Additional file 1: Table A3. All analyses were performed using SAS® 9.4 (SAS Institute Inc., Cary, NC, USA).

Results

Between 1998 and 2008, 26 491 unique cases of chronic HCV were identified in the MADO database. Of these, 20,862 cases were included in the final cohort; 1922 cases (9.2%) in immigrants and 18 940 cases (90.8%) in non-immigrants (Fig. 1). A total of 5255 (19.8%) cases did not link due to anonymous reporting by certain clinics or missing demographic or RAMQ numbers. Additional cases were excluded because episodes occurred during a period of ineligibility for RAMQ of > 6 months or prior to permanent resident status (immigrants). Unlinked cases (19.8%) were slightly younger (41 vs 43 years), more likely to be male and to reside in certain regions such as Montreal, than linked cases (Additional file 1: Table A4). They were not found to be differentially distributed between immigrants and non-immigrants after imputing with inverse probability weighting. The RR was similar for unweighted and weighted incidence; 0.85 (0.81–0.90) vs 0.87 (0.84–0.91) (Additional file 1: Table A3). All reported rates are therefore likely to be 20% higher than estimated for both groups.

Demographic characteristics and comorbidities of HCV cases are shown in Table 1. Cases in immigrants were older than in non-immigrants and were less likely to be male. Immigrant cases originated mainly from East Asia and the Pacific region (23%), Eastern Europe and Central Asia (14.7%), and the Middle East and North Africa (13%). The mean time to diagnosis of HCV after

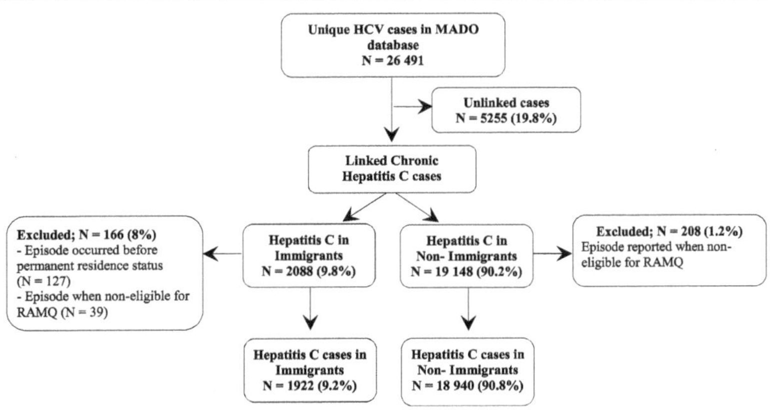

Fig. 1 Flow chart for hepatitis C cases identification and Cohorts' creation

Table 1 Demographic characteristics of chronic hepatitis C cases (1998–2008) in immigrants and non-immigrants

Characteristics	Immigrants (*N* = 1922)	Non-immigrants (*N* = 18 940)	*P*-value
Age at time of HCV diagnosis (years)			
Mean (SD)	47.5 (15.1)	43.2 (13.3)	<0.001
Age group (years)			
< 15	11 (0.6)	104 (0.5)	<0.001
15–19	17 (0.9)	297 (1.6)	
20–29	133 (6.9)	2040 (10.8)	
30–39	452 (23.5)	5114 (27.0)	
40–49	588 (30.6)	6666 (35.2)	
50–59	324 (16.9)	2705 (14.3)	
60–69	193 (10.0)	1022 (5.4)	
≥ 70	203 (10.6)	991 (5.2)	
Sex			
Female	891 (46.4)	6004 (31.7)	<0.001
Male	1031 (53.6)	12,936 (68.3)	
Residence area by public health region			
Montréal	1488 (77.4)	7104 (37.5)	<0.001
Montérégie	157 (8.2)	2674 (14.1)	
Laval	105 (5.5)	747 (3.9)	
Capitale-Nationale	52 (2.7)	1713 (9.0)	
Laurentides	28 (1.5)	1582 (8.4)	
Outaouais	32 (1.7)	905 (4.8)	
Estrie	25 (1.3)	694 (3.7)	
Mauricie et du Centre-du-Québec	8 (0.4)	1132 (5.9)	
Other regions	35 (1.8)	2389 (12.6)	
Immigration category			
Permanent residents[a]	1209 (62.9)		
Refugee	522 (27.2)		
Missing	191 (9.9)		
Region of origin[b]			
East Asia and Pacific	443 (23.0)		
Eastern Europe and Central Asia	287 (14.9)		
Middle East and North Africa	255 (13.3)		
Latin America and Caribbean	205 (10.7)		
South Asia	181 (9.4)		
Western Europe	167 (8.7)		
Sub-Saharan Africa	152 (7.9)		
US, Australia, and New Zealand	22 (1.1)		
Missing	209 (10.9)		
Mean Time to diagnosis after arrival (years) (SD)	9.8 (7.0)		
Co-morbidities prior to diagnosis			
Problematic alcohol use	29 (1.5)	2419 (12.8)	<0.001
Alcohol-related liver disease	30 (1.6)	581 (3.1)	0.0003
Problematic drug abuse	47 (2.5)	4520 (23.9)	<0.001
HIV	23 (1.2)	874 (4.6)	<0.001

[a]Other categories included permanent residents who were workers, spouses, children, and students
[b]Countries of origin regrouped according to the World Bank criteria [27]. Top 10 countries were Vietnam (226), Pakistan (128), Cambodia (123), Romania (118), Haiti (111), Morocco (92), France (90), Egypt (60), Congo (55), and Russia (36) accounting for 54% of all cases

arrival in Quebec was 9.8 ± 7.0 years. There were significant differences between the prevalence of comorbidities. The Canadian born population was significantly more likely than immigrants to have behavioral co-morbidities such as problematic alcohol or drug use and to be HIV co-infected (Table 1). The prevalence of problematic drug use in immigrants was not significantly different by country/region of origin or immigration categories: the frequency of problematic drug use ranged between 1% in East Asia to 4% in the Middle East and North Africa, and was 2% overall for both refugees and other immigrants.

Rates of reported cases of chronic hepatitis C

The rate of reported cases of HCV was higher in non-immigrants compared to all immigrants [27.1 vs 23.2/100,000, RR 0.85 (95% CI 0.80, 0.90)] (Table 2). Immigrants from low/intermediate income countries (ie. excluding immigrants from Western Europe, the US, Australia and New Zealand) however, had higher rates compared to non-immigrants; 32.3/100,000 with a RR of 1.19 (95% CI 1.13, 1.25). Rates of reported HCV cases adjusted for age and sex decreased by 4.89% per year in non-immigrants between 1998 and 2008 whereas it increased slightly by 0.27% per year in all immigrants (Fig. 2). The proportion of all HCV cases occurring in immigrants doubled during the study period; they accounted for 5.1% of all cases in 1998 and 11.1% of all cases in 2008. The overall reported rate of all HCV cases present in the MADO database (includes both linked and unlinked cases) between 1998 and 2008 was 33.9/100,000 (95% CI 33.5, 34.3). Supplemental data for all cases in the MADO database from 1991 to 2008 are presented in the Additional file 1: Table A5.

Reported rates of all hepatitis C cases per year stratified by sex are shown in Additional file 1: Figure A1. Reported HCV rates in all immigrant females were slightly higher over the study period compared to non-immigrant females with overall rates of 21.1 and 17/100,000 respectively [RR 1.25 (1.17–1.35)] (Table 2). HCV rates were lower in all immigrant males compared to non-immigrant males with overall rates of 25.3 and

Table 2 Rates of Reported Cases of HCV per 100,000 from 1998 to 2008 (95% CI)

Characteristic	Immigrants		Non-immigrants		RR[a] (95% CI)
	N	Reported rate (95% CI)	N	Reported rate (95% CI)	
Overall	1922	23.2 (22.1–24.2)	18 940	27.1 (26.7–27.5)	0.85 (0.8–0.9)
Low/Intermediate income source countries[b]	1733	32.3 (30.8–33.8)			1.2 (1.1–1.3)
Age groups (years)					
< 15	12	2.08 (0.90–3.26)	105	0.79 (0.64–0.94)	2.63 (1.45–4.77)
15–19	17	5.15 (2.70–7.60)	297	6.28 (5.56–6.99)	0.82 (0.50–1.34)
20–29	133	14.1 (11.7–16.5)	2040	22.6 (21.6–23.5)	0.62 (0.52–0.74)
30–39	452	28.4 (25.8–31.2)	5114	53.1 (51.7–54.6)	0.54 (0.49–0.59)
40–49	588	38.3 (35.2–41.4)	6666	56.9 (55.6–58.3)	0.67 (0.62–0.73)
50–59	324	24.2 (21.5–26.8)	2705	28.5 (27.5–29.6)	0.85 (0.75–0.95)
60–69	193	19.6 (16.8–22.4)	1022	16.5 (15.5–17.5)	1.19 (1.02–1.38)
≥ 70	203	20.5 (17.7–23.4)	991	17.1 (16.1–18.2)	1.20 (1.03–1.39)
Sex					
Female	891	21.1 (19.8–22.5)	60,004	17.0 (16.4–17.3)	1.25 (1.17–1.35)
Male	1031	25.3 (23.7–26.8)	12,936	37.8 (37.2–38.5)	0.67 (0.63–0.71)
Region of origin					
Sub-Saharan Africa	152	47.2 (39.7–54.7)			1.7 (1.5–2.0)
East Asia and Pacific	443	43.7 (39.6–47.8)			1.6 (1.5–1.8)
Eastern Europe and Central Asia	287	43.1 (38.1–48.1)			1.6 (1.4–1.8)
South Asia	181	41.5 (35.4–47.5)			1.5 (1.3–1.8)
Middle East and North Africa	255	19.0 (16.7–21.4)			0.7 (0.6–0.8)
Latin America and Caribbean	205	14.1 (12.2–16.0)			0.5 (0.5–0.6)
US, Australia, and New Zealand	22	7.8 (4.5–11.1)			0.3 (0.2–0.4)
Western Europe	167	6.6 (5.6–7.6)			0.2 (0.2–0.3)
Countries of origin[c]					
Viet Nam	226	53.0 (45.9–60.1)			1.9 (1.7–2.2)
Pakistan	128	123.1 (101.6–144.6)			4.5 (3.8–5.4)
Cambodia	123	116.6 (95.6–137.5)			4.3 (3.6–5.1)
Romania	118	39.3 (31.9–46.6)			1.4 (1.2–1.7)
Haiti	111	13.0 (10.5–15.4)			0.5 (0.4–0.6)
Morocco	92	24.0 (19.0–29.0)			0.9 (0.7–1.1)
France	90	10.0 (7.8–12.1)			0.4 (0.3–0.5)
Egypt	60	21.7 (15.2–27.2)			0.8 (0.6–1.0)
Congo	55	151.0 (110.0–192.0)			5.6 (4.3–7.3)
Russia	36	53.5 (40.7–66.3)			2.0 (1.4–2.7)

[a]Rate ratio comparing immigrants to non-immigrants, overall and in each category
[b]Immigrants from Western Europe, USA, Australia and New Zealand were excluded
[c]Top 10 Countries of Origin with the largest number of cases accounting for 54% of all immigrant cases

37.8/100,000 respectively [RR 0.67; 95% CI 0.63–0.71]. Rates of HCV in non-immigrants males and females both decreased over the study period whereas HCV rates did not change in immigrant males and females (Fig. 3). Reported HCV rates also differed by age group between immigrants and non-immigrants; in immigrants cases were found in all age groups. Those who were younger (<15 years) and older (≥60 years) were more likely to be immigrants whereas young and middle aged adults (20–50 years) were more likely to be non-immigrants (Table 2). Reported HCV rates were higher in immigrants from Sub-Saharan Africa, East Asia and Pacific, Eastern Europe and Central Asia, and South Asia (47.2, 43.7, 43.1 and 41.5/100,000 respectively) compared to those in non-immigrants (27.1/100,000). Rate ratios ranged from 1.5 to 1.7 in these immigrant groups compared to non-

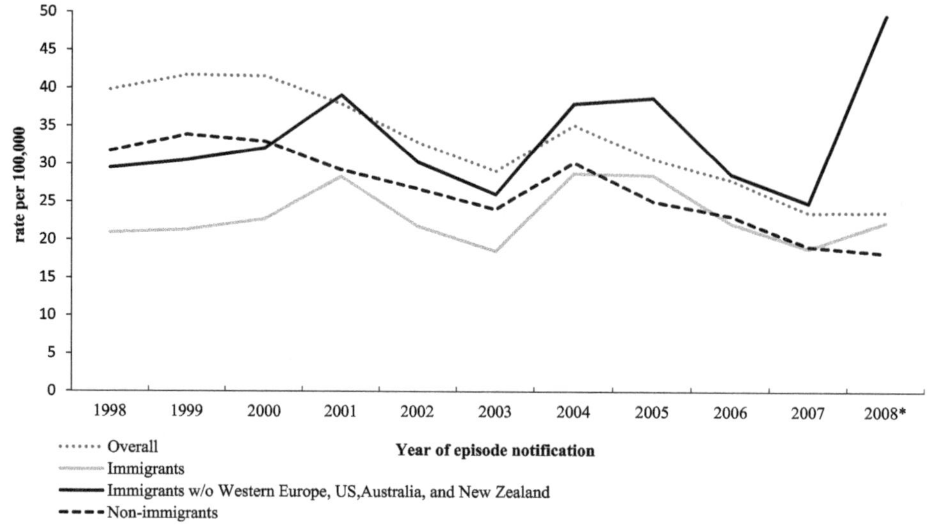

Fig. 2 Reported rates of HCV Cases/100,000 overall and in immigrants and non-immigrants (1998–2008). Between 1998 and 2008, the rate of reported HCV cases adjusted for age and sex decreased by 4.89% per year in non-immigrants (95% CI = 4.85–4.93; p <0.001) compared to a 0.27% annual increase in immigrants (95% CI = 0.03–0.51; p = 0.028)

immigrants (Table 2, Fig. 4). Reported HCV rates were particularly high in immigrants from Congo, Pakistan, Cambodia, Russia and Vietnam (Table 2).

Discussion

Immigrants from intermediate and high HCV prevalence regions of Sub-Saharan Africa, Asia and Eastern Europe had a 1.5–1.7-fold higher risk of HCV compared to non-immigrants. Immigrants were older and less likely to be male compared to non-immigrants cases and were diagnosed a mean of almost 10 years after arrival. Non-immigrant cases were more likely than immigrant cases to have behavioral co-morbidities such as problematic alcohol or drug use, and to be HIV co-infected. The age and sex adjusted HCV annual notification rate decreased by almost 5% per year in non-immigrants but remained relatively unchanged in immigrants between 1998 and 2008. As a consequence, the proportion of HCV cases

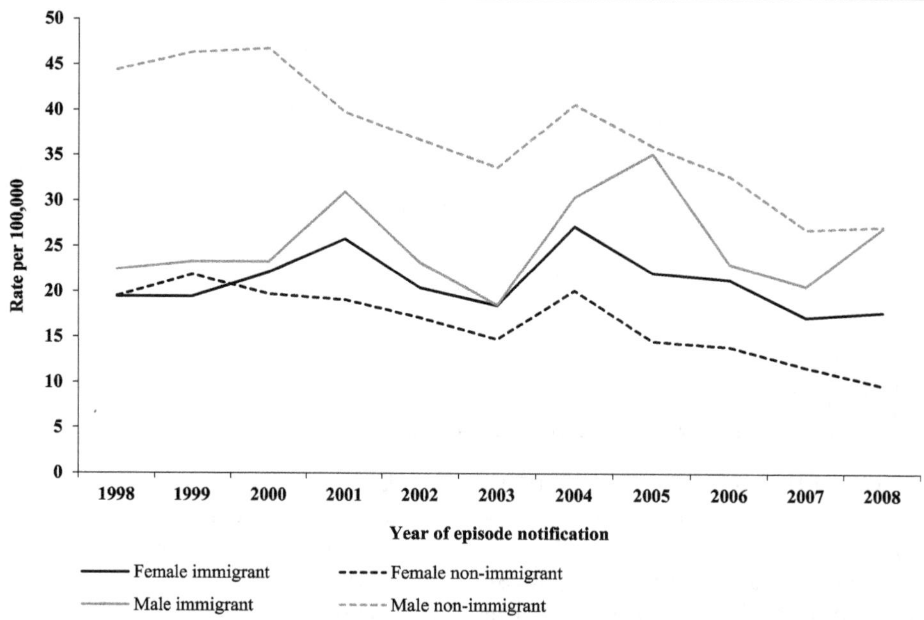

Fig. 3 Reported rates of HCV cases/100,000 by sex and immigrant status (1998–2008). Between 1998 and 2008, the annual HCV cumulative incidence adjusted for age decreased by 5.21% per year in non-immigrant females and by 4.72% in non-immigrant males compared to 0.60% decrease in immigrant females and 1.18% annual increase in immigrant males (p <0.001)

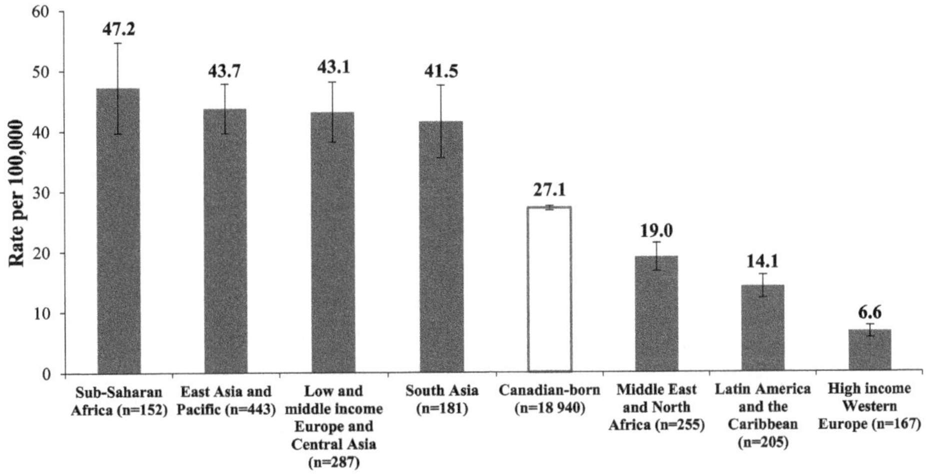

Fig. 4 Reported rates of HCV cases /100,000 (95% CI) by region of origin

occurring in immigrants doubled over the study period from 5 to 11%.

In our study, immigrants from Sub-Saharan Africa, Asia and Eastern Europe had a higher HCV risk compared to non-immigrants whereas immigrants from North Africa and the Middle East and Latin America and the Caribbean had a lower risk. The pattern of the magnitude of HCV risk by region of origin in immigrants in our study reflects published epidemiology of HCV in immigrants after arrival in host countries as well as in their countries of origin [18, 24, 32]. HCV seroprevalence is a reasonable surrogate measure for the magnitude of HCV risk by region of origin and was used as there were no comparative studies on HCV notification rates in immigrants. HCV seroprevalence in Asia, Africa, and Central and Eastern Europe is intermediate to high (2 to 4%) whereas it is low (1–2%) in Canada, Western Europe, the US, Latin America and the Caribbean and most countries in North Africa except Egypt and Iraq [15, 19, 32]. Furthermore, high HCV reported rates in immigrants from Congo (151/100,000 and RR 5.6), Pakistan (123; 4.5), and Cambodia (117; 4.3) and are also consistent with global epidemiology as these countries all have a high HCV seroprevalence ranging from 2.3 to 6.7% [32].

We found major demographic and behavioral differences between immigrants and non-immigrants with HCV. The demographic and behavior characteristics of HCV in non-immigrants is consistent with the characteristics of HCV cases in Canadian surveillance data [15, 33]. HCV cases in Canada occur more frequently in males and in current and previous intravenous drug users and have a high risk of HIV co-infection [15, 33]. There is little data on HCV-infected immigrants in Canada or other high income countries. Our findings are similar to two other Canadian studies that also found that immigrants with HCV were older, and were less likely to be male or to have problematic drug use compared to non-immigrants [34, 35]. In our study there were significant differences in the HCV risk by age group for immigrants and non-immigrants. Male and female immigrants of all ages were found to have HCV, likely reflecting the fact that exposure to contaminated blood or unsafe medical procedures can occur at any age and equally by gender. In non-immigrants, cases were more likely to occur in young and middle age adults and reflects the age group at highest risk for initiation and active intravenous drug use [21]. Although the numbers are small, immigrants <15 years of age were more likely to have HCV than non-immigrants and may, in part, be due to perinatal transmission.

The decreasing trend of reported HCV cases seen in non-immigrants of 4.9% per year between 1998 and 2008 is consistent with the trends of notified HCV cases in Canada, the US and Australia over this same period [9, 33]. In contrast, rates of reported cases in immigrants during this same period remained unchanged. This could be explained by increased screening or reporting of HCV in immigrants, newly acquired infections after arrival, increased numbers of immigrants from at risk countries arriving over the study period, or a steady rate of imported HCV cases acquired in their country of origin in the setting of no routine post-arrival screening. The latter is the most likely explanation given that HCV screening in Canada during the study period was focussed on those with risk factors for HCV exposure such as intravenous drug use and did not identify immigrants as a high risk group [16, 36]. Furthermore, immigrants are at low risk for HCV transmission after arrival in Canada given the low prevalence of problematic drug use in this group and the fact that the number of new immigrants from at risk countries was stable during the study period [20]. With this dataset we cannot eliminate the possibility that immigrants may have become infected with HCV after arrival in Canada during periods of travel back to their countries of origin. Canadian immigrants are less likely to access health care due to several barriers including language, cultural difference or infrastructure [37, 38]. This coupled with the lack of a targeted HCV screening program may explain the 10-year timeframe to diagnosis after arrival. These findings, taken together, support the hypothesis that immigrants are most likely to have been infected with HCV in their countries of origin through unscreened blood products or unsafe medical procedures rather than through injecting drugs in Canada. The long asymptomatic period of chronic HCV and lower health care access may explain the long delay in diagnosis after arrival.

The major strengths of this study are that it is a large population based sample spanning almost a 10-year period in which immigration status was accurately assigned through linkage with the landed immigration database. All notified HCV cases were ascertained, were laboratory confirmed, and acute and chronic cases were identified and differentiated with standardized case definitions. This study has some limitations including the well-known underestimation of cases in a passive surveillance system such as MADO. These data are also influenced by health seeking behavior, non-nominal reporting for some groups, and increased screening of those at increased risk of hepatitis such as drug users. Due to the anonymous reporting of certain cases or due to missing demographic information or RAMQ numbers, almost 20% of cases did not link. Unlinked cases were not differentially distributed between immigrants and non-immigrants, thus calculated rates in this study are under estimated by 20% in both groups, but without misclassification between these groups. The increased reported HCV rate observed between 2002 and 2004 is likely due to the fact that HCV became reportable in Quebec in 2002 and that there was enhanced surveillance during this period of time [39]. We only have access to data up until 2008 however, we expect that the trends in case rates, underlying co-morbidities and time to diagnosis after arrival for immigrants found in our study would be similar to that after 2008. This is because there are no targeted HCV screening programs for immigrants in Quebec or Canada and this was the case both before and 2008. The accuracy of diagnostic codes to detect co-morbidities in RAMQ databases has not been validated, however good accuracy has been shown in other administrative databases [29]. Administrative coding for problematic drug use is limited by the fact that it is not possible to determine if drug use was intravenous or by another route and cases of prior drug use (in those not actively using drugs), may not be detected. We used the same codes for problematic drug use as were used in a recently published study [28]. Despite these limitations our data show important trends in HCV in immigrants compared to non-immigrants that are both plausible and are externally validated.

Untreated HCV is an enormous health and economic burden in Canada and other low HCV prevalence countries. This burden is projected to increase over the next decade unless the large pool of asymptomatic infected individuals are detected and treated prior to developing end stage liver disease [40, 41]. Eradication of HCV is now within reach given the recent availability of highly effective, well tolerated, short course, direct acting antiviral treatments [12]. Identifying all asymptomatic HCV-infected individuals and successfully linking them to care is a critical issue that will need to be addressed in order to decrease the rising economic and individual burden from HCV.

Conclusions

Immigrants born in intermediate and high HCV prevalence countries living in Canada are at increased risk for HCV, less likely to have behavioral risk factors for HCV and in the absence of a routine screening program were diagnosed a mean of almost 10 years after arrival. These immigrants are an important group to consider for targeted HCV screening and early linkage to care.

Abbreviations

CI: Confidence interval; HCV: Hepatitis C virus; ICD: International classification of disease; IDU: Intravenous drug use; MADO: Maladies à declaration obligatoire; The Quebec public health mandatory reportable infectious disease; MED-ECHO: Maintenance et exploitation des données pour l'étude de la clientèle hospitalière; the Quebec hospital discharge database; MIDI: Ministère de l'Immigration, de la Diversité et de l'Inclusion; Provincial Ministry of immigration; RAMQ: The Régie de l'assurance maladie du Québec; Administers the provincial public health and prescription drug insurance plans; RAMQ-PB: RAMQ Physician billing; the physician reimbursement claims; RAMQ-Pharm: RAMQ Pharmacy billing; RR: Rate ratio

Acknowledgments

Not applicable.

Funding

This study was funded in full by Fonds de recherche du Québec-Santé (FRQS), grant #14364.

Authors' contributions

CG designed the study, supervised the analyses, interpreted the data, drafted and reviewed the manuscript. LA, RA, JC, RS, MK provided advice on the methods, interpreted the data and reviewed the manuscript. VAT performed the analyses. CNAC performed analyses and drafted the manuscript. All authors read and approved the final manuscript.

Authors' information
Not applicable.

Competing interests
The authors declare that they have no competing interests.

Consent for publication
Not applicable.

Ethics approval and consent to participate
This study received ethics approval from; 1) the Table de concertation nationale en maladies infectieuses to access the Quebec public health mandatory reportable infectious disease data (MADO) from all the public health regions in Quebec (Abitibi-Témiscamingue, Bas-Saint-Laurent, Capitale-Nationale, Chaudière-Appalaches, Côte-Nord, Estrie, Gaspésie-Îles-de-la-Madeleine, Lanaudière, Laurentides, Laval, Mauricie et du Centre-du-Québec Montréal, Montérégie, Nord-du-Québec, Nunavik, Outaouais, Saguenay - Lac-Saint-Jean, and Terres-Cries-de-la-Baie-James), 2) the Ministère de l'Immigration, de la Diversité et de l'Inclusion (MIDI) to access the Quebec Immigration database, and 3) the Commission d'accès à l'information of Quebec to access and link the MADO and MIDI databases with the RAMQ Health services databases. Finally, we received approval from the Research Ethics Committee of the Jewish General Hospital to store the anonymous database and conduct the study at the Centre for Clinical Epidemiology at the Jewish General Hospital, the primary institution of Dr C Greenaway (the study PI).

Author details
[1]Division of Infectious Diseases, Jewish General Hospital, McGill University, 3755 Côte St. Catherine Road, Room E-0057, Montreal PQ H3T 1E2, Canada. [2]Centre for Clinical Epidemiology, Lady Davis Research Institute for Medical Research, Jewish General Hospital, McGill University, Montreal, Canada. [3]Department of Oncology, McGill University, Montreal, Canada. [4]Montreal Public Health Department, Montreal, Canada. [5]Sexually Transmitted Infections Division, Montreal Public Health Department, Montreal, Canada. [6]Department of Mathematics and Statistics, McGill University, Montreal, Canada. [7]Division of Infectious Diseases, McGill University Health Center, McGill University, Montreal, Canada.

References
1. Stanaway JD, Flaxman AD, Naghavi M, et al. The global burden of viral hepatitis from 1990 to 2013: findings from the Global Burden of Disease Study 2013. Lancet. 2016;38(10049):1081–8.
2. Ly KN, Hughes EM, Jiles RB, Holmberg SD. Rising mortality associated with hepatitis C virus in the United States, 2003–2013. Clin Infect Dis. 2016;62(10): 1287–8.
3. Kwong JC, Ratnasingham S, Campitelli MA, et al. The impact of infection on population health: results of the Ontario burden of infectious diseases study. PLoS One. 2012;7(9):e44103.
4. Mühlberger N, Schwarzer R, Lettmeier B, Sroczynski G, Zeuzem S, Siebert U. HCV-related burden of disease in Europe: a systematic assessment of incidence, prevalence, morbidity, and mortality. BMC Public Health. 2009;9: 34. doi:10.1186/1471-2458-9-34.
5. Mathurin P. HCV burden in Europe and the possible impact of current treatment. Dig Liver Dis. 2013;45 Suppl 5:S314–7.
6. Galbraith JW, Donnelly JP, Franco R, Overton T, Rodgers JB, Wang HE. National estimates of healthcare utilization by individuals with hepatitis C virus infection in the United States. Clin Infect Dis. 2014;59(6):755–64.
7. Myers RP, Krajden M, Bilodeau M, et al. Burden of disease and cost of chronic hepatitis C virus infection in Canada. Can J Gastroenterol. 2014; 28(5):243–50.
8. El Khoury AC, Wallace C, Klimack WK, Razavi H. Economic burden of hepatitis C-associated diseases: Europe, Asia Pacific, and the Americas. J Med Econ. 2012;15(5):887–96.
9. Hajarizadeh B, Grebely J, Dore G. Epidemiology and natural history of HCV infection. Nat Rev Gastroenterol Hepatol. 2013;10:553–62.
10. Canadian Liver Foundation. Liver disease in Canada: a crisis in the making. 2013.
11. Thuluvath PJ, Guidinger MK, Fung JJ, Johnson LB, Rayhill SC, Pelletier SJ. Liver transplantation in the United States, 1999–2008. Am J Transplant. 2010;10(4p2):1019.
12. Feeney E, Chung R. Antiviral treatment of hepatitis C. BMJ. 2014;349:g3308.
13. Simmons B, Saleem J, Heath K, Cooke GS, Hill A. Long-term treatment outcomes of patients infected with hepatitis C virus: a systematic review and meta-analysis of the survival benefit of achieving a sustained virological response. Clin Infect Dis. 2015;61(5):730–40.
14. Holmberg SD, Spradling PR, Moorman AC, Denniston MM. Hepatitis C in the United States. N Engl J Med. 2013;368(20):1859–61.
15. Trubnikov M, Yan P, Archibald C. Estimated prevalence of Hepatitis C Virus infection in Canada, 2011. Can Commun Dis Rep. 2014;40(19):421–9.
16. Health Canada. Hepatitis C prevention and control: a public health consensus. Can Commun Dis Rep. 1999;25(S2):1–23.
17. Centrers for Disease Control and Prevention. Recommendations for prevention and control of Hepatitis C Virus (HCV) infection and HCV-related chronic disease. MMWR Recomm Rep. 1998;47(RR19):1–39.
18. European Centre for Disease Prevention and Control. Hepatitis B and C in the EU neighbourhood: prevalence, burden of disease and screening policies. Stockholm: European Centre for Disease Prevention and Control (ECDC). 2010. http://ecdc.europa.eu/en/publications/publications/ter_100914_hep_b_c%20_eu_neighbourhood.pdf.
19. European Centre for Disease Prevention and Control. Epidemiological assessment of hepatitis B and C among migrants in the EU/EEA - Technical Report. 2016.
20. Citizenship and Immigration Canada. Canada facts and figures. Immigrant overview permanent residents. 2014.
21. Pepin J, Abou Chakra CN, Pepin E, Nault V, Valiquette L. Evolution of the global burden of viral infections from unsafe medical injections, 2000–2010. PLoS One. 2014;9(6):e99677. doi:10.1371/journal.pone.0099677.
22. Montella M, Crispo A, Grimaldi M, et al. Prevalence of hepatitis C virus infection in different population groups in southern Italy. Infection. 2005; 33(1):9–12.
23. Montella M, Crispo A, Serraino D, Rezza G, Franceschi S. Is the spread of HCV in Southern Italy attributable to iatrogenic transmission through unsterile injections? Eur J Cancer Prev. 2003;12(1):85–6.
24. Greenaway C, Thu Ma A, Kloda LA, et al. The seroprevalence of hepatitis C antibodies in immigrants and refugees from intermediate and high endemic countries: a systematic review and meta-analysis. PLoS One. 2015; 10(11):e0141715. doi:10.1371/journal.pone.0141715.
25. Ministère de la Santé et des Services sociaux. Surveillance des maladies a déclaration obligatoire au Québec. Définitions nosologiques de Maladies d'origine infectieuse. 5th ed. 2005.
26. Turcotte N. Tableaux sur l'immigration permanente au Québec 2006–2010. In: Direction de la recherche et de l'analyse prospective du ministère de l'Immigration et des Communautés culturelles, ed. Quebec: Gouvernement du Québec. 2011. http://www.midi.gouv.qc.ca/publications/fr/recherches-statistiques/Portraits_categories_2006_2010_1.pdf.
27. World Bank. How we classify countries. 2011. https://datahelpdesk.worldbank.org/knowledgebase/articles/906519. Accessed 11 Feb 2011.
28. Janjua NZ, Yu A, Kuo M, et al. Twin epidemics of new and prevalent hepatitis C infections in Canada: BC Hepatitis Testers Cohort. BMC Infect Dis. 2016;16:334. doi:10.1186/s12879-016-1683-z.
29. Quan H, Li B, Duncan Saunders L, et al. Assessing validity of ICD-9-CM and ICD-10 administrative data in recording clinical conditions in a unique dually coded database. Health Serv Res. 2008;43(4):1424–41.
30. Seaman SR, White IR. Review of inverse probability weighting for dealing with missing data. Stat Methods Med Res. 2013;22(3):278–95.
31. Cole SR, Hernan MA. Constructing inverse probability weights for marginal structural models. Am J Epidemiol. 2008;168(6):656–64.
32. Gower E, Estes C, Blach S, Razavi-Shearer K, Razavi H. Global epidemiology and genotype distribution of the hepatitis C virus infection. J Hepatol. 2014; 61(1 Suppl):S45–57.
33. Payne E, Totten S, Archibald C. Hepatitis C surveillance in Canada. Can Commun Dis Rep. 2014;40(19):1–25.
34. Giordano C, Druyts EF, Garber G, Cooper C. Evaluation of immigration

status, race and language barriers on chronic hepatitis C virus infection management and treatment outcomes. Eur J Gastroenterol Hepatol. 2009; 21(9):963–8. doi:10.1097/MEG.0b013e328326f598.
35. Chen W, Tomlinson G, Krahn M, Heathcote J. Immigrant patients with chronic hepatitis C and advanced fibrosis have a higher risk of hepatocellular carcinoma. J Viral Hepat. 2012;19(8):574–80.
36. Public Health Agency of Canada, The College of Family Physicians of Canada. Primary care management of chronic hepatitis C: professional desk reference. 2009.
37. McDermott S, Gupta S, DesMeules M, et al. Health services use among immigrants and refugees to Canada. Health Policy Res Bull. 2010;17:37–40.
38. Subedi RP, Rosenberg MW. Determinants of the variations in self-reported health status among recent and more established immigrants in Canada. Soc Sci Med. 2014;115(6):103–10.
39. Cox J, Maurais E, Hu L, et al. Correlates of drug use cessation among participants in the Canadian HIV-HCV Co-infection Cohort. Drug Alcohol Depend. 2014;1(137):121–8.
40. Razavi H, Waked I, Sarrazin C, et al. The present and future disease burden of hepatitis C virus (HCV) infection with today's treatment paradigm. J Viral Hepat. 2014;21:34–59.
41. Kershenobich D, Razavi HA, Cooper CL, et al. Applying a system approach to forecast the total hepatitis C virus-infected population size: model validation using US data. Liver Int. 2011;31:4–17.

2

Optimising diagnosis of viraemic hepatitis C infection: the development of a target product profile

Elena Ivanova Reipold[1*], Philippa Easterbrook[4], Alessandra Trianni[1], Nivedha Panneer[2], Douglas Krakower[3], Stefano Ongarello[1], Teri Roberts[1], Veronica Miller[2] and Claudia Denkinger[1,3]

Abstract

Background: The current low access to virological testing to confirm chronic viraemic HCV infection in low- and middle-income countries (LMIC) is limiting the rollout of hepatitis C (HCV) care. Existing tests are complex, costly and require sophisticated laboratory infrastructure. Diagnostic manufacturers need guidance on the optimal characteristics a virological test needs to have to ensure the greatest impact on HCV diagnosis and treatment in LMIC. Our objective was to develop a target product profile (TPP) for diagnosis of HCV viraemia using a global stakeholder consensus-based approach.

Methods: Based on the standardised process established to develop consensus-based TPPs, we followed five key steps. (i) Identifying key potential global stakeholders for consultation and input into the TPP development process. (ii) Informal priority-setting exercise with key experts to identify the needs that should be the highest priority for the TPP development; (iii) Defining the key TPP domains (scope, performance and operational characteristics and price). (iv) Delphi-like process with larger group of key stakeholder to facilitate feedback on the key TPP criteria and consensus building based on pre-defined consensus criteria. (v) A final consensus-gathering meeting for discussions around disputed criteria. A complementary values and preferences survey helped to assess trade-offs between different key characteristics.

Results: The following key attributes for the TPP for a test to confirm HCV viraemic infection were identified: The scope defined is for both HCV detection as well as confirmation of cure. The timeline of development for tests envisioned in the TPP is 5 years. The test should be developed for use by health-care workers or laboratory technicians with limited training in countries with a medium to high prevalence of HCV (1.5–3.5% and >3.5%) and in high-risk populations in low prevalence settings (<1.5%). A clinical sensitivity at a minimum of 90% is considered sufficient (analytical sensitivity of the equivalent of 3000 IU/ml), particularly if the test increases access to testing through an affordable price, increase ease-of-use and feasibility on capillary blood. Polyvalency would be optimal (i.e. ability to test for HIV and others). The only characteristic that full agreement could not be achieved on was the price for a virological test. Discussants felt that to reach the optimal target price substantial trade-offs had to be made (e.g. in regards to sensitivity and integration).

Conclusion: The TPP and V&P survey results define the need for an easy-to-use, low cost test to increase access to diagnosis and linkage to care in LMIC.

* Correspondence: elena.ivanova@finddx.org
[1]FIND, MSF Access Campaign, Geneva, Switzerland
Full list of author information is available at the end of the article

Background

Hepatitis C virus (HCV) causes both acute and chronic infection, and is a leading cause of liver-related mortality worldwide [1]. Spontaneous clearance of acute HCV infection occurs in between 15 and 45% of infected individuals in the absence of treatment [2]. The remaining 55–85% of persons who do not clear HCV within six months are defined as having chronic viraemic infection and require treatment to prevent the substantial liver-related morbidity and mortality. It is estimated that 71 million people are living with chronic viraemic HCV infection [3].

The treatment landscape for HCV has undergone a dramatic transformation in recent years, from the use of complex interferon-based regimens with low cure rates and significant rates of adverse effects, to availability of short all-oral direct acting antiviral (DAA) regimens, which are both well tolerated and offer very high cure rates of >90% across different HCV genotypes after 12 weeks of treatment [4]. There has also been recent expansion of access in low- and middle income countries (LMIC) as a result of the availability of generic DAAs [5–7] resulting in substantial price reductions and price of US $ 100–250 for a 2-drug treatment course is within reach [8, 9].

Despite these opportunities for treatment, a major bottleneck to appropriate HCV care is diagnosis [10]. It is estimated that around 20% of infected persons globally have been tested and are aware of their diagnosis [3], but this is much lower in LMICs [11]. There are several key reasons for this low uptake: lack of awareness about HCV among population, exiting diagnostic algorithms are complex, laboratory capacity to diagnose hepatitis C in LMIC remains very low and is largely located in the private sector, and available tests are costly [12–14]. The current diagnostic algorithm first requires screening for evidence of past or current HCV infection with a serological assay that detects hepatitis C antibody (either an enzyme immunoassay (EIA) or by a rapid diagnostic test (RDT)). Those with positive serology will need further testing to confirm the presence of HCV viraemia, and need for treatment, by nucleic acid testing (NAT) detection HCV RNA (either quantitative or qualitative) or antigen detection targeting HCV (p22) core antigen (HCV cAg) [15–17].

Currently available commercial quantitative and qualitative HCV RNA or HCV cAg assays are focused on centralized laboratory infrastructure (e.g. Roche COBAS Taqman HCV assay, Abbott RealTime HCV assay, Hologic Aptima® HCV Quant Dx Assay) [13]. While such platforms may play an important role in countries that favour a centralized infrastructure, and have the appropriate specimen referral system in place, improvements are necessary on the specimen collection and transport (e.g. through Dried Blood Spots) and on reaching affordability. Recently, one integrated platform for decentralized use has entered the market (i.e. Cepheid GeneXpert) and has also received WHO pre-qualification [18]. Other promising diagnostics are under development, but manufacturers need further guidance on the optimal characteristics of the tests that can be implemented in LMIC. An HCV RNA or HCV cAg test that can be performed near or at the site of patient care (point-of-care [POC] testing) may help increase access to HCV care especially in resource-limited settings and hard to reach populations. Also, the advantages of rapid turn-around times offered by near-patient or POC platforms may reduce loss to follow-up and allow for immediate treatment decisions [19]. In addition, if these tests can be made affordable, it may be possible to dispense with the need for an initial serological screening test and have a single test strategy to diagnose viraemic infection (Fig. 1).

A target product profile (TPP) is a tool that has been used widely to support and guide drug, and diagnostic development in various fields of health [20, 21]. This article describes the development of a TPP for a near-patient test for diagnosis of HCV viraemia using a global stakeholder consensus-based approach. The TPP process was complemented by a comprehensive survey of values and preferences (V&P survey) to seek additional perspectives on the TPP criteria and capture acceptable trade-offs between test price, performance and operational characteristics. This TPP is intended to inform test developers as well as donors and provide a tool for communication in accelerating the path towards HCV diagnostic tests suitable for scale-up of HCV care in LMIC.

Methods

Developing target product profiles for drugs and diagnostics

A target product profile (TPP) is a strategic planning tool – usually in the form of a document that provides a clear statement of desired outcome of product development [22]. There have been several TPPs for diagnosis of tuberculosis, sexually transmitted diseases and others [21, 23–25]. A TPP aims to (i) Define the medical/public health need; (ii) Make the need transparent to test developers to increase interest in the field by defining features and characteristics of the desired test; and (iii) Outline features that would provide a competitive advantage, utilizing the input of key stakeholders in the field. The standard categories of criteria included in a TPP are scope, performance and operational characteristics and price.

Methodology for development of TPPs for HCV RNA and core antigen tests

There were five key steps in the process of developing this TPP.

1. *Identifying key potential global stakeholders for consultation and input into the TPP development*

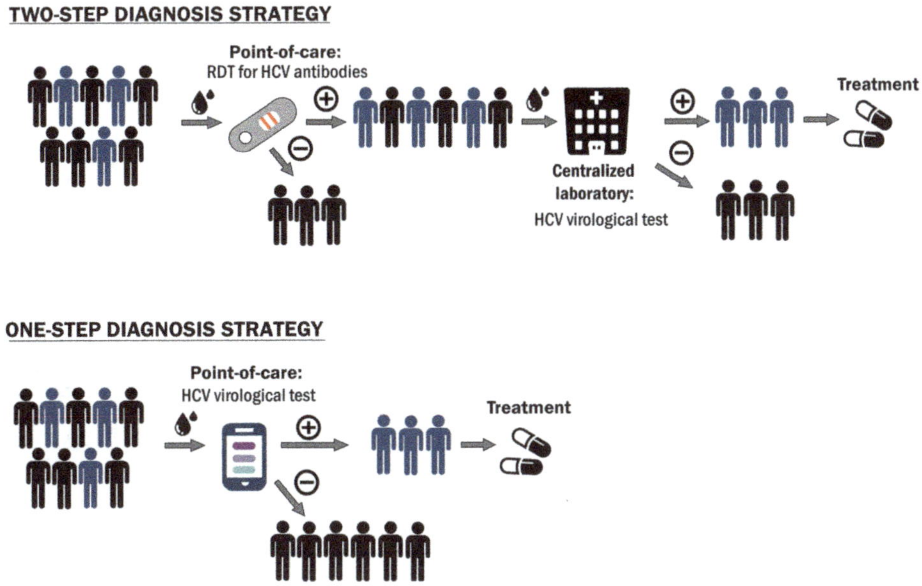

Fig. 1 One-step and two-step testing strategy for HCV diagnosis. RDT states for rapid diagnostic test; POC – point-of-care (i.e. test can be performed at any level of patient care)

process. A list of 50 potential stakeholders were identified for consultation and input into the TPP development process. The stakeholders were chosen to provide a representation from (i) National Hepatitis programs; (ii) Implementers and Clinicians (including from NGOs); (iii) Technical agencies and researchers; (iv) International organizations; (v) Advocacy organizations/Civil society; (vi) industry (pharmaceutical and IVD-manufacturers)

2. *Informal priority-setting exercise with key experts.* Second, we undertook an informal priority-setting exercise with key stakeholders to identify the needs that should be the highest priority in the TPP development. Given the availability of centralized platforms to diagnose viraemic infection, it was decided to focus this TPP development on point-of-care or near-patient diagnostic tests that detect the presence of HCV RNA or HCV cAg. Such diagnostic tests were considered to play an important role in settings with challenges in specimen and results transfer and high loss-to-follow-up after initial diagnosis [26, 27].
3. *Defining the key TPP domains (scope, performance and operational characteristics and price).* Third, we defined the domains and characteristics of a comprehensive TPP. The domains included (i) Scope (characteristics: goal of the test, target population, level of the health-care system where the test could be run and intended end user(s) and lowest setting for implementation); (ii) Performance (characteristics: clinical and analytical sensitivity and specificity, polyvalency and quantitation); (iii) Operational (characteristics: specimen type and preparation steps, time to result, specimen through-put and capacity, biosafety and waste disposal, instrumentation, power requirements, maintenance calibration, data analysis, connectivity, result capture, operating temperature/humidity, reagent kit transport/storage and stability, internal quality control); (iv) price (characteristics: maximum price per test and for instrumentation), as well as the most important performance and operational characteristics and prices (Table 1). These characteristics were described in terms of both minimal and optimal characteristics, which defined a range, where "minimal" referred to the lowest acceptable output for a characteristic and "optimal" to the ideal target (preferable/ideal). The original TPPs were developed by FIND and the Forum for Collaborative HIV Research ("the Forum"), in collaboration with WHO's Global Hepatitis Programme. Additional input was sought from experts in the field at the U.S. Center for Disease Control and Prevention (CDC), Médecins Sans Frontières (MSF), the Treatment Action Group (TAG), and WHO's Prequalification Program.
4. *Delphi-like process with larger group of key stakeholder to facilitate feedback on the key TPP criteria and consensus building based on pre-defined consensus criteria.* Fourth, a Delphi process [28] was used to facilitate anonymous feedback on the key TPP criteria and consensus building. Organizations/individuals that were invited and agreed to participate were asked to provide a statement on their level of agreement with each of the proposed characteristics for each TPP. Agreement was scored on a Likert scale ranging from 1

Table 1 Combined HCV RNA and cAg TPP for an HCV test

Characteristic	Optimal	Minimal	Rationale and evidence
Scope			
Goal of test	The goal of the test is two-fold: 1. To diagnose active viraemic HCV infection (new or reinfection) and provide baseline virological assessment (quantitative or qualitative); 2. To confirm cure upon treatment completion. Ideally, the test would be done with the purpose of initiating treatment within the same clinical encounter or the same day. Not intended for blood screening. The timeline of development for tests envisioned in the TPP is 5 years.	The goal of the test is two-fold: 1. To diagnose active HCV viraemic infection (new or reinfection) and provide baseline virological assessment (qualitative) with the purpose of initiating treatment; 2. To confirm cure upon treatment completion. Not intended for blood screening. The timeline of development for tests envisioned in the TPP is 5 years.	Detection can be performed by HCV RNA test or by HCV cAg detection. Presence of HCV RNA or cAg in a patient is indicative of active HCV infection. Currently, the HCV RNA or cAg test is performed after a positive anti-HCV serological test (i.e. two-step algorithm). Conceivably, provided the prevalence is substantial and the cost of the HCV RNA or cAg test is low, either test could be used in a one-step algorithm.
Target population	Countries with a medium to high prevalence of HCV (1.5–3.5% and >3.5%) High-risk populations in low prevalence settings (<1.5%).		High-risk populations include: persons who inject drugs or have used intranasal drugs (PWID), people living with HIV (PLWH), men who have sex with men (MSM), prisoners, people with tattoos, sex workers, people with frequent contact with the health-care system (i.e. chronically ill) and children born to HCV-infected mothers. In order to achieve the long-term goal of HCV elimination, optimally the test should be performed on all patients in primary care settings, antenatal clinics and in community screening programmes.
Target operator of test	Community workers with minimal training	Health-care workers or laboratory technicians with limited training (i.e. able to operate an integrated test with minimal additional steps)	
Lowest level of setting for implementation (public & private)	Community centres	District hospital (Level II)	
Performance characteristics			
Diagnostic sensitivity*	>99%	90%–95%	Rationale of optimal test: Ideally a test should be as sensitive and specific as available plasma-based HCV RNA tests. A commonly used reference standard is the VERSANT HCV RNA Qualitative Assay, which is FDA-approved for diagnosis of active HCV infection (although the VERSANT HCV RNA Qualitative Assay is being taken off the market, it remains the most analytically sensitive assay and was used as the gold standard in most instances). Rationale of minimal: If a test is easier to implement at lower levels of the health care system without requiring substantial technical expertise or complex laboratory infrastructure, and is less costly, then a compromise can be made on sensitivity. A test with a suboptimal sensitivity of 90–95% with improved operational characteristics was considered acceptable by stakeholders as it would improve rates of diagnosis substantially over what is currently possible. However, no studies or modelling have been done on the minimal acceptable sensitivity and the

Table 1 Combined HCV RNA and cAg TPP for an HCV test *(Continued)*

Characteristic	Optimal	Minimal	Rationale and evidence
			optimal other characteristics needed by a test for HCV diagnosis to lead to substantial improvement in HCV detection on a population level. Modelling work for TB has provided insights that could potentially be applicable for HCV as well. A model showed that for the WHO Southeast Asia Region a POC biomarker test with a sensitivity of 50% for smear-negative TB, if employed at the most peripheral health-care setting, would result in a similar reduction in TB incidence as a test with 70% sensitivity for smear-negative TB that would be employed at the district level (e.g. Xpert MTB/RIF) [17]. However, the exact trade-off between a lower sensitivity (for smear-negative TB) and an increase in access to testing is setting dependent. Under the minimal scenario, some patients would be incorrectly diagnosed as not having active HCV infection, What impact that would have on patient and provider behaviour is unclear.
Analytical sensitivity (comparison with HCV RNA test reference standard)	200 IU/ml	1000–3000 IU/ml	Among the majority of infected individuals with chronic HCV infection, HCV RNA viral loads are between 10^4 and 10^7 IU/ml [13]. In studies of viral dynamics during acute infection, viral loads as low as 3 log IU/ml (or 1000 IU/ml) were seen during the first four months after infection [13]. The optimal LOD of 200 IU/ml should therefore detect most patients (>99%). At a minimum, analytical sensitivity of 1000–3000 IU/ml or 3 fmol cAg/l (current LOD of the Abbott HCV cAg assay), the corresponding clinical sensitivity should be 90–95%. Upper limit of the dynamic range should be equivalent to that of current laboratory-based quantitative HCV RNA tests. An HCV RNA test should be standardized with the WHO International Standard for Hepatitis C Virus RNA, as has been done with current FDA-approved and CE-marked qualitative and quantitative HCV RNA assays. Interestingly, HCV cAg test have been shown to be negative among a portion of untreated individuals with high HCV RNA levels, indicating the likely presence of mutant variants [18]. The limitation of the cAg assay to accurately detect these variants may present a challenge to elimination. Data from patients who relapsed after treatment with peg-interferon and ribavirin therapy indicate that HCV rebounds quickly to high levels (10^3 IU/ml and greater) within a few weeks after the end of treatment [19]. Early data from DAA-based therapy suggests that an even more rapid relapse would happen (unpublished data; communication with A. Hill). Given the high correlation between HCV cAg and HCV RNA levels, either test would likely be suitable for monitoring virologic

Table 1 Combined HCV RNA and cAg TPP for an HCV test *(Continued)*

Characteristic	Optimal	Minimal	Rationale and evidence
			response after treatment completion several weeks after completion of therapy.
Diagnostic specificity (comparison with HCV RNA reference standard)*	>99%	>98%	Since the test is a test for detection of active HCV infection, it should be as specific as current commercially available and FDA-approved HCV RNA tests to avoid false positive results.
Analytical specificity – HCV detection	No cross reactivity with endogenous substance and exogenous factors (e.g. HIV-1, HIV-2, HBV, HEV, antimalarials, anti-TB, ART)	No cross reactivity with endogenous substance and exogenous factors (e.g. HIV-1, HIV-2, HBV, HEV, antimalarials, anti-TB, ART)	
Polyvalency	Ability to detect HIV, hepatitis B on the same instrument		
Quantitation	Quantitative	Qualitative	Treatment monitoring is not considered necessary or feasible with novel DAA agents [14], therefore a qualitative test result is preferred. According to stakeholder opinion, a quantitative result would be beneficial as it allows research questions to be investigated; however, it cannot come at an increased cost.
Operational Characteristics			
Specimen type	Capillary whole blood	Venous whole blood or plasma	The emphasis is for the use of capillary whole blood that can diagnose infection in the clinic without requiring additional laboratory equipment such as a bench top centrifuge. The need for phlebotomy to draw venous whole blood would limit the applicability of the test in lower settings of care as per stakeholder opinion. If plasma is to be a specimen type (minimal criteria), the plasma separation step should be integrated into the instrument.
Specimen prep (total steps)	Integrated specimen preparation (including plasma separation if needed); less than 2 steps required (no precision volume control and precision time steps)	Maximally 2 steps (no precision volume control and precision time steps)	Equipment such as a centrifuge or heat block are available only infrequently at level 1 health centres and some district hospitals, and therefore should not be required for novel assays. Expertise to operate a precision pipette is also often lacking [21]. For the detection of cAg, several specimen preparation steps are needed: i) to dissociate antibody-bound cAg; ii) to lyse viral particles and expose cAg; and iii) to inactivate antibody. These should also optimally be integrated with the test of detection.
Time to result	< 15 min	< 60 min	The need for a rapid turn-around time, the possibility for batching and/or random access for testing, and the testing of multiple specimens at the same time are interrelated. The time to result is probably the most important parameter, as extending the wait time for patients will possibly result in loss to follow-up [22, 23]. Most current immune-chromatographic rapid tests produce results within 20 min.

Table 1 Combined HCV RNA and cAg TPP for an HCV test *(Continued)*

Characteristic	Optimal	Minimal	Rationale and evidence
			The ideal time to result has not been studied and might vary largely between countries and between settings where the patient is tested. But in order to be deployable as a test for POC, the result should be available within the same visit.
Specimen capacity and throughput	Multiple at a time; random access/parallel processing	One at a time (any external reagents should be aliquoted for one time use)	Preferred that one specimen does not occupy the instrument at a time - i.e., random access/parallel analysis. If the platform is multi-analyte, then running different assays should be feasible at the same time.
Biosafety + waste disposal	Mostly simple waste; minimal biosafety waste; no sharps	No need for a biosafety cabinet; consumables should be able to be disposed of as biosafety waste; simple trash.	Increased biosafety of a novel test will enhance acceptability of the test by providers. Further information provided in WHO Laboratory Biosafety Manual [24].
Instrumentation	Instrument-free	Allow for separate specimen preparation device (e.g. mini-centrifuge)	The simpler, more portable and durable/robust the test is, the more likely it will be implemented in peripheral settings. Ideally an instrument free test (e.g. immunochromatographic test) would be the preferred optimal solution but this is likely not feasible with the analytical sensitivity that is necessary and a small specimen volume from a fingerstick.
Power requirements	If device necessary then: battery-operated with recharging solution (e.g. solar) and circuit protector lasting up to 3 days of constant use and able to run off standard electricity	Rechargeable battery or solar power lasting at least 8 h.	Continuous power is not always available at the level of a health and microscopy centre and even less likely at primary care clinics, therefore a battery-operated device with charge possibility conceivably through solar power would be most ideal in order for a test to fit into the entire breadth of settings [21, 23]
Maintenance/ calibration	Disposable, no maintenance or calibration required If device necessary then: preventative maintenance at 2 years or >5000 specimens; include maintenance alert; remote calibration	Preventative maintenance at 1 year or >1000 specimens; only simple tools/minimal expertise required; include maintenance alert. Swap-out of platforms permitted.	If a device is anticipated to have a longer lifespan, then a maintenance alert is essential to ensure proper functionality in settings where it is unlikely that the same person will always handle the device and records will be kept on duration of use. It is essential that only simple tools/minimal expertise are necessary to do the maintenance given that service visits are difficult outside of urban settings.
Data analysis	Integrated data analysis	Integrated data analysis (no requirement for PC); exported data capable of being analysed on a separate or networked PC.	
Connectivity	If device necessary then integrated connectivity; if no device necessary, then the test should allow data export via a separate reader. Full data export (on usage of device, error/invalid rates, and personalized, protected results data) over USB port and network. Network connectivity through Ethernet, WiFi, and/or GSM/UMTS mobile broadband modem. Results should be encoded using a documented standard (such as HL7) and be formatted as JSON text. JSON data should be transmitted	Full data export (on usage of device, error/invalid rates, and personalized, protected results data) over USB port and network. Network connectivity through Ethernet, WiFi, and/or GSM/UMTS mobile broadband modem. Results should be encoded using a documented standard (such as HL7) and be formatted as JSON text. JSON data should be transmitted through http(s) to a local or remote server as results are generated. Results should be locally stored and	Data export will enhance surveillance, device and operator management and allow for supply chain management.

Table 1 Combined HCV RNA and cAg TPP for an HCV test *(Continued)*

Characteristic	Optimal	Minimal	Rationale and evidence
	through http(s) to a local or remote server as results are generated. Results should be locally stored and queued during network interruptions and sent as a batch when connectivity is restored.	queued during network interruptions and sent as a batch when connectivity is restored.	
Result capture, documentation, data display	If instrument-free: ability to save results via separate reader. If device necessary: integrated results screen and ability to save and print results; USB port. On-instrument visual readout and the ability to add information (patient ID, operator ID, date location, etc.)	Ability to save results The test menu should be simple with integrated LCD screen; simple key pad or touch screen.	Results should be simple to interpret (positive/negative for HCV detection).
Operating temperature/humidity/altitude	Between +5 to +40° C at 90% humidity and at an altitude of 3000 m	Between +10° to +35° C at 70% humidity and at an altitude of 2000 m	High environmental temperatures and high humidity are often a problem in countries where HCV is endemic.
Reagent kit transport	No cold chain required; tolerance of transport stress for a minimum of 72 h at -15° to +40 °C	No cold chain required; tolerance of transport stress for a minimum of 48 h at -15° to +40° C	Refrigerated transport is costly and often cannot be guaranteed during the entire transportation process. Frequent delays in transport are commonplace.
Reagent kit storage/stability	2 years at +5 °C to +40° C at 90% humidity & transport stress (72 h at 50° C); no cold chain required	12 months at +5 °C to 35° C, 70% humidity, including transport stress (48 h at 50° C); no cold chain required	High environmental temperatures and high humidity is often a problem in many countries where HCV is prevalent.
Internal process quality control	Internal full-process control, positive control & negative controls	External positive control	In addition to compatibility with existing external quality assessment schemes
Pricing			
Maximum price for individual test (reagent costs only; at scale; ex-works)	< US $ 5	< US $ 15	For a one-step solution, the cost needs to be low, as a trade-off in the ease-of-use/performance for price would not be accepted. Conversely, in a two-step solution, a higher cost is more likely to be accepted, as people would be willing to make a trade-off provided the overall cost of the algorithm remains low. Cost-benefit analyses are needed to explore different options. Trade-offs between optimal characteristics may be necessary to achieve optimal pricing. Preferences about acceptable trade-offs need to be further defined.
Maximum price for instrumentation	< US $ 2000	< US $ 20,000	The lower the price for instrumentation, the lower the up-front cost to a health-care system would be and thus the lower the barrier to implementation. Further modelling is necessary to confirm the maximal price estimated. Price should include warranties, service contracts and technical support. Alternatively, rental agreements for equipment should be an option.

The TPP was finalized using input from the Delphi-like survey and discussion at the consensus meeting (April 22, 2015, Vienna, Austria). TPPs were combined because characteristics were similar for both, independent of whether the test envisioned was a RNA or cAg-based test. The TPP needs to be considered in the context of different types of testing strategies (one-step versus two-step)

*Compared to a HCV RNA reference test performed on plasma

**Ex-works, including proprietary reagents and consumables cost only (without instrumentation), produced at scale to 5 (1 = disagree, 2 = mostly disagree, 3 = do not agree or disagree, 4 = mostly agree, 5 = fully agree). Consensus was pre-defined as more than 50% of respondents providing a score of at least four on the Likert scale (as per WHO policy for expert group consensus). Initially, one round was planned followed by an anonymous summary of the experts' opinion, followed again by a second survey round. However, since predefined consensus for all characteristics was reached after the first round, a second round was not initiated and thus a "Delphi-like" method was used.

5. *A final consensus-gathering meeting for further discussions around disputed characteristics.* A consensus-gathering meeting was convened by FIND and the Forum, in collaboration with WHO, on April 22, 2015, prior to the European Association for the Study of the Liver's annual meeting in Vienna, Austria. The invitation to the meeting was sent to 50 organizations/individuals who participated in the TPP survey (step 4) and 35 people were able to attend. No financial support was provided to participants at the meeting. Given the high level of consensus in the Delphi-like process, the main purpose of this meeting was to discuss issues on which fewer than 75% of the respondents agreed, or on which a distinct subgroup disagreed, or on which further need for clarification and discussion was considered useful. If any voting was necessary throughout the consensus-gathering meeting, >75% was considered a majority.

Values and preferences survey of implementers and users of hepatitis C tests

In the development of the WHO 2017 guidelines on hepatitis B and C testing, the GRADE system (Grading of Recommendations, Assessment, Development and Evaluation) was used to categorise both the strength of recommendations as strong or conditional (based on consideration of the quality of evidence, balance of benefits and harms, acceptability or values and preferences of end-users, resource use and programmatic feasibility). To assess the values and preferences for trade-offs between different test characteristics in the TPP, different testing strategies and approaches, a four-part online survey tool was developed by FIND and WHO with input from MSF, CDC and Médecins du Monde using SurveyMonkey software (SurveyMonkey Inc., Palo Alto, California, USA) Ivanova et al [35]. Survey questions were designed as multiple-choice with comments sections where appropriate (see Additional file 1; only the questions relevant to further the understanding around user preferences in regards to the TPP for HCV diagnostics are listed). The survey was undertaken in September 2015, and the invitation to participate was sent via email to 306 people on the WHO Hepatitis database and included in the FIND and Forum newsletters, and included clinicians, patient organizations, civil society representatives, national hepatitis programme managers, policy-makers and diagnostics and pharmaceutical industry employees. Responses were exported into a Microsoft Excel table (Microsoft Office 2010, Microsoft Corporation). A descriptive analysis was performed using R statistical software (version 3.2, R Foundation for Statistical Computing). Responders were not required to answer to all questions, thus the denominator for each response are the number of responders to the specific question. Only findings relevant to user preferences in regards to the TPP for HCV diagnostics are presented here.

Results

Stakeholder participants in TPP development

Of the 50 organizations/individuals invited to participate in the Delphi-like TPP consultation, 36 responded to the HCV RNA TPP and 26 to the cAg TPP, and 35 attended the consensus meeting in Vienna. About half of responders were from the in vitro diagnostics industry or product development partnerships/technical agencies/researchers (27% and 25% respectively), 14% were from advocacy organizations and the same from the pharmaceutical industry, 11% were implementers/clinicians and the remainder (3% each) represented national hepatitis programmes, international bodies and consultants (Fig. 2).

Consensus on TPP characteristics

The consensus process was used to define the characteristics within the four categories of the TPP: scope, performance, operational characteristics and price. Of the 27 characteristics across the four categories, there was greater than 50% agreement on all of the TPP characteristics. There was even greater than 75% agreement for all characteristics except the minimum clinical sensitivity and the price. All stakeholders agreed that the TPP for HCV RNA and for HCV cAg test could be combined into one TPP for a near-patient HCV virological test.

Target specifications for key characteristics of TPP for HCV virological test

The final characteristics in the TPP are summarized in Table 1. Key characteristics are described below.

Scope of the test

Goal of the test The near-patient test defined in the TPP is for diagnosis of active, viraemic HCV infection. Two testing strategies are considered: (i) a one-step strategy using a single HCV RNA or cAg test (ii) a two-step strategy using an HCV antibody screening test followed by a confirmatory HCV RNA or cAg test, if antibody positive (Fig. 1). Conceivably, provided the prevalence is substantial and the cost of the test is sufficiently low, it could be used in a one-step

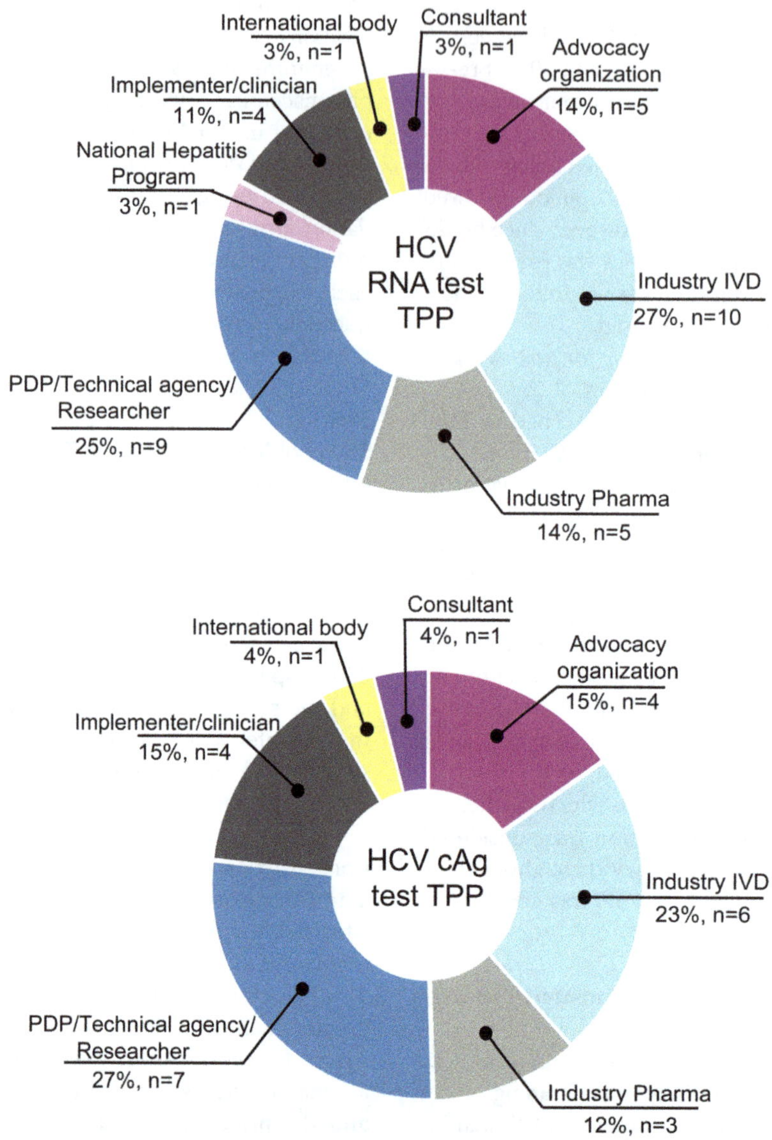

Fig. 2 Information about respondents. Professional profiles of 36 respondents to the HCV RNA and cAg TPPs

diagnostic strategy, thus obviating the need for an upfront antibody screening test. Additionally, since the risk of re-infection is substantial in some population groups, this means that certain high risk groups who have been treated for HCV infection in the past should be tested again for HCV RNA or HCV cAg directly as HCV antibody screening test is expected to be positive.

Furthermore, the test should be also usable to confirm cure upon treatment completion.

Target population The target population for the test was considered to be all persons in countries with a medium to high prevalence of HCV (1.5–3.5% and >3.5%) as well as high-risk populations in low prevalence settings (<1.5%).

Target operator The target operator of a test optimally was considered to be a community worker with minimal training particularly in the context of a one-step testing strategy, where easy-to-use testing close to the patient is paramount to increase access to care. At a minimum the test should be easy enough to perform by a health-care workers or laboratory technicians with limited training (i.e. the test would need to be integrated test with minimal additional and no precision steps; see operational characteristics below).

Performance characteristics

Analytical and clinical sensitivity The analytical sensitivity or the lower limit of detection (LOD) describe the smallest concentration of an analyte that can be reliably measured by an analytical procedure. Current available HCV RNA assays are able to detect as low as 5 IU/ml [18]. Trade-offs such as cost and ease-of use have to be considered in setting targets for analytical sensitivity. If the optimal specimen type (i.e. capillary blood; see below) or a simplified transport tool (e.g. dried blood spots, DBS) were considered, a lower analytical sensitivity (<1000 IU/ml) would be technically difficult to achieve.

In the proposed TPP, the optimal analytical sensitivity was defined as 200 IU/mL for both HCV RNA and cAg tests, while the minimum acceptable level was 1000–3000 IU/mL. Translating the proposed minimal analytical sensitivity into clinical sensitivity (i.e. the probability that the test will correctly identify an infected individual), the LOD would result in >95% of viraemic patients correctly diagnosed based on available limited data on distribution of viral load measurements in those diagnosed with viraemic HCV infection [29, 30]. The majority of stakeholders felt that from a population perspective any test with 95% sensitivity that would substantially improve access to diagnosis and treatment would be a step forward. Further, it was suggested that an optimal sensitivity of 200 IU/ml would likely be sufficient to detect >99% of viraemic patients. Both limits of detection need to be validated in larger surveillance studies on quantitative viral load measurement.

Polyvalency (i.e., same device can be used for different tests) Polyvalency was considered a key characteristic to increase affordability of and access to a diagnostic test by the stakeholder group. Given that polyvalency was initially not voted upon in the Delphi-like survey, a vote was taken in the consensus-meeting. More than three-quarters of stakeholders supported the development of polyvalent platforms that integrate diagnosis of multiple diseases such as HIV, TB and hepatitis B with HCV as an optimal characteristic. Multiplexing (i.e. detecting different analytes in a single sample at the same time) was seen as advantageous for some tests by but not considered as essential by the majority.

Quantitation The majority of stakeholders (>85%) thought that a quantitative test is no longer required if DAA regimens are used, as a decision to treat and confirmation of cure is based on presence of viraemia, and response-guided therapy is likely no longer required or feasible [31]. However, several stakeholders highlighted that a quantitative test is still advantageous to address specific research questions. Furthermore, diagnostic manufacturers suggested that there is only a small cost differential for the development of a qualitative and quantitative test. Therefore, quantitation was integrated as an optimal target.

Operational characteristics

Specimen type All stakeholders (100%) agreed that the optimal test is the one that can be performed on capillary whole blood without any requirement for any additional laboratory equipment as the need for phlebotomy to draw venous whole blood would limit the applicability of the test in lower settings of care. If plasma is to be a specimen type (minimal criteria), the plasma separation step should be integrated into the instrument.

Specimen preparation For the specimen preparation, the majority (>86%) of stakeholders suggested that an integrated specimen preparation (including plasma separation if needed) would be optimal. At a minimum, less than 2 steps should be required (with no steps being precision volume control and precision time steps). These requirements are in line with the skills set a test operator would be expected to have at the settings of intended use [32].

Time to result/throughput The optimal turnaround time defined in the TPP is less than 15 minutes and, at a minimum, the test results should be delivered within 1 hour. The need for a rapid turn-around time, the possibility for batching and/or random access for testing, and the testing of multiple specimens at the same time are interrelated. The time to result is probably the most important parameter, as extending the wait time for patients will possibly result in loss to follow-up [33, 34]. The ideal time to result might vary largely between settings where the patient is tested and has been further evaluated in the values and preferences survey. In order to be deployable as a test for point-of-care, the result should be available within the same visit. Most current immune-chromatographic rapid tests produce results within 20 minutes.

Instrumentation and power requirements The ideal test was considered to be an instrument-free test. If an instrument is necessary, then it needs to be battery operated, ideally with a recharging solution (e.g. solar) and circuit protector lasting up to 3 days of constant use.

For the description of other performance and operational characteristics please refer to the Table 1.

Price of the test

The specification on the ex-works test price (i.e. price of test at the manufacturing factory) at scale had the lowest level of agreement among stakeholders (only 58% agreement for minimal price for HCV RNA test at <US $ 15 and 73% for HCV cAg test at <US $ 10), while 75% agreed on an optimal cost of an HCV RNA of <7 $ US and 85% agreed on an optimal cost of a HCV cAg test at <US $ 3. The opinions on the minimal cost were split between

stakeholders, with many considering the price was too low and others the price was too high. During the discussion, the main factors raised by the stakeholders that would influence the price of tests included the following: (i) the complexity of the test, for example, if there was complex specimen preparation required for the release and detection of HCV cAg; and (ii) the volume of tests undertaken, which was expected to be lower initially given the anticipated lower demand for HCV diagnostics, as compared to diagnostics for other diseases such as HIV due to the lack of hepatitis C care services in LMICs. Furthermore, stakeholders highlighted that the ex-works price, while better compared to other diagnostics, would not be the price seen by the end-user as shipping costs, import taxes, customs charges and local distribution costs would be added on. The control and limitation of these add-on costs was considered paramount to enable the scale up of testing. Ultimately the cost was set at US $ 5 optimally and US $ 15 minimally and the majority of stakeholders (>75%) agreed under the precondition that substantial trade-offs would have to be accepted (e.g. in regards to sensitivity) with a test at US $ 5.

Values and preferences (V&P) survey

The V&P survey questionnaire covered current hepatitis B and C testing practices and preferences for future testing diagnostics. Only the findings relevant to further the understanding around user preferences in regards to the TPP for HCV diagnostics are presented here (see Additional file 1), while the major part of the survey results is reported separately [35].

In total, 104 respondents from 43 countries (56 respondents from 20 high-income countries and 48 respondents from 23 LMIC) participated in the survey. The absolute majority of respondents (94 out of 104) were implementers (i.e. people working in projects for HCV care in countries either within governmental or non-governmental organizations) and IVD industry employees accounted for only 5.8% (6/104). More than a half of the respondents (65 out of 104) had more than 10 years of experience in the field of viral hepatitis.

Responses to survey questions on several key TPP characteristics were as follows:

Test of cure: Almost half of the respondents (47 out of 99) considered that the diagnostic test for HCV viraemic diagnosis should the same as the one for test of cure (Fig. 3). Of these forty-seven, 90% preferred a HCV RNA test (decentralized or laboratory-based) primarily because of its high accuracy over a cAg test.

To explore preferences for future HCV diagnostics in resource-limited settings, the survey specifically collected opinions of stakeholders from LMIC on desired performance and operational characteristics of future HCV test and acceptable trade-offs.

Sensitivity: Half of the respondents (23 out of 46 LMIC respondents) considered that 95% was the lowest acceptable level of clinical sensitivity (Fig. 4b), and 43% (20 out of 46) preferred a sensitivity of 98%. However, when asked about the price for tests with different sensitivity, most of the respondents (83%) indicated that a test with 95% sensitivity is acceptable if the price is lower than US $ 10 (Fig. 4c and d). Only 7% (3 out of 46) felt that a 95% sensitivity would be unacceptably low.

Specimen type: Half of respondents (21 out of 45) expressed a preference for a test that can be performed on capillary blood even if this was at the expense of sensitivity (Fig. 5a). The majority (75%) also considered the ability of the test to use dried blood spots (DBS) as important or very important particularly for centralized testing (Fig. 5b).

Turnaround time: 21% of respondents considered 30 minutes the optimal turnaround time, while 14% and 16% were willing to accept 1 or 2 hours, respectively. Twenty-seven percent were willing to accept a turnaround time of 1 day and 14% allowed even for the next day (Fig. 6).

Price: The majority of respondents considered current prices of virological tests as a barrier to implementation, particularly for HCV RNA tests (77%) and less so for cAg tests (60%) (Fig. 4a). When asked about a maximum acceptable price per test (ex-works and at scale), 52% (24 out of 46) of respondents indicated US $ 1–10 for a test with 98% sensitivity, while 41% (19 out of 46) were ready to pay up to US $ 20 (Fig. 4c). Half of respondents (21 out of 46) would also accept a 95% sensitive test at the cost of US $ 1–10, while 37% (17 out of 46) considered that such a test should cost < US $ 1 (Fig. 4d).

Testing strategy: When asked about preferred testing strategy (Fig. 1), half of respondents (50%) considered a two-step approach with an HCV serological test followed by confirmatory HCV virological test to be an optimal testing strategy. Almost the same number of respondents (48%) expressed preference for a one-step testing strategy that implies a single HCV virological POC. They explained their preference by the simplicity of the algorithm and reduced rate of loss-to-follow-up (Fig. 7a). If a one-step strategy is used, 52% of the respondents (24 out of 46) preferred an HCV RNA test as a single virological test, while 35% (16 out of 46) considered that an HCV cAg test would be an optimal diagnostic solution (Fig. 7b).

Discussion and conclusions

For the next generation of near-patient/point-of-care diagnostic tests for HCV viraemia based on HCV RNA or HCV cAg detection to succeed in improving access to care, certain key specifications need to be met. We report on these key specifications for scope, performance, operational characteristics and price in a TPP utilizing a consensus-based process with key global stakeholders.

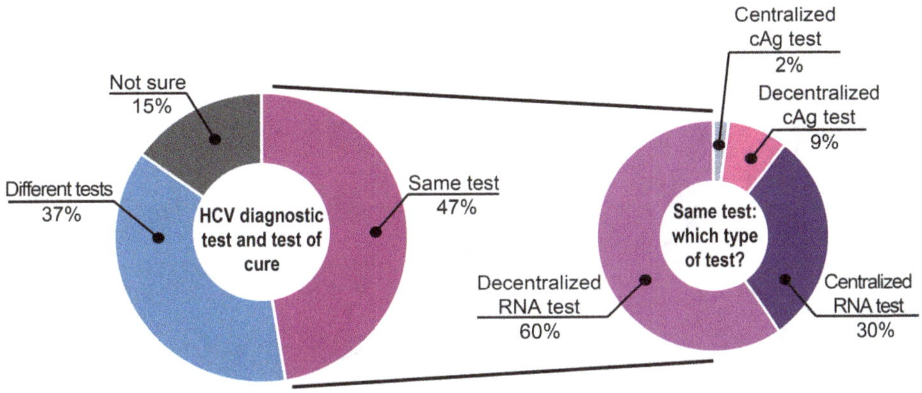

Fig. 3 Preference for the HCV diagnostic test and the test of cure to be the same or different. Almost half of respondents preferred that the diagnostic test and test of cure be the same and about two thirds of these preferred that it be a decentralized (i.e. near-patient) HCV RNA test

The most critical features of the assay identified are sensitivity, specimen type, steps required to perform the test and price. The additional V&P survey that was performed to understand the values and preferences of end users and implementers around specifications set in the TPP, highlights potential compromises on performance features to achieve lower cost and ease-of-use.

The TPP sets high requirements for optimal test accuracy (>99%) but set a lower target under minimal criteria (90–95%). The V&P survey showed that a majority of end-users and implementers considered a test with 95% sensitivity to be acceptable while 90% sensitivity was considered to be insufficient. Modelling studies are required in order to determine the minimum sensitivity that is needed for the point-of-care test to lead to the substantial improvement in HCV detection on a population level. Also, only limited data are available to understand the limit of detection that corresponds to 90–95% clinical sensitivity. Available data show that the majority of infected individuals with chronic HCV infection have

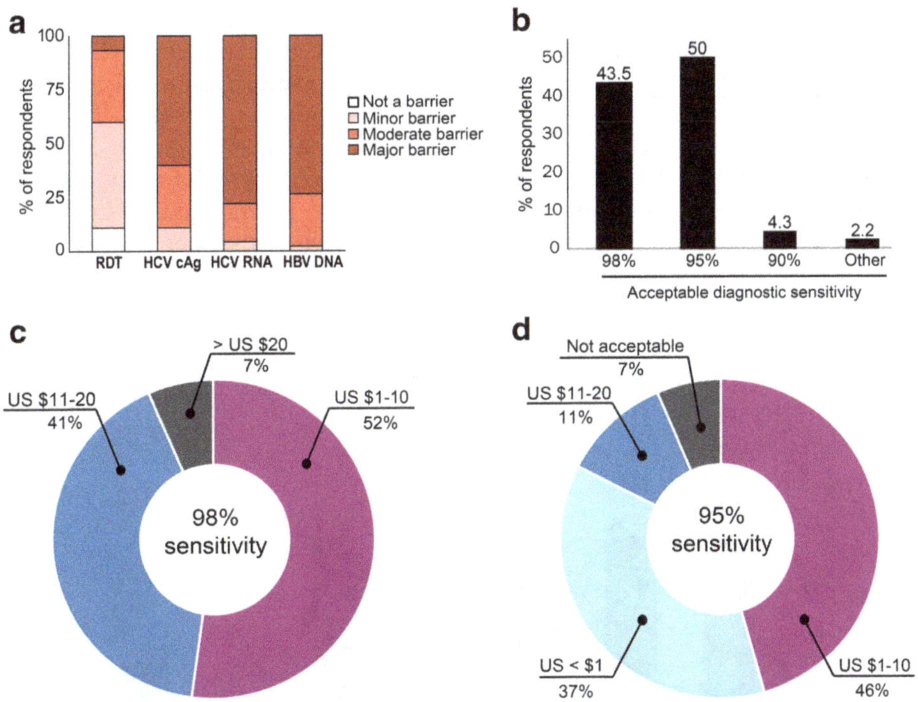

Fig. 4 Preferred sensitivity and acceptable trade-offs between sensitivity and price. Over 50% of respondents see current price of HBV DNA, HCV RNA, and to a lesser extent HCV cAg, is seen as a major barrier to scale up the testing **a**. Half of respondents consider that 95% as an acceptable diagnostic sensitivity for a one-step diagnostic test whereas 43% prefer 98% **b**. Respondents were willing to pay more for a higher sensitivity and were willing to compromise on sensitivity for a cheap test **c** and **d**

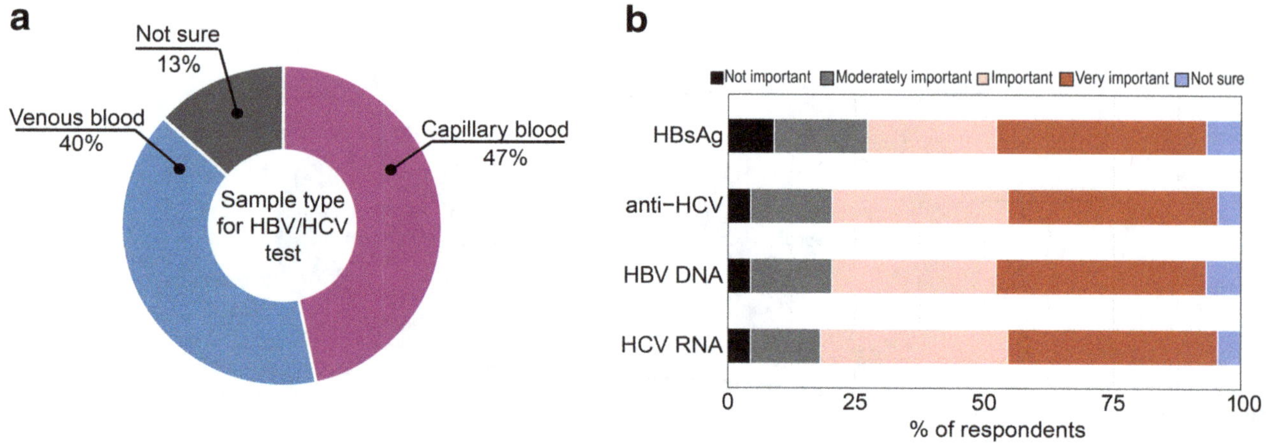

Fig. 5 The importance of specimen type and the ability to use dried blood spots. Capillary and venous blood are the preferred specimen types **a** and most respondents consider the ability to use DBS as a specimen type important or very important **b**

viral loads between 10^4 and 10^7 IU/mL, however a transient dip to values below 10^3 IU/ml can be observed in patients with partial viral control within the first 6 months [29]. Thus, the optimal limit of detection of 200 IU/mL set in the proposed TPP should detect almost all viraemic patients (i.e. >99%(LOD) i.e. optimal). However, the data are limited in terms of capturing different populations, stages of disease and genotypes and further comprehensive studies are needed to confirm the acceptable LOD. The V&P survey indicated that many stakeholders would be willing to compromise on sensitivity if such a test could be achieved at decreased cost and increased ease-of-use. Certainly, test design decisions such as the use of capillary blood for a specimen will limit the ability to achieve a LOD below 1000 IU/mL. The detection of cAg instead of RNA will also limit the ability to reach an optimal analytical sensitivity, as even laboratory-based assays that include complex specimen preparation (i.e. Abbott Architect) can detect femtomolar amounts of cAg and have a LOD equivalent to about 3000 IU/ml for an RNA assay.

The TPP also sets challenging operational characteristics to ensure the usability of the test in low levels of the healthcare system, close to where the patients first present. Capillary blood is defined as an optimal specimen type as it greatly reduces the need for skilled workers, precision pipetting, centrifugation or nearby complex laboratory infrastructure, which is particularly beneficial at lower levels of the healthcare system where these resources and skills are lacking [32, 34]. The acceptable and optimal turnaround time will enable diagnostic decision making possibly on the same day, reduce costs of transportation for patients and so in turn loss to follow-up [33]. However, results of the V&P survey suggest that an even longer turn-around time would be acceptable in some settings. Other operational characteristics, such as

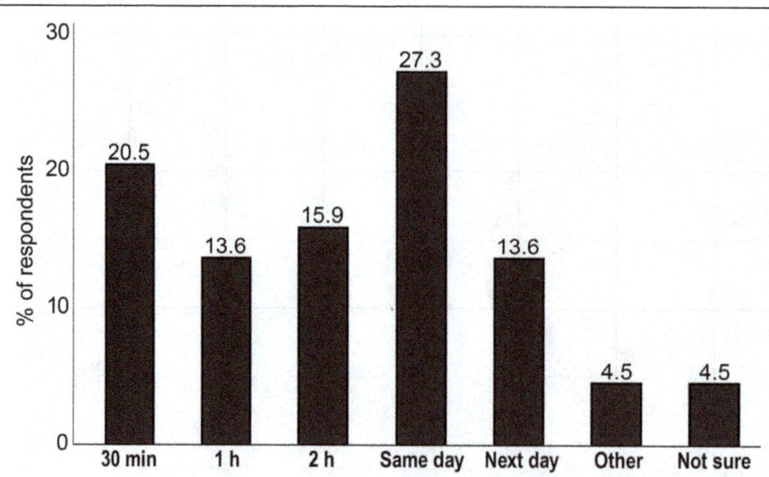

Fig. 6 Acceptable turn around times between taking the specimen and returning the result to the service provider. A maximum of a same day result is preferred

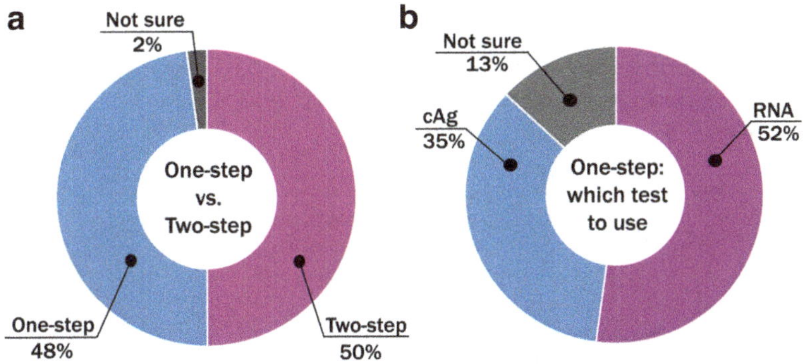

Fig. 7 Preferences for HCV testing strategy. Half of respondents consider two-step testing strategy (see Figure 1) to be an optimal future testing approach in LMIC, while the other half prefer currently used two-step approach **a**. If one-step testing strategy is implemented, more than a half of respondents prefer to use HCV RNA test **b**

the requirement for an instrument to run of battery power, the need for stability in wide ranges of temperature and humidity reflect upon the possible settings the test could be used in LMIC.

A further consensus conclusion is that on-treatment monitoring does not appear to be necessary or useful with DAA regimens as the early reduction in viral load does not correlate with cure [31]. However a test of cure is still important. Given the high correlation between HCV cAg and HCV RNA levels [36], either test would likely be suitable as a test-of-cure. Again, limited data is available on the required analytical sensitivity for a test of cure. Cohn et al. have suggested that 3000 IU/mL is likely suffice for this indication [37], however further data are needed about the rapidity and trajectory of a viral load rebound after treatment failure across different populations, fibrosis stages and genotypes particularly with new DAA regimens. The WHO guidelines recommend a single test of cure performed either at 12 weeks or 24 weeks after the end of treatment [1].

The topic on which unsurprisingly there was the least consensus between stakeholders in the meeting as well as in the V&P survey was the price per test, with end-users and manufactures disagreeing on acceptable prices. A key conclusion was the need for greater transparency, both from the manufacturers themselves on cost of goods and volume-based price-breaks, but also from implementers on cost of distribution so that costs can be disaggregated and end-users can gauge what a fair price should be for the goods purchased. Approaches to reducing costs include (i) countries and donors coming together to pool procurement and forecasting; (ii) launch of competitive tenders; (iii) request bundled pricing on the back of HIV and TB test roll-out; (iv) exploration of different supply chain models for LMIC to reduce the distribution costs incurred; and (v) integrate HCV care within programs for other diseases, such as HIV, TB and hepatitis B, to leverage investments made in polyvalent platforms and care infrastructure. Particularly for the pooled procurement and forecasting there are many lessons learned from the HIV experience.

The strengths of this work include:- (i) it followed a formalized step-wise process established for the development of consensus-based TPPs prior; (ii) It included a broad group of stakeholders; (iii) the TPP process was complementary by a survey that was able to elucidate trade-offs between characteristics. However, we also have to acknowledge limitations. The TPP reflects the opinion of the stakeholders represented in the Delphi-like survey and at the meeting. While we attempted to have a large group of stakeholders that was representative of all the different groups (national Hepatitis programs; implementers and clinicians (including from NGOs); technical agencies and researchers; international organizations; advocacy organizations/civil society; industry (pharmaceutical and IVD-manufacturers), not everybody was able to participate. It also has to be noted that industry representatives accounted for a large percentage of the stakeholders however an analysis of the TPP survey excluding the responses from industry representatives showed minimal differences to an overall analysis (data not shown).

As part of the discussion the following key research questions were identified, that should be addressed to inform future test development and guidelines:

1. Improve understanding on what clinical sensitivity would be achieved with an optimal analytical sensitivity of 200 IU/ml and a minimum analytical sensitivity of 1000–3000 IU/ml. Also, what are the characteristics of HCV-infected individuals with a viraemia of <1000–3000 IU/ml who are missed by an assay with minimum sensitivity? Are they less prone to develop substantial HCV disease? Are they more likely to resolve their infection?

2. What should be the sensitivity of a test of cure and when should such a test be best performed to optimize feasibility, ideally with the same platform as used for detection and minimize loss-to-follow up.
3. What is the cost effectiveness of a one-step approach versus a conventional two-step approach (with HCV serological test first followed by HCV RNA or cAg test) in different prevalence settings?

The ability to diagnose HCV infection in LMIC near to the patient or at the point of care is an important aspect of scaling up access to HCV care. While centralized platforms are already available, an accurate, easy-to-use and affordable diagnostic solution to confirm active HCV infection near to the patient is lacking and urgently needed in LMIC. Independently, such a test would likely be of use in expanding diagnostic testing in resource-rich settings. In considering the needs in resource limited settings, the stakeholder community and donors need to come together to now translate this high priority TPP into actual tests that can help to curb the HCV epidemic and ensure affordable and accessible diagnosis for HCV.

Acknowledgements
Grateful thanks to the late Dr. Samuel Lattimore.

Funding
Publication of this article was funded by the World Health Organization.

About this supplement
This article has been published as part of BMC Infectious Diseases Volume 17 Supplement 1, 2017: Testing for chronic hepatitis B and C – a global perspective. The full contents of the supplement are available online at https://bmcinfectdis.biomedcentral.com/articles/supplements/volume-17-supplement-1.

Authors' contributions
TPP development: Claudia Denkinger, Philippa Easterbrook, Alessandra Trianni, Nivedha Panneer, Veronica Miller; The V&P survey: Elena Ivanova Reipold, Douglas Krakower, Stefano Ongarello, Teri Roberts; Drafting of manuscript: Claudia Denkinger, Philippa Easterbrook, Elena Ivanova, Teri Roberts; Critical revision of manuscript: Claudia Denkinger, Philippa Easterbrook; All authors read and approved the final manuscript.

Consent for publication
Not Applicable.

Competing interests
The authors declare that they have no competing interests.

Author details
[1]FIND, MSF Access Campaign, Geneva, Switzerland. [2]Forum for Collaborative HIV Research, Washington D.C, USA. [3]Beth Israel Deaconess Medical Center, Harvard Medical School, Boston, MA, USA. [4]Global Hepatitis Programme, HIV Department, World Health Organization, Geneva, Switzerland.

References

1. Guidelines on hepatitis B and C testing. Geneva: World Health Organization; 2017. http://apps.who.int/iris/bitstream/10665/254621/1/9789241549981-eng.pdf?ua=1. Accessed June 2017.
2. Mohd Hanafiah K, Groeger J, Flaxman AD, Wiersma ST. Global epidemiology of hepatitis C virus infection: New estimates of age-specific antibody to HCV seroprevalence. Hepatology. 2013;57:1333–42.
3. Global Hepatitis Report 2017. Geneva: World Health Organization; 2017. http://apps.who.int/iris/bitstream/10665/255016/1/9789241565455-eng.pdf?ua=1. Accessed June 2017.
4. Pol S, Corouge M, Vallet-Pichard A. Daclatasvir-sofosbuvir combination therapy with or without ribavirin for hepatitis C virus infection: from the clinical trials to real life. Hepat Med. 2016;8:21–6.
5. Andrieux-Meyer I, Cohn J. Affonso de Araujo E, Hamid S. Disparity in market prices for hepatitis C virus direct-acting drugs. Lancet. 2015;3:e676–7.
6. Gilead. Chronic Hepatitis C Treatment Expansion Generic Manufacturing for Developing Countries. August. 2015. p. 2. http://www.gilead.com/~/media/Files/pdfs/other/HCVGenericAgreementFactSheet.pdf. Accessed June 2017.
7. The Medicines Patent Pool Signs First Sub-licences for Hepatitis C Medicine Daclatasvir. Available from https://medicinespatentpool.org/mpp-media-post/the-medicines-patent-pool-signs-licence-with-bristol-myers-squibb-to-increase-access-to-hepatitis-c-medicine-daclatasvir/. 2016. Accessed June 2017.
8. Hill A, Bryony S, Dzintars G, Joseph F. Rapid reductions in prices for generic sofosbuvir and daclatasvir to treat hepatitis C Rapid reductions in prices for generic sofosbuvir and daclatasvir to treat hepatitis C. J Virus Erad. 2016;2:28–31.
9. Hill A, Khoo S, Fortunak J, Simmons B, Ford N. Minimum costs for producing Hepatitis C Direct Acting Antivirals, for use in large-scale treatment access programs in developing countries. Clin Infect Dis. 2015;61:1174–82.
10. Denkinger CM, Kessel M. Diagnostics for hepatitis C: an urgent need for action. Lancet Glob Heal. Denkinger et al. Open access article distributed under the terms of CC BY; 2015;3:e195.
11. Vos T, Barber RM, Bell B, Bertozzi-Villa A, Biryukov SBI, et al. Global, regional, and national incidence, prevalence, and years lived with disability for 301 acute and chronic diseases and injuries in 188 countries, 1990–2013: a systematic analysis for the Global Burden of Disease Study 2013. Lancet. 2015;386:743–800.
12. Murtagh M. UNITAID Hepatitis C Diagnostics Technology Landscape 1st Edition. Geneva: 2015. http://unitaid.org/images/marketdynamics/publications/UNITAID-HCV_Diagnostic_Landscape-1st_edition.pdf. Accessed June 2017.
13. Putting HIV and HCV to the Test: A Product Guide for Point-of-Care CD4 and Laboratory-Based and Point-of-Care Virological HIV and HCV Tests. Geneva: Médecins Sans Frontières (MSF); 2015:1–100. http://www.msfaccess.org/sites/default/files/HIV_HCV_Report_Diagnostic_Guide_2015.pdf. Accessed Nov 2016.
14. Roberts T, Cohn J, Bonner K, Hargreaves S. Scale-up of Routine Viral Load Testing in Resource-Poor Settings: Current and Future Implementation Challenges. Clin Infect Dis. 2016;62:1043–8.
15. Peterson J, Green G, Lida K, Lee S. Detection of Hepatitis C Core Antigen in the Antibody Negative "Window" Phase of Hepatitis C Infection. Vox Sang. 2000;78:80–5.
16. Chevaliez S, Feld J, Cheng K, Wedemeyer H, Sarrazin C. Clinical utility of Hepatitis C virus core antigen detection and quantification in the diagnosis and management of patients with chronic hepatitis C receiving an all-oral, interferon-free regimen. Antivir Ther. 2016. doi:10.3851/IMP3042. [Epub ahead of print]
17. Medici MC, Furlini G, Rodella A, Fuertes A, Monachetti A, Calderaro A, et al. Hepatitis C virus core antigen: Analytical performances, correlation with viremia and potential applications of a quantitative, automated immunoassay. J Clin Virol. 2011;51:264–9.
18. Cepheid, Sunnyvale U. Cepheid brochure: Xpert HCV Viral load. http://www.cepheid.com/administrator/components/com_productcatalog/library-files/611eae732b51634d8a7e64878d8222a1-615085cee2245c0c5e547ebff505211 9-Xpert-HCV-Viral-Load-Brochure-CEIVD-3043-02.pdf. Accessed Oct 2016.
19. Price CP. Point-of-care testing. Impact on medical outcomes. Clin Lab Med. 2001;21:285–303.

20. Target product profiles and priority digital health products for TB. Geneva: World Health Organization; 2015. http://www.who.int/tb/areas-of-work/digital-health/target-product-profiles/en/. Accessed June 2017.
21. High-priority target product profiles for new tuberculosis diagnostics: report of a consensus meeting. Geneva: World Health Organization; 2014. http://apps.who.int/iris/bitstream/10665/135617/1/WHO_HTM_TB_2014.18_eng.pdf?ua=1&ua=1. Accessed June 2017.
22. U.S. Department of Health and Human Services, Food and Drug Administration, Center for Drug Evaluation and Research (CDER). Guidance for Industry and Review Staff: Target Product Profile — A Strategic Development Process Tool. Rockville MD. 2007. Available from http://www.fda.gov/downloads/drugs/guidancecomplianceregulatoryinformation/guidances/ucm080593.pdf. Accessed June 2017.
23. STI POCT Meeting report: Point of Care Tests –Target Product Profiles and Research Questions, May 6–8, Annecy, France. http://who.int/reproductivehealth/POTC-TPPs-2016.pdf?ua=1. Accessed June 2017.
24. Denkinger CM, Dolinger D, Schito M, Wells W, Cobelens F, Pai M, et al. Target product profile of a molecular drug-susceptibility test for use in microscopy centers. J Infect Dis. 2015;211:S39–49.
25. Porrás AI, Yadon ZE, Altcheh J, Britto C, Chaves GC, Flevaud L, et al. Target Product Profile (TPP) for Chagas Disease Point-of-Care Diagnosis and Assessment of Response to Treatment. Debrabant A, editor. PLoS Negl Trop Dis Public Libr Sci; 2015;9:e0003697.
26. Price CP. Medical and Economic Outcomes of Point-of-Care Testing. Clin Chem Lab Med. 2002;40:246–51.
27. Hyle EP, Jani I V., Lehe J, Su AE, Wood R, Quevedo J, et al. The Clinical and Economic Impact of Point-of-Care CD4 Testing in Mozambique and Other Resource-Limited Settings: A Cost-Effectiveness Analysis. Sansom SL, editor. PLoS Med Public Libr Sci; 2014;11:e1001725.
28. Rowe G, Wright G. The Delphi technique as a forecasting tool: issues and analysis. Int J Forecast. 1999;15:353–75.
29. Glynn SA, Wright DJ, Kleinman SH, Hirschkorn D, Tu Y, Heldebrant C, et al. Dynamics of viremia in early hepatitis C virus infection. Transfusion. 2005;45:994–1002.
30. Fytili P, Tiemann C, Wang C, Schulz S, Schaffer S, Manns MP, et al. Frequency of very low HCV viremia detected by a highly sensitive HCV-RNA assay. J Clin Virol. 2007;39:308–11.
31. Sidharthan S, Kohli A, Sims Z, Nelson A, Osinusi A, Masur H, et al. Utility of Hepatitis C Viral Load Monitoring on Direct-Acting Antiviral Therapy. Clin Infect Dis. 2015;60:1743–51.
32. Denkinger C, Nicolau I, Ramsay A, Chedore P, Pai M. Are peripheral microscopy centres ready for next generation molecular tuberculosis diagnostics? Eur Respir J. 2013;42:544–7.
33. Sreeramareddy CT, Kishore PV, Menten J, Van den Ende J. Time delays in diagnosis of pulmonary tuberculosis: a systematic review of literature. BMC Infect Dis. 2009;9:91.
34. Usdin M, Guillerm M, Calmy A. Patient needs and point-of-care requirements for HIV load testing in resource-limited settings. J Infect Dis. 2010;201:S73–7.
35. Ivanova E, Trianni A, Krakower D, Ongarello S, Roberts T, Easterbrook P and Denkinger C. Values, preferences and current hepatitis B and C testing practices in low- and middle-income countries: results of a survey of end users and implementers. BMC Infect Dis. 2017;17:(Suppl 1). doi:10.1186/s12879-017-2769-y.
36. Hadziyannis E, Minopetrou M, Georgiou A, Spanou F, Koskinas J. Is HCV core antigen a reliable marker of viral load? An evaluation of HCV core antigen automated immunoassay. Ann Gastroenterol. 2013;26:146–9.
37. Cohn J, Roberts T, Amorosa V, Lemoine M, Hill A. Simplified diagnostic monitoring for Hepatitis C, in the era of Direct Acting Antiviral treatment. Curr Opin HIV AIDS. 2015;10:369–73.

3

Hepatitis C testing and re-testing among people attending sexual health services in Australia, and hepatitis C incidence among people with human immunodeficiency virus: analysis of national sentinel surveillance data

David C. Boettiger[1*], Matthew G. Law[1], Gregory J. Dore[1], Rebecca Guy[1], Denton Callander[1], Basil Donovan[1,2], Catherine C. O'Connor[3,4], Christopher K. Fairley[5], Margaret Hellard[6] and Gail Matthews[1]

Abstract

Background: Direct acting antivirals are expected to drastically reduce the burden of hepatitis C virus (HCV) in people living with Human Immunodeficiency Virus (HIV). However, rates of HCV testing, re-testing and incident infection in this group remain uncertain in Australia. We assessed trends in HCV testing, re-testing and incident infection among HIV-positive individuals, and evaluated factors associated with HCV re-testing and incident infection.

Methods: The study population consisted of HIV-positive individuals who visited a sexual health service involved in the Australian Collaboration for Coordinated Enhanced Sentinel Surveillance (ACCESS) between 2007 and 2015. Poisson regression was used to assess trends and to evaluate factors associated with HCV re-testing and incident HCV infection.

Results: There were 9227 HIV-positive individuals included in our testing rate analysis.
Of 3799 HIV-positive/HCV-negative people that attended an ACCESS sexual health service more than once, 2079 (54.7%) were re-tested for HCV and were therefore eligible for our incidence analysis. The rate of HCV testing increased from 17.1 to 51.4 tests per 100 patient years between 2007 and 2015 (p for trend <0.01). Over the same period, HCV re-testing rates increased from 23.9 to 79.7 tests per 100 person years (p for trend <0.01). A clear increase in testing and re-testing began after 2011. Patients who identified as men who have sex with men and those with a history of injecting drug use experienced high rates of HCV re-testing over the course of the study period. Among those who re-tested, 157 incident HCV infections occurred at a rate of 2.5 events per 100 person years. Between 2007 and 2009, 2010–2011, 2012–2013 and 2014–2015, rates of incident HCV were 0.8, 1.5, 3.9 and 2.7 events per 100 person years, respectively (p for trend <0.01). Incident HCV was strongly associated with a history of injecting drug use.

Conclusions: High rates of HCV testing and re-testing among HIV-positive individuals in Australia will assist strategies to achieve HCV elimination through rapid treatment scale up. Continued monitoring of HCV incidence in this population is essential for guiding both HCV prevention and treatment strategies.

Keywords: Hepatitis C virus, Human immunodeficiency virus, Sexual health, Australia

* Correspondence: dboettiger@kirby.unsw.edu.au
[1]The Kirby Institute, UNSW Sydney, Sydney, NSW, Australia
Full list of author information is available at the end of the article

Background

Hepatitis C virus (HCV) is a major contributor to morbidity and mortality in people living with Human Immunodeficiency Virus (HIV) [1–3]. In Australia, it is estimated that around 3000 individuals are HIV/HCV co-infected [4, 5]. Interferon-based therapies for HCV have exhibited poor efficacy and significant toxicity in this population, limiting the capacity for large scale treatment delivery and success. However, current evidence indicates that direct acting antivirals (DAAs) exhibit excellent safety and efficacy in HIV-positive and HIV-negative individuals [6]. Moreover, the first DAAs became available under government subsidy to all HCV infected Australian adults in March 2016 [7].

Australia has one of the highest rates of HCV screening globally with an estimated 80% of the HCV infected population having been tested and diagnosed [5]. While current guidelines recommend HCV antibody testing for all HIV-positive people at initial presentation and at least annually thereafter (with a follow up HCV RNA test to confirm chronic infection if antibody testing is positive) [8], true rates of testing and incident infection in this group remain uncertain.

To allow monitoring of changes in HCV incidence after the introduction of DAA therapies it is important to evaluate past incidence trends. This will also facilitate the development of mathematical models to investigate the likely impact of DAA treatment scale-up and identify factors that could reduce the anticipated benefit of DAAs. Such work could have substantial public health implications as it is anticipated that appropriate use of DAAs in the HIV-positive population will lead to eventual elimination of HIV/HCV co-infection [9].

This paper assesses trends in HCV testing and re-testing among people attending Australian sexual health services, and evaluates trends in incident HCV infection among HIV-positive individuals. It also explores factors associated with HCV re-testing and incident infection among HIV-positive individuals.

Methods

Study population

The study population consisted of patients attending sexual health services participating in the Australian Collaboration for Coordinated Enhanced Sentinel Surveillance (ACCESS) project. ACCESS is a HIV/sexually transmitted infection sentinel surveillance network of sexual health services, general practice clinics, infectious diseases hospital outpatient clinics, and pathology laboratories. The methods behind this collaboration have been described in detail elsewhere [10]. For this analysis, de-identified demographic, behavioral, and clinical data were extracted from the patient management systems of 42 sexual health services using customized extraction scripts. Services were located in New South Wales, Victoria, Western Australia, Queensland, and the Northern Territory.

The ACCESS sexual health services network is broadly representative of sexual health services across the country. In Australia, sexual health services frequently manage the care of men who have sex with men (MSM) and people living with HIV. Nevertheless, a recent study of gay and bisexual men attending ACCESS general practice clinics found that about half were tested for a sexually transmitted infection between 2011 and 2015 [5]. The current analysis precedes a wider investigation of HCV testing and incidence across both sexual health services and general practice clinics which is currently being planned.

Data analysis

Data on patient demographics, HIV and HCV testing were analyzed for patients who attended an ACCESS sexual health service between 2007 and 2015. Three main analyses were undertaken: (i) trends in HCV testing; (ii) trends in, and factors associated with, HCV re-testing; and (iii) trends in, and factors associated with, incident HCV infection. HCV testing/re-testing could consist of HCV antibody or RNA testing, and HCV positivity could include a positive HCV antibody or RNA test. Incident HCV infection was defined as a negative antibody test followed by either a positive antibody test or a positive RNA test, or a negative RNA test followed by a positive RNA test. Factors associated with HCV testing were not evaluated because of the bias introduced by high-risk individuals knowing their HCV status before attending an ACCESS sexual health service and therefore not undergoing testing.

HCV testing: Patients were included in the HCV testing rate population if they had at least one clinic visit after their first visit and were not known to be HCV-positive. Baseline was defined as the date of the first clinic visit. Annual rates of HCV testing were stratified by HIV status (HIV-negative individuals were retained as a comparison group). Follow up was censored at the time of testing HCV-positive, at HIV seroconversion, or 3 months after the last clinic visit. Those that were censored because of HIV seroconversion could re-enter the analysis as long as they had documentation of at least one further clinic visit after their date of HIV seroconversion.

HCV re-testing: Patients were only included in the HCV re-testing rate population if they had documentation of a negative HCV test and at least one further clinic visit. Baseline was defined as the date the first negative HCV test was undertaken. Annual rates of re-testing were stratified by HIV status. Censoring was as per the testing rate analysis. Those that were censored because of HIV seroconversion could re-enter the analysis as long as they had documentation of a negative HCV test while HIV-positive and at least one further clinic visit.

HCV incidence: HIV-positive individuals in our re-testing rate analysis were included in our HCV incidence population if they had at least one HCV test after a negative HCV antibody test, or at least one HCV RNA test after a negative HCV RNA test. The date of HCV infection was taken as the mid-point between the last negative HCV test and the first positive HCV test. Follow up was censored 3 months after the last negative HCV test for those that never returned a positive result.

Statistics: Poisson regression was used to assess the significance of time trends in HCV testing, re-testing and incidence, and to evaluate factors associated with HCV re-testing and incident HCV infection. Our analysis of factors associated with HCV re-testing was split by calendar year (between 2007 and 2011 and between 2012 and 2015). Baseline age, sex, country of birth, place of residence, sexual orientation, history of sex work (at any stage of study period), history of injecting drug use (at any stage of study period), and Aboriginal and Torres Strait Islander status were considered fixed covariates. CD4 cell count, HIV viral load, antiretroviral therapy use and calendar year were evaluated as time-updated covariates. Undetectable HIV viral load was defined as <200 copies/ml. Covariates were considered for inclusion in our multivariate models if they exhibited a univariate p-value <0.2. They were retained in the multivariate models if they exhibited an adjusted p-value <0.05. Patients with missing data for any of the covariates analyzed were included in all analyses, but incidence rate ratios (IRRs) for missing covariate categories are not reported. Stata (StataCorp, College Station, TX) version 14.1 was used for all statistical analysis.

Sensitivity analyses: We chose to include HCV RNA in our primary definitions of HCV testing/re-testing and incident HCV infection to account for the fact that HCV testing is often not performed as recommended [11]. Others have defined incident infection as seroconversion only [12, 13]. To enhance the comparability of our findings we repeated our main analyses using only antibody testing/re-testing and seroconversion as our definitions of HCV testing/re-testing and HCV positivity, respectively.

Results

Of 362,341 patients who attended a sexual health service contributing data to ACCESS, there were 198,050 who contributed follow up time in our testing rate analysis. However, since 2073 patients contributed data to both our HIV-positive and HIV-negative study populations (i.e., they seroconverted during follow up), the total number of HIV-negative and HIV-positive individuals contributing to each group was 190,896 and 9227, respectively. In our re-testing rate analysis, 25,248 patients contributed follow up – 21,945 HIV-negative and 3799 HIV-positive. Of the 3799 HIV-positive patients in our re-testing rate analysis, 2079 were re-tested at least once for HCV after their initial negative test and were therefore included in our incidence analysis. Figure 1 provides a comprehensive breakdown of the patient selection process.

HCV testing

Baseline characteristics of the HCV testing rate population (HIV-positive and HIV-negative) are presented in Additional file 1: Table S1. In the HIV-positive group, median age was 40 years (interquartile range [IQR] 31–48)

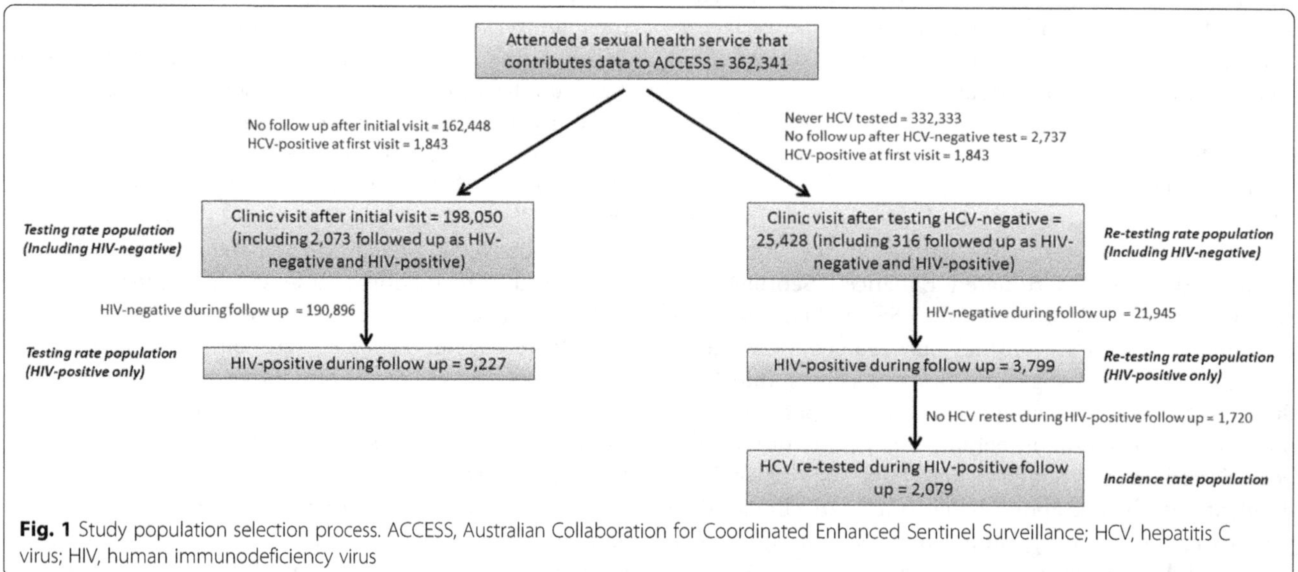

Fig. 1 Study population selection process. ACCESS, Australian Collaboration for Coordinated Enhanced Sentinel Surveillance; HCV, hepatitis C virus; HIV, human immunodeficiency virus

and 85.5% were male. In the HIV-negative group, median age was 27 years [IQR 23–36] and 58.0% were male.

Figure 2 shows that, among HIV-positive individuals, the rate of HCV testing increased from 17.1 tests per 100 person years (95% confidence interval [CI] 15.2–19.1) in 2007 to 51.4 tests per 100 person years (95% CI 49.2–53.8) in 2015 (*p* for trend <0.01). In HIV-negative individuals, the rate increased from 6.5 tests per 100 person years (95% CI 6.1–6.9) in 2007 to 15.2 tests per 100 person years (95%CI 14.6–15.8) in 2015 (*p* for trend <0.01). A steady increase in HCV testing began after 2011 in both groups.

Similar trends were found in our sensitivity analyses focusing on HCV antibody testing. In HIV-positive individuals, the rate of HCV antibody testing increased from 7.9 tests per 100 person years (95% CI 6.7–9.3) to 39.4 tests per 100 person years (95%CI 37.4–41.4) between 2007 and 2015 (*p* for trend <0.01). Among HIV-negative individuals over the same period, the rate increased from 2.3 tests per 100 person years (95% CI 2.1–2.6) to 11.1 tests per 100 person years (95% CI 10.6–11.6; *p* for trend <0.01).

HCV re-testing

Baseline characteristics of the HCV re-testing rate population (HIV-positive and HIV-negative) are presented in Additional file 1: Table S2. Among the HIV-positive group, median age was 39 years (IQR 30–48) and 88.2% were male. In the HIV-negative group, median age was 29 years [IQR 23–38] and 61.7% were male.

In HIV-positive individuals, the rate of HCV re-testing increased from 23.9 tests per 100 person years (95% CI 17.9–32.0) in 2007 to 79.7 tests per 100 person years (95% CI 75.7–83.8) in 2015 (*p* for trend <0.01). Among HIV-negative individuals, the rate increased from 26.5 tests per 100 person years (95% CI 23.5–29.8) in 2007 to 52.4 tests per 100 person years (95% CI 49.6–55.3) in 2015 (*p* for trend <0.01). An increase in HCV re-testing began after 2011 (see Fig. 3).

Table 1 shows that, among HIV-positive individuals, a history of injecting drug use and identifying as MSM were the only factors significantly associated with a shorter time to HCV re-testing between both 2007–2011 and 2012–2015. Country of birth other than Australia, residing in a regional/remote location, and identifying as Aboriginal or Torres Strait Islander were associated with a greater rate of HCV re-testing between 2007 and 2011 and younger age, residing in a major city, and later calendar year were associated with a greater rate of HCV re-testing between 2012 and 2015.

Similar results were found in our sensitivity analyses. In HIV-positive individuals, the rate of HCV re-testing increased from 21.2 tests per 100 person years (95% CI 13.3–33.6) to 76.9 tests per 100 person years (95% CI 72.2–81.8) between 2007 and 2015 (*p* for trend <0.01). Among HIV-negative individuals over the same period, the rate increased from 17.9 tests per 100 person years (95% CI 13.9–23.2) to 49.3 tests per 100 person years (95% CI 45.9–52.9; *p* for trend <0.01). A history of injecting drug use and identifying as MSM remained important factors associated with HCV re-testing between both 2007–2011 (IRR 2.1, 95% CI 1.6–2.9, $p < 0.01$ for history of injecting versus no history and IRR 1.8, 95% CI 1.2–2.9, $p = 0.01$ for MSM versus heterosexual male) and 2012–2015 (IRR 1.2, 95% CI 1.0–1.5, $p = 0.09$ for

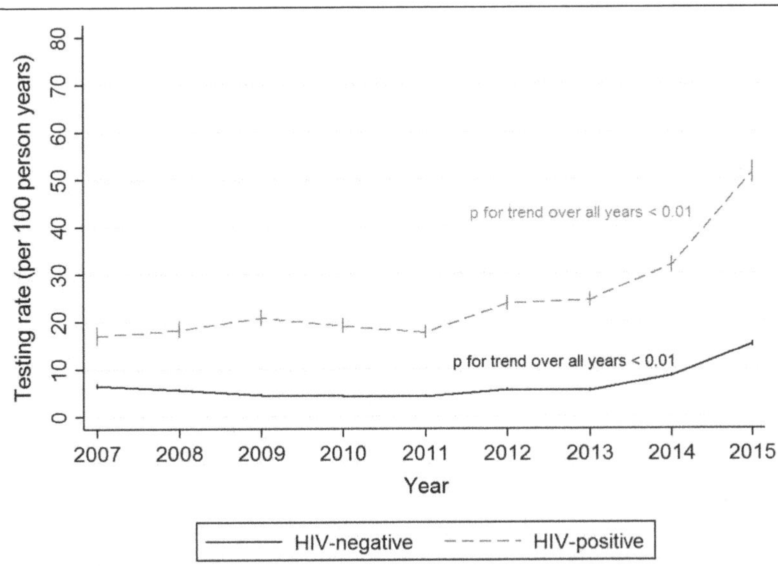

Fig. 2 Rates of HCV testing in HIV-positive ($n = 9227$) and HIV-negative ($n = 190{,}896$) people. There were 2073 individuals who HIV seroconverted during follow up and contributed person years to both HIV-positive and HIV-negative study populations. Error bars represent 95% confidence interval. HCV, hepatitis C virus; HIV, human immunodeficiency virus

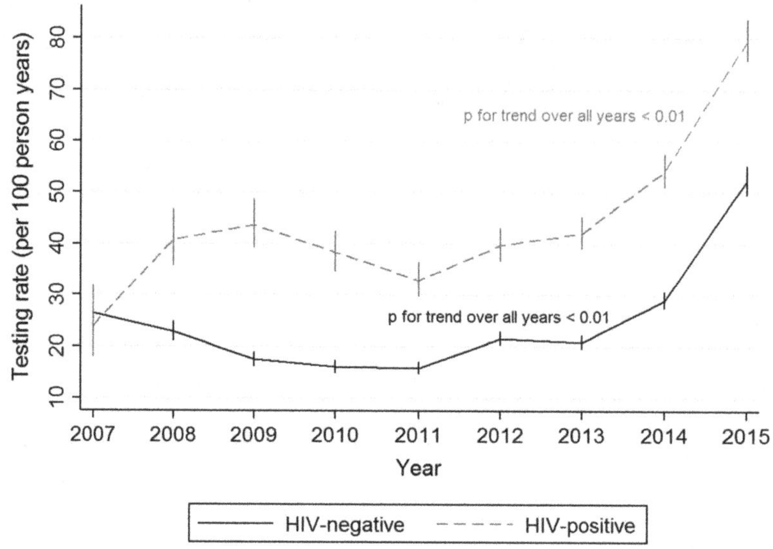

Fig. 3 Rates of HCV re-testing in HIV-positive ($n = 3799$) and HIV-negative ($n = 21{,}945$) people. There were 316 individuals who HIV seroconverted during follow up and contributed person years to both HIV-positive and HIV-negative study populations. Error bars represent 95% confidence interval. HCV, hepatitis C virus; HIV, human immunodeficiency virus

history of injecting versus no history and IRR 1.3, 95% CI 1.1–1.6, $p = 0.01$ for MSM versus heterosexual male). Those residing in a major city were also subject to a higher rate of re-testing between 2012 and 2015 (IRR 0.7, 95% CI 0.6–0.8, $p < 0.01$ for regional/remote versus major city).

HCV incidence

Characteristics of the HCV incidence rate population at the time of their first negative HCV test are presented in Additional file 1: Table S3. The median age was 41 years (IQR 32–50) and 90.7% were male. Median CD4 cell count was 510 cells/mm^3 (IQR 356–672), 74.9% of patients with a known treatment status were using antiretroviral therapy, and 50.2% of patients with a documented HIV viral load had a level that was undetectable.

Over the study period, 157 incident HCV infections occurred at a rate of 2.5 events per 100 person years (95% CI 2.1–2.9). Between 2007 and 2009, 2010–2011, 2012–2013 and 2014–2015, rates of incident HCV were 0.8 (95% CI 0.4–1.6), 1.5 (95% CI 1.0–2.3), 3.9 (95% CI 3.1–4.9) and 2.7 (95% CI 2.0–3.5) events per 100 person years, respectively (p for trend <0.01). During the same periods, rates among those who identified as MSM without a history of injecting drug use were 0.4 (95% CI 0.1–1.4), 1.2 (95% CI 0.6–2.1), 3.0 (95% CI 2.2–4.1) and 2.5 (95% CI 1.8–3.5) events per 100 person years, respectively (p for trend <0.01). Among MSM with a history of injecting drug use, rates were 1.8 (95% CI 0.5–7.4), 2.6 (95% CI 1.0–6.7), 10.7 (95% CI 6.9–16.3) and 2.7 (95% CI 1.1–6.6) events per 100 person years, respectively (p for trend = 0.24). In our final model adjusted for calendar year, incident HCV infection was associated with younger age, living in a major city, being a heterosexual male, having a history of injecting drug use, and being an Aboriginal or Torres Strait Islander (Table 2). When sexual orientation and injecting drug use were included as an interaction term, there was no difference in the rate of incident HCV infection between non-injecting MSM and non-injecting male heterosexuals (IRR 1.4 with non-injecting MSM as the reference group, 95% CI 0.8–2.4, $p = 0.25$), but a substantial difference between injecting MSM and injecting male heterosexuals (IRR 3.1 with injecting MSM as the reference group, 95% CI 1.5–6.1, $p < 0.01$).

In our sensitivity analysis focusing on HCV antibody testing, 14 incident HCV infections occurred at a rate of 0.4 events per 100 person years (95% CI 0.2–0.6). Between 2007 and 2009, 2010–2011, 2012–2013 and 2014–2015, rates of incident HCV were 0.2 (95% CI 0.0–1.6), 0.1 (95% CI 0.0–1.0), 0.6 (95%CI 0.3–1.2) and 0.3 (95% CI 0.1–0.8) events per 100 person years, respectively (p for trend = 0.59). The low number of seroconversions observed precluded us from developing a meaningful multivariate model, however, a history of injecting drug use was strongly associated with incident HCV infection in our univariate model (IRR 8.4, 95% CI 2.9–24.2, $p < 0.01$ versus no history).

Discussion

HCV testing and re-testing in Australian sexual health services has increased substantially among HIV-positive (and HIV-negative) people since 2011. Rates of re-testing were consistently high among MSM and injecting

Table 1 Factors associated with HCV re-testing in HIV-positive people ($n = 3799$)

	Between 2007 and 2011							Between 2012 and 2015						
	HCV re-tested	Person years	Rate per 100 person years (95% CI)	Univariate IRR (95% CI)	*p*	Multivariate IRR (95% CI)	*p*	HCV re-tested	Person years	Rate per 100 person years (95% CI)	Univariate IRR (95% CI)	*p*	Multivariate IRR (95% CI)	*p*
Age														
Every additional 5 years	666	2001.5	33.3 (30.8–35.9)	1.0 (0.9–1.0)	0.07			1323	2862.2	46.2 (43.8–48.8)	0.9 (0.9–1.0)	<0.01	1.0 (0.9–1.0)*	<0.01
Sex														
Male	606	1762.8	34.4 (31.7–37.2)	1.0				1195	2456.3	48.6 (46.0–51.5)	1.0			
Female	60	238.8	25.1 (19.5–32.4)	0.7 (0.6–1.0)	0.02			128	405.9	31.5 (26.5–37.5)	0.6 (0.5–0.8)	<0.01		
Country of birth														
Australia	449	1397.4	32.1 (29.3–35.2)	1.0		1.0		871	1903.0	45.8 (42.8–48.9)	1.0			
Other	217	604.1	35.9 (31.4–41.0)	1.1 (1.0–1.3)	0.18	1.3 (1.1–1.6)	<0.01	452	959.2	47.1 (43.0–51.7)	1.0 (0.9–1.2)	0.62		
Place of residence														
Major city	339	1092.4	31.0 (27.9–34.5)	1.0		1.0		944	1726.4	54.7 (51.3–58.3)	1.0		1.0	
Regional/ remote	316	878.1	36.0 (32.2–40.2)	1.2 (1.0–1.4)	0.06	1.3 (1.1–1.5)	<0.01	367	1085.6	33.8 (30.5–37.4)	0.6 (0.5–0.7)	<0.01	0.7 (0.6–0.8)	<0.01
Unknown	11	31.0	35.5 (19.7–64.1)	–		–		12	50.2	23.9 (13.6–42.1)	–		–	
Sexual orientation														
MSM	528	1416.0	37.3 (34.2–40.6)	1.7 (1.3–2.1)	0.00	1.8 (1.4–2.3)	<0.01	996	1941.6	51.3 (48.2–54.6)	1.3 (1.1–1.5)	<0.01	1.2 (1.0–1.4)	0.03
Heterosexual male	78	346.7	22.5 (18.0–28.1)	1.0		1.0		198	512.7	38.6 (33.6–44.4)	1.0		1.0	
Unknown	60	238.8	25.1 (19.5–32.4)	–		–		129	407.9	31.6 (26.6–37.6)	–		–	
Ever performed sex work														
No	649	1942.7	33.4 (30.9–36.1)	1.0				1278	2783.7	45.9 (43.5–48.5)	1.0			
Yes	17	58.8	28.9 (18.0–46.5)	0.9 (0.5–1.4)	0.56			45	78.5	57.3 (42.8–76.8)	1.2 (0.9–1.7)	0.14		
Ever injected drugs														
No	507	1649.6	30.7 (28.2–33.5)	1.0		1.0		1126	2513.1	44.8 (42.3–47.5)	1.0		1.0	
Yes	109	223.9	48.7 (40.3–58.7)	1.6 (1.3–1.9)	<0.01	1.7 (1.4–2.1)	<0.01	148	256.6	57.7 (49.1–67.8)	1.3 (1.1–1.5)	<0.01	1.3 (1.1–1.5)	0.01
Unknown	50	128.0	39.1 (29.6–51.5)	–		–		49	92.5	52.9 (40.0–70.1)	–		–	
Aboriginal or Torres Strait Islander														
No	629	1915.1	32.8 (30.4–35.5)	1.0		1.0		1270	2748.6	46.2 (43.7–48.8)	1.0			
Yes	37	86.4	42.8 (31.0–59.1)	1.3 (0.9–1.8)	0.12	1.4 (1.0–2.0)	0.04	53	113.6	46.6 (35.6–61.1)	1.0 (0.8–1.3)	0.95		
Current CD4 cell count (cells/mm^3)														

Table 1 Factors associated with HCV re-testing in HIV-positive people ($n = 3799$) *(Continued)*

	Between 2007 and 2011							Between 2012 and 2015						
	HCV re-tested	Person years	Rate per 100 person years (95% CI)	Univariate IRR (95% CI)	*p*	Multivariate IRR (95% CI)	*p*	HCV re-tested	Person years	Rate per 100 person years (95% CI)	Univariate IRR (95% CI)	*p*	Multivariate IRR (95% CI)	*p*
≥ 500	164	596.3	27.5 (23.6–32.1)	1.0				501	1107.2	45.2 (41.5–49.4)	1.0			
< 500	158	567.2	27.9 (23.8–32.6)	1.0 (0.8–1.3)	0.91			340	786.7	43.2 (38.9–48.1)	1.0 (0.8–1.1)	0.51		
Unknown	344	838.1	41.0 (36.9–45.6)	–				482	968.3	49.8 (45.5–54.4)	–			
Current HIV RNA														
Undetectable	299	898.5	33.3 (29.7–37.3)	1.0				758	1585.1	47.8 (44.5–51.3)	1.0			
Detectable	167	536.3	31.1 (26.8–36.2)	0.9 (0.8–1.1)	0.49			243	465.2	52.2 (46.1–59.2)	1.1 (0.9–1.3)	0.23		
Unknown	200	566.7	35.3 (30.7–40.5)	–				322	811.9	39.7 (35.6–44.2)	–			
Current ART use														
Yes	366	1121.3	32.6 (29.5–36.2)	1.0				919	1851.9	49.6 (46.5–52.9)	1.0			
No	100	313.5	31.9 (26.2–38.8)	1.0 (0.8–1.2)	0.84			82	198.5	41.3 (33.3–51.3)	0.8 (0.7–1.0)	0.11		
Unknown	200	566.7	35.3 (30.7–40.5)	–				322	811.9	39.7 (35.6–44.2)	–			
Current calendar year~														
2007 / 2012	74	236.7	31.3 (24.9–39.3)	1.0		1.0		279	760.9	36.7 (32.6–41.2)	1.0		1.0	
2008 / 2013	167	424.3	39.4 (33.8–45.8)	1.3 (1.0–1.7)	0.10	1.3 (1.0–1.7)	0.07	361	819.4	44.1 (39.7–48.8)	1.2 (1.0–1.4)	0.02	1.2 (1.0–1.4)	0.02
2009 / 2014	155	487.2	31.8 (27.2–37.2)	1.0 (0.8–1.3)	0.90	1.1 (0.8–1.4)	0.66	414	808.1	51.2 (46.5–56.4)	1.4 (1.2–1.6)	<0.01	1.4 (1.2–1.6)	<0.01
2010 / 2015	158	487.3	32.4 (27.7–37.9)	1.0 (0.8–1.4)	0.80	1.1 (0.8–1.4)	0.52	269	473.8	56.8 (50.4–64.0)	1.5 (1.3–1.8)	<0.01	1.5 (1.3–1.8)	<0.01
2011 / -	112	366.0	30.6 (25.4–36.8)	1.0 (0.7–1.3)	0.89	1.1 (0.8–1.4)	0.74	–	–	–	–		–	

Missing categories were included in models but coefficients are not shown. *IRR (95%CI) to two decimal places was 0.96 (0.94–0.98); ~Calendar year for 2007–2011 model / calendar year for 2012–2015 model. Despite calendar year not reaching significance in the multivariate 2007–2011 model, it was retained to allow comparison with the unadjusted testing rates in Fig. 2; HCV, hepatitis C virus; HIV, human immunodeficiency virus; CI, confidence interval; IRR, incidence rate ratio; MSM, men who have sex with men; ART, antiretroviral therapy

Table 2 Factors associated with incident HCV infection in HIV-positive people ($n = 2079$)

	Incident infections	Person years	Rate per 100 person years (95% CI)	Univariate IRR (95% CI)	*p*	Multivariate IRR (95% CI)	*p*
Age							
Every additional 5 years	157	6279.7	2.5 (2.1–2.9)	0.8 (0.8–0.9)	<0.01	0.9 (0.8–0.9)	<0.01
Sex							
Male	141	5772.2	2.4 (2.1–2.9)	1.0			
Female	16	507.5	3.2 (1.9–5.1)	1.3 (0.8–2.2)	0.33		
Country of birth							
Australia	99	4316.1	2.3 (1.9–2.8)	1.0			
Other	58	1963.6	3.0 (2.3–3.8)	1.3 (0.9–1.8)	0.13		
Place of residence							
Major city	132	3795.0	3.5 (2.9–4.1)	1.0		1.0	
Regional/remote	25	2414.6	1.0 (0.7–1.5)	0.3 (0.2–0.5)	<0.01	0.3 (0.2–0.5)	<0.01
Unknown	0	70.1	–	–		–	
Sexual orientation							
MSM	115	4950.0	2.3 (1.9–2.8)	0.7 (0.5–1.1)	0.15	0.5 (0.4–0.8)	0.01
Heterosexual male	26	820.5	3.2 (2.2–4.7)	1.0		1.0	
Unknown	16	509.1	3.1 (1.9–5.1)	–		–	
Ever performed sex work							
No	151	6086.7	2.5 (2.1–2.9)	1.0			
Yes	6	192.9	3.1 (1.4–6.9)	1.3 (0.6–2.8)	0.59		
Ever injected drugs							
No	111	5249.1	2.1 (1.8–2.5)	1.0		1.0	
Yes	46	795.6	5.8 (4.3–7.7)	2.7 (1.9–3.9)	<0.01	2.5 (1.8–3.5)	<0.01
Unknown	0	234.9	–	–		–	
Aboriginal or Torres Strait Islander							
No	146	5992.9	2.4 (2.1–2.9)	1.0		1.0	
Yes	11	286.8	3.8 (2.1–6.9)	1.6 (0.9–2.9)	0.15	2.0 (1.1–3.7)	0.03
Current CD4 cell count (cells/mm^3)							
≥ 500	34	1648.2	2.1 (1.5–2.9)	1.0			
< 500	17	1116.1	1.5 (0.9–2.5)	0.7 (0.4–1.3)	0.31		
Unknown	106	3515.4	3.0 (2.5–3.6)	–			
Current HIV RNA							
Undetectable	63	2647.6	2.4 (1.9–3.0)	1.0			
Detectable	21	869.0	2.4 (1.6–3.7)	1.0 (0.6–1.7)	0.95		

Table 2 Factors associated with incident HCV infection in HIV-positive people (n = 2079) *(Continued)*

	Incident infections	Person years	Rate per 100 person years (95% CI)	Univariate IRR (95% CI)	*p*	Multivariate IRR (95% CI)	*p*
Unknown	73	2763.1	2.6 (2.1–3.3)	–			
Current ART use							
Yes	74	3008.6	2.5 (2.0–3.1)	1.0			
No	10	508.0	2.0 (1.1–3.7)	0.8 (0.4–1.5)	0.51		
Unknown	73	2763.1	2.6 (2.1–3.3)	–			
Current time period							
2007–09	8	1027.6	0.8 (0.4–1.6)	1.0		1.0	
2010–11	21	1385.5	1.5 (1.0–2.3)	1.8 (0.8–4.1)	0.15	1.7 (0.8–3.9)	0.19
2012–13	77	1960.5	3.9 (3.1–4.9)	4.5 (2.2–9.4)	<0.01	4.1 (2.0–8.5)	<0.01
2014–15	51	1906.0	2.7 (2.0–3.5)	2.6 (1.2–5.4)	0.01	2.2 (1.1–4.7)	0.04

Missing categories were included in models but coefficients are not shown. HCV, hepatitis C virus; HIV, human immunodeficiency virus; CI, confidence interval; IRR, incidence rate ratio; MSM, men who have sex with men; ART, antiretroviral therapy

drug users between 2007 and 2015, however, there was a marked increase in testing rates during the latter years of the study period among those residing in a major city. The rate of incident HCV infection increased between 2007 and 2013 but remained stable between 2014 and 2015. Incident HCV was associated with a history of injecting drug use, particularly among heterosexual males.

HIV-positive MSM have an increased risk of HCV infection compared with HIV-negative MSM, possibly due to higher rates of high-risk sexual behavior [14]. Current Australian guidelines recommend routine HCV testing among HIV-positive MSM [15]. This explains why HCV testing and re-testing rates were consistently higher over time among our HIV-positive group. The increasing rates of HCV testing and re-testing observed are probably linked to a growing awareness of sexual HCV transmission [16] and, more recently, increasing awareness of DAA availability [17]. The number of state and national campaigns aiming to increase HCV and DAA awareness has increased substantially over the past decade [18, 19]. Moreover, national advisory groups such as the Australasian Society for HIV, Viral Hepatitis and Sexual Health Medicine have actively sought to keep prescribers informed about DAA availability [20]. Given that non-sterile injecting practices and sexual behaviors that increase the potential for exposure to blood increase the possibility of transmitting HCV, it was unsurprising to find that injecting drug users and MSM were subject to high rates of HCV re-testing. Of note, however, the increase in HCV re-testing rates between the periods 2007–2011 and 2012–2015 among patients living in a major city was contrasted by a small decline in testing among those living in regional/remote locations. This suggests that knowledge of DAA availability may be lacking outside of Australia's main urban centers.

Other recent studies from Australia and abroad have described an overall HCV incidence rate in HIV-positive people similar to that reported here (2.5 events per 100 person years) [12, 13, 21–27]. In contrast to our findings, however, which show HCV incidence increased between 2007 and 2013 then plateaued, data from the Swiss HIV Cohort suggests HCV incidence has increased consistently since 2000 among MSM [13] and results from the UK Collaborative HIV Cohort indicate that HCV incidence remained stable between 2004 and 2011 among MSM [12]. There are two important methodological differences between these two studies and ours. Firstly, unlike our study, patients enrolled in the Swiss and UK cohorts underwent routine HCV testing. The low rates of testing/re-testing during the earlier years of our study period could have caused us to underestimate HCV incidence. However, given HCV diagnoses were uncommon and that all patients in our incidence analysis were tested at least twice for HCV, it is unlikely that testing rates substantially influenced our results. The other main difference is that the Swiss and UK studies defined incident infection as HCV seroconversion. Unfortunately, a preliminary assessment of our data indicated that, consistent with findings from the US [11], HCV testing was often not performed as recommended. This meant that the group of patients we identified as having experienced an incident HCV infection included an unknown number of re-infected patients. Nevertheless, our main and sensitivity analyses showed similar trends in both HCV testing and incident infection rates.

Interestingly, another Australian study recently found no change in HCV incidence between 2008 and 2016 among MSM [21]. Of note, this single-center study specifically asked HCV cases about injecting drug use and excluded those reporting a positive history of injecting regardless of what was noted in their records. Our analysis relied upon routinely collected surveillance data in which injecting drug use was probably under-reported. This is supported by the results of our incidence model. While those with a history of injecting drug use had a high risk of incident HCV infection, it is likely that the other significantly associated factors (younger age, living in a major city, being a heterosexual male, and being Aboriginal and Torres Strait Islander) were largely the result of residual confounding. Each of these additional factors are known to be associated with injecting drug use [28, 29]. This implies that the increase in HCV incidence among Australia's HIV-positive population may have been driven by injecting drug use and that sexual transmission has not changed substantially. This could be related to increased rates of unsafe injecting among sub-populations of the HIV-positive community. For example, between 2011 and 2014, the proportion of HIV infections attributable to IDU increased dramatically among Aboriginal and Torres Strait Islanders [5]. Importantly, heterosexual males that inject drugs appear to be at especially high risk of contracting HCV. This finding warrants further investigation.

There are several limitations to bear in mind when evaluating the results of this work. Firstly, we were unable to link records between the sexual health services involved. Therefore, patients could have re-entered the analysis at multiple services. Additionally, we had limited information on sexual risk behavior and there is a high likelihood that injecting drug use was under-reported. Our analysis populations represent only a sample of the approximately 21,000 HIV patients who are currently diagnosed and in care in Australia [5], which means our rate estimates reflect only a subset of the total number of tests and diagnoses carried out nationwide. As mentioned earlier, an analysis of HCV testing and incidence across both sexual health services and general practice clinics involved in ACCESS is currently being planned. We were not able to conduct an appropriate analysis of factors associated with HCV testing because of the bias introduced by high-risk individuals knowing their HCV status prior to enrolment and therefore not undergoing testing. Further details on HCV testing rates and factors associated with HCV testing should form the topic of future investigation. Finally, while our testing and re-testing rate sensitivity analyses supported our main findings, our incidence rate sensitivity analyses were impeded by a very low number of outcomes.

Conclusions

The increasing rates of HCV testing and re-testing reported here are encouraging. High rates of HCV testing and re-testing among high-risk groups in Australia will assist strategies to achieve HCV elimination through rapid treatment scale up. Continued monitoring of HCV incidence in the HIV-positive population, particularly those with a history of injecting drug use, is essential for guiding both HCV prevention and treatment strategies.

Additional file

Additional file 1: Table S1. Characteristics of the HIV-positive and HIV--negative HCV testing rate populations at the time of their first clinic visit. Values are presented as n (% of patients) unless otherwise indicated. *2073 individuals HIV seroconverted during follow up and contributed person years to both HIV-positive and HIV-negative study populations; HIV, human immunodeficiency virus; HCV, hepatitis C virus; IQR, interquartile range; MSM, men who have sex with men. **Table S2.** Characteristics of the HIV-positive and HIV-negative HCV re-testing rate populations at the time of their first documented HCV test. Values are presented as n (% of patients) unless otherwise indicated. *316 individuals HIV seroconverted during follow up and contributed person years to both HIV-positive and HIV-negative study populations; HIV, human immunodeficiency virus; HCV, hepatitis C virus; IQR, interquartile range; MSM, men who have sex with men. **Table S3.** Characteristics of the HCV incidence population at the time of their first negative HCV test. Values are presented as n (% of patients) unless otherwise indicated. HCV, hepatitis C virus; IQR, interquartile range; MSM, men who have sex with men; HIV, human immunodeficiency virus; ART, antiretroviral therapy. (DOCX 34 kb)

Abbreviations

ACCESS: Australian Collaboration for Coordinated Enhanced Sentinel Surveillance; CI: Confidence interval; DAA: Direct acting antiviral; HCV: Hepatitis C Virus; HIV: Human Immunodeficiency Virus; IQR: Interquartile range; IRR: Incidence rate ratio; MSM: Men who have sex with men

Acknowledgements

The authors would like to acknowledge the participants that contribute data to ACCESS.

Consent to publication

Not applicable

Funding

This work was supported by a grant awarded to DCB by Gilead Sciences. Gilead Sciences played no role in the design of the study, data collection, data analysis, interpretation of data, or in the writing of the manuscript.

Authors' contributions

DCB conceived and carried out the analysis, and drafted the final manuscript. MGL, GJD, RG, DC, BD, CCOC, CKF, MH and GM participated in the design of the analysis and drafting of the final manuscript. All authors have read and approved the final manuscript.

Ethics approval and consent to participate

Approval for the sexual health services network of ACCESS was granted by the Human Research Ethics Committees of St Vincent's Hospital, Sydney (reference number 08/051) with further approval granted by the separate Human Research Ethics Committees responsible for each participating service. De-identified demographic, behavioral, pathology and diagnoses data were extracted from patient management systems using customized extraction scripts. Therefore, individual patient consent was waived.

Competing interests

DCB has received grant funding from Gilead Sciences. MGL has received unrestricted grants from Boehringer Ingelhiem, Gilead Sciences, Merck Sharp & Dohme, Bristol-Myers Squibb, Janssen-Cilag, ViiV HealthCare, and consultancy fees from Gilead Sciences, and DSMB sitting fees from Sirtex Pty Ltd. GJD is an advisory board member and receives honorarium from Gilead Sciences, Merck Sharpe & Dohme, Abbvie, and Bristol-Myers Squibb, has received research grant funding from Gilead Science, Merck Sharp and Dohme, Abbvie, and Bristol-Myers Squibb, and travel sponsorship from Gilead Science, Merck Sharp and Dohme, Abbvie, and Bristol-Myers Squibb. MH has received funding for investigator initiated research from Gilead Sciences, Bristol-Myers Squibb and Abbvie. GM has received research funding and consultancy fees for Gilead Sciences and Abbvie. All other authors report no competing interests.

Author details

[1]The Kirby Institute, UNSW Sydney, Sydney, NSW, Australia. [2]Sydney Sexual Health Centre, Sydney, NSW, Australia. [3]The Kirby Institute, UNSW Sydney and Sexual Health Service, Sydney Local Health District, Sydney, NSW, Australia. [4]Central Clinical School, Sydney University, Sydney, NSW, Australia. [5]Melbourne Sexual Health Centre, Alfred Health and Monash University, Melbourne, Victoria, Australia. [6]Viral Hepatitis Elimination Program, Burnet Institute, Melbourne, Victoria, Australia.

References

1. Greub G, Ledergerber B, Battegay M, Grob P, Perrin L, Furrer H, Burgisser P, Erb P, Boggian K, Piffaretti JC, et al. Clinical progression, survival, and immune recovery during antiretroviral therapy in patients with HIV-1 and hepatitis C virus coinfection: the Swiss HIV Cohort Study. Lancet. 2000; 356(9244):1800–5.
2. Sulkowski MS, Mast EE, Seeff LB, Thomas DL. Hepatitis C virus infection as an opportunistic disease in persons infected with human immunodeficiency virus. Clin Infect Dis. 2000;30(Suppl 1):S77–84.
3. Thein HH, Yi Q, Dore GJ, Krahn MD. Natural history of hepatitis C virus infection in HIV-infected individuals and the impact of HIV in the era of highly active antiretroviral therapy: a meta-analysis. AIDS. 2008;22(15):1979–91.
4. The Australian HIV Observational Database Annual report 2016.
5. The Kirby Institute. HIV, viral hepatitis and sexually transmissible infections in Australia. Annual Surveillance Report 2017. The Kirby Institute, UNSW Australia, Sydney NSW 2052.
6. Arends JE, Lieveld FI, Boeijen LL, de Kanter CT, van Erpecum KJ, Salmon D, Hoepelman AI, Asselah T, Ustianowski A. Natural history and treatment of HCV/HIV coinfection: is it time to change paradigms? J Hepatol. 2015;63(5): 1254–62.
7. Australian Government: Turnbull govt invests over $1B to cure Hep C - media release. (2015).
8. Gastroenterological Society of Australia: Australian recommendations for the management of hepatitis C virus infection: a consensus statement (2017). Available from: https://www.asid.net.au/documents/item/1208 [accessed: 08 Mar 2017].
9. Aitken S. ASHM Report Back - Elimination of Hepatitis C and HIV coinfection in Australia. Available from: http://ashm.info/hiv-co-infections/elimination-of-hepatitis-c-and-hiv-coinfection-in-australia [accessed: 10 Mar 2017].

10. Guy RJ, Kong F, Goller J, Franklin N, Bergeri I, Dimech W, Reilly N, Sullivan E, Ward J, Kaldor JM, et al. A new national Chlamydia sentinel surveillance system in Australia: evaluation of the first stage of implementation. Commun Dis Intell Q Rep. 2010;34(3):319–28.
11. Centers for Disease Control and Prevention. Hepatitis C. Available from: https://www.cdc.gov/vitalsigns/hepatitisc/index.html [accessed: 08 Mar 2017].
12. Martin NK, Thornton A, Hickman M, Sabin C, Nelson M, Cooke GS, Martin TC, Delpech V, Ruf M, Price H, et al. Can hepatitis C virus (HCV) direct-acting antiviral treatment as prevention reverse the HCV epidemic among men who have sex with men in the United Kingdom? Epidemiological and modeling insights. Clin Infect Dis. 2016;62(9):1072–80.
13. Salazar-Vizcaya L, Kouyos RD, Zahnd C, Wandeler G, Battegay M, Darling KE, Bernasconi E, Calmy A, Vernazza P, Furrer H, et al. Hepatitis C virus transmission among human immunodeficiency virus-infected men who have sex with men: modeling the effect of behavioral and treatment interventions. Hepatology. 2016;64(6):1856–69.
14. van de Laar TJ, Matthews GV, Prins M, Danta M. Acute hepatitis C in HIV-infected men who have sex with men: an emerging sexually transmitted infection. AIDS. 2010;24(12):1799–812.
15. National HCV Testing Policy Expert Reference Committee. National Hepatitis C Testing Policy v1.2. Available from: http://testingportal.ashm.org.au/images/HCV/HCV_TESTING_POLICY_Mar_2017.pdf [accessed: 03 Nov 2017].
16. Jin FY, Matthews GV, Grulich AE. Sexual transmission of hepatitis C virus among gay and bisexual men: a systematic review. Sex Health. 2017; 14(1):28–41.
17. Higgs P, Hsieh K, Hellard M. "You're better off waiting": knowledge and awareness of hepatitis C direct-acting antivirals in a cohort of people who inject drugs (P1269). J Hepatol. 2015;62:S834.
18. Hepatitis Australia. Love your liver. Available from: http://loveyourliver.com.au/ [accessed: 06 Nov 2017].
19. New South Wales Health. Enter the party. Available from: http://hepc.health.nsw.gov.au/ [accessed: 06 Nov 2017].
20. ASHM. Australasian Society for HIV, Viral Hepatitis and Sexual Health Medicine. Available from: http://www.ashm.org.au/ [accessed: 06 Nov 2017].
21. Medland NA, Chow EP, Bradshaw CS, Read TH, Sasadeusz JJ, Fairley CK. Predictors and incidence of sexually transmitted hepatitis C virus infection in HIV positive men who have sex with men. BMC Infect Dis. 2017;17(1):185.
22. Hagan H, Jordan AE, Neurer J, Cleland CM. Incidence of sexually transmitted hepatitis C virus infection in HIV-positive men who have sex with men. AIDS. 2015;29(17):2335–45.
23. Wandeler G, Gsponer T, Bregenzer A, Gunthard HF, Clerc O, Calmy A, Stockle M, Bernasconi E, Furrer H, Rauch A, et al. Hepatitis C virus infections in the Swiss HIV cohort study: a rapidly evolving epidemic. Clin Infect Dis. 2012;55(10):1408–16.
24. Gamage DG, Read TR, Bradshaw CS, Hocking JS, Howley K, Chen MY, Fairley CK. Incidence of hepatitis-C among HIV infected men who have sex with men (MSM) attending a sexual health service: a cohort study. BMC Infect Dis. 2011;11:39.
25. Vanhommerig JW, Stolte IG, Lambers FA, Geskus RB, van de Laar TJ, Bruisten SM, Schinkel J, Prins M. Stabilizing incidence of hepatitis C virus infection among men who have sex with men in Amsterdam. J Acquir Immune Defic Syndr. 2014;66(5):e111–5.
26. Witt MD, Seaberg EC, Darilay A, Young S, Badri S, Rinaldo CR, Jacobson LP, Detels R, Thio CL. Incident hepatitis C virus infection in men who have sex with men: a prospective cohort analysis, 1984-2011. Clin Infect Dis. 2013; 57(1):77–84.
27. van Santen DK, van der Helm JJ, Del Amo J, Meyer L, D'Arminio Monforte A, Price M, Beguelin CA, Zangerle R, Sannes M, Porter K, et al. Lack of decline in hepatitis C virus incidence among HIV-positive men who have sex with men during 1990-2014. J Hepatol. 2017;67(2):255–62.
28. Memedovic S, Iversen J, Geddes L, Maher L. Australian Needle Syringe Program Survey National Data Report 2011–2015: Prevalence of HIV, HCV and injecting and sexual behaviour among NSP attendees. Available from: https://kirby.unsw.edu.au/report-type/australian-nsp-survey-national-data-report. [accessed: 09 Mar 2017].
29. Sundquist K, Frank G. Urbanization and hospital admission rates for alcohol and drug abuse: a follow-up study of 4.5 million women and men in Sweden. Addiction. 2004;99(10):1298–305.

4

Estimating the scale of chronic hepatitis C virus infection in the EU/EEA: a focus on migrants from anti-HCV endemic countries

A. M. Falla[1,2*†], A. A. Ahmad[3,4†], E. Duffell[5], T. Noori[5] and I. K. Veldhuijzen[2,6]

Abstract

Background: Increasing the proportion diagnosed with and on treatment for chronic hepatitis C (CHC) is key to the elimination of hepatitis C in Europe. This study contributes to secondary prevention planning in the European Union/ European Economic Area (EU/EEA) by estimating the number of CHC (anti-HCV positive and viraemic) cases among migrants living in the EU/EEA and born in endemic countries, defining the most affected migrant populations, and assessing whether country of birth prevalence is a reliable proxy for migrant prevalence.

Methods: Migrant country of birth and population size extracted from statistical databases and anti-HCV prevalence in countries of birth and in EU/EEA countries derived from a systematic literature search were used to estimate caseload among and most affected migrants. Reliability of country of birth prevalence as a proxy for migrant prevalence was assessed via a systematic literature search.

Results: Approximately 11% of the EU/EEA adult population is foreign-born, 79% of whom were born in endemic (anti-HCV prevalence ≥1%) countries. Anti-HCV/CHC prevalence in migrants from endemic countries residing in the EU/EEA is estimated at 2.3%/1.6%, corresponding to ~580,000 CHC infections or 14% of the CHC disease burden in the EU/EEA. The highest number of cases is found among migrants from Romania and Russia (50–60,000 cases each) and migrants from Italy, Morocco, Pakistan, Poland and Ukraine (25–35,000 cases each). Ten studies reporting prevalence in migrants in Europe were identified; in seven of these estimates, prevalence was comparable with the country of birth prevalence and in three estimates it was lower.

Discussion: Migrants are disproportionately affected by CHC, account for a considerable number of CHC infections in EU/EEA countries, and are an important population for targeted case finding and treatment. Limited data suggest that country of birth prevalence can be used as a proxy for the prevalence in migrants.

Keywords: Chronic viral hepatitis, Hepatitis C virus (HCV), Migrants, Epidemiology, Europe

Background

Chronic infection with the hepatitis C virus (HCV) is a global public health challenge and a leading cause of liver disease-related morbidity and mortality. The epidemiology remains poorly understood, however, and global, national and risk group-specific anti-HCV and viraemic prevalence estimates vary considerably. Recent studies suggest that between 105 million and 185 million people are anti-HCV positive worldwide and that global anti-HCV prevalence in adults could be as high as 2% [1, 2]. The Global Burden of Disease study estimated that chronic HCV (CHC) infection causes almost half a million deaths annually and is the 25th leading cause of death worldwide [3].

Chronic HCV infection affects the liver and has a mostly asymptomatic onset, but can lead to cirrhosis and hepatocellular carcinoma (HCC) decades later [4]. The asymptomatic nature of infection and the lack of adequate screening programmes means that the majority of people infected with CHC are unaware of their

* Correspondence: am.falla@rotterdam.nl; abby.falla@gmail.com
†Equal contributors
[1]Department of Public Health, Erasmus MC, University Medical Center Rotterdam, Rotterdam, the Netherlands
[2]Division of Infectious Disease Control, Municipal Public Health Service Rotterdam-Rijnmond, PO Box 70032, 3000, LP, Rotterdam, The Netherlands
Full list of author information is available at the end of the article

infection and only around one third of all estimated CHC infections in Europe have been diagnosed [5–7]. Effective antiviral treatment can prevent the development of cirrhosis and HCC and, with newer direct acting antivirals (DAAs) reporting cure rates in more than 90% of cases, [8] the elimination of HCV infection is now possible in Europe [9]. This will require continued primary prevention of new infections in parallel with expansion of secondary prevention through effective screening, linkage to care and treatment.

Primary prevention measures in Europe, including a safe blood supply, improved infection control practices and harm reduction programmes, have led to a significant reduction of HCV transmission in many countries and a mathematical modelling study shows incident cases are declining [10]. Incident data is not systematically collected and reported in most EU/EEEA countries hampering a good understanding of time trends although iatrogenic and nosocomial transmission is reported to be rare in most EU/EEA countries [11]. However, models predict that the peak in the mortality is yet to be reached [9, 10, 12]. An estimated 7.4 million people are anti-HCV positive in the European Union/European Economic area (EU/EEA), although prevalence varies from 0.9% in Western Europe to 3.3% in Eastern Europe [1, 13]. Deaths from viral hepatitis now exceed those from HIV and tuberculosis combined and latest published estimates show that 96,000 people die each year in EU/EEA countries from HBV and HCV-related liver disease [3]. Some populations are disproportionately affected and have a high prevalence of chronic infection. One such population is migrants born in high anti-HCV prevalence countries [10, 14–16], although estimates of the number of cases and the most affected migrant populations in Europe are lacking.

This epidemiological study seeks to inform targeted screening, linkage to care and treatment in the EU/EEA by: providing estimates, across and within all 31 EU/EEA countries, of the number of CHC cases among migrants from countries where anti-HCV prevalence is ≥1%; providing an estimate of the relative contribution of migrants to the overall burden of disease; and comparing the reported in-country of birth prevalence with that found among migrants living in European countries. In a sister paper to this, we conduct a similar analysis for chronic hepatitis B among migrants from endemic countries.

Methods

The data retrieval and analysis process are described in detail below and in a schematic representation (Fig. 1). Demographic data on the size of and countries of birth of migrant populations were extracted from statistical databases. Country of birth-specific and EU/EEA country general population anti-HCV prevalence estimates were derived from a systematic literature search. To assess the reliability of using country of birth-derived prevalence as a proxy for the prevalence among migrants, a systematic literature search was conducted to identify prevalence estimates among migrants in Europe to compare with country of birth-derived prevalence.

Definitions

Migrant

An adult 15 years old or above, born in a country other than the current country of residence. Children are excluded due to the dominance of older age populations in sero-prevalence studies and the higher prevalence reported among adults than among children [1]. The use of the term 'migrant' in this study therefore refers to adult (foreign-born) migrants only. The study accounts for and includes migration from outside the EU/EEA and migration within the EU/EEA, but excludes undocumented migrants.

Anti-HCV prevalence

The common measure of exposure to HCV/endemicity used in sero-prevalence studies. Anti-HCV prevalence can include exposed individuals with a resolved infection.

Chronic hepatitis C (CHC)

Refers to viraemic infection, i.e. anti-HCV and HCV-RNA positivity. Endemic country: the anti-HCV prevalence in the general adult population is ≥1%. This relatively low threshold was chosen to take into account migrants from countries where prevalence is higher than that of the EU/EEA as a whole.

Part 1: The contribution of migrants from endemic countries to the burden of CHC in the EU/EEA

Demographic data (Step 1)

The size and country of birth of the migrant population was obtained for all 31 EU/EEA countries from Eurostat for 2013, if available [17]. Where data were unavailable, either the 'EU 2011 – Housing and Population Census', the most recent demographic data from the Organisation for Economic Co-operation and Development (OECD) Stats website or national statistics were used, in that order [18–20]. The data source is indicated in footnotes in Table 1. For each EU/EEA country, the countries of birth of migrants were sorted into descending order of magnitude of the number of migrants, and the top 50 countries of birth by migrant population size were then selected for estimating the CHC burden.

Country-specific anti-HCV prevalence (Step 2)

The online databases Medline, Embase, the Cochrane library, Web of Science, Scopus, PubMed publisher and

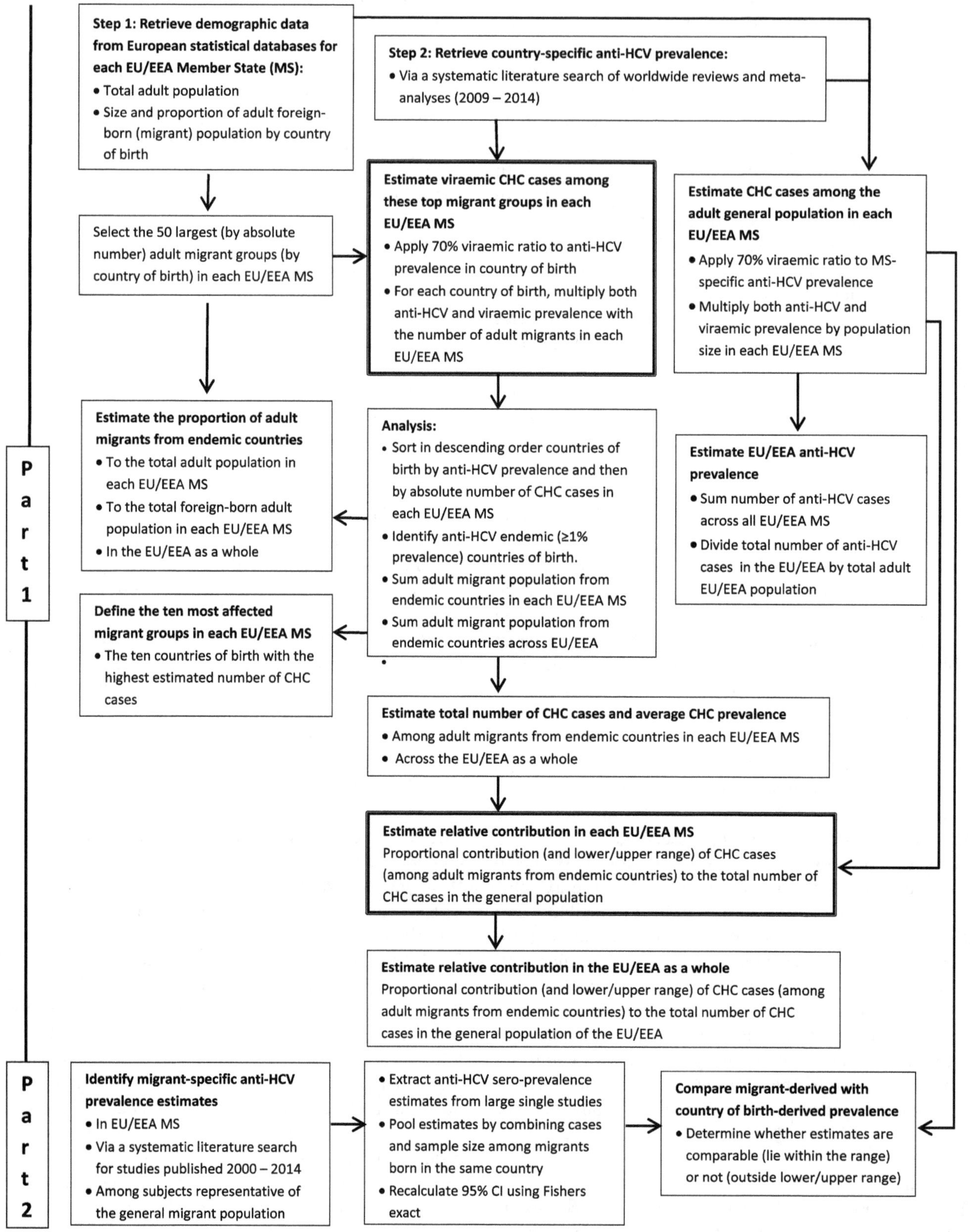

Fig. 1 Schematic methodological representation to estimating the burden of CHC among migrants in the EU/EEA

Table 1 Demographic data and CHC epidemiology in the general population and among migrants in EU/EEA countries

Country (anti-HCV prevalence; range)	General Adult Population				Migrants from endemic countries						
	Total Population[a]	Estimated no. of CHC cases			Number	Proportion (of the total population)	Estimated number of CHC cases			CHC prevalence	Relative contribution (and range) to burden of CHC
		Central estimate	Lower estimate	Upper estimate			Central Estimate	Lower Estimate	Upper Estimate		
Austria (0.5%; 0.1–0.7)	7,232,026	25,312	5062	35,437	883,345	12.2%	11,753	8243	15,117	1.3%	46% (15% - 77%)
Belgium (0.9%; 0.1–1.2)	9,263,570	58,360	6484	77,814	1,054,155	11.4%	18,607	9729	32,764	1.8%	32% (4% - 60%)
Bulgaria (1.1%; 0.3–2.4)	6,294,563	48,468	13,219	105,749	62,941	1.0%	1366	605	1836	2.2%	3% (0% - 6%)
Croatia (1.3%; 1.1–1.6)	3632,461[b,c]	33,055	27,970	40,684	524,609	14.4%	4901	4058	6081	0.9%	15% (10% - 22%)
Cyprus (0.6%; 0.5–0.7)	705,459[b]	2963	2469	9383	128,712	18.2%	2740	1821	3567	2.1%	92% (<0% - >100%)[f]
Czech Republic (0.7%; 0.2–0.7)	8,955,829	43,884	12,538	43,884	331,840	3.7%	5937	2596	8219	1.8%	14% (6% – 22%)
Denmark (0.7%; (0.5–0.7)	4,625,032	22,663	16,188	22,663	278,041	6.0%	3894	2244	5194	1.4%	17% (10% - 24%)
Estonia (3.3%; 1.6–4.5)	1,113,355	25,719	12,470	35,071	189,495	17.0%	5090	1625	7033	2.7%	20% (6% - 33%)
Finland (0.7%; 0.6–0.9)	4,535,282	22,223	19,048	28,572	176,980	3.9%	3383	1682	4826	1.9%	15% (7% - 23%)
France (0.7%) (0.5–0.8)	52,901,411[b]	259,217	185,155	296,248	5,714,076	10.8%	88,799	37,816	154,348	1.6%	34% (11% - 58%)
Germany (0.5%; 0.3–0.9)	69,414,404[b]	242,950	145,770	437,311	8,888,710	12.8%	128,809	61,796	193,947	1.4%	53% (11% - 95%)
Greece (1.9%; 0.5–2.6)	9464,000[c]	125,871	33,124	172,245	588,275	6.2%	12,959	9854	15,519	2.2%	10% (4% -16%)
Hungary (0.8%; 0.4–2.7)	8,477,933	47,476	23,738	160,233	336,360	4.0%	6548	4980	7889	1.9%	14% (0% - 34%)
Iceland (0.9%; 0.7–1.5)	255,391	1609	1251	2682	18,311	7.2%	206	111	307	1.1%	13% (4% - 21%)
Ireland (1.1%; 0.7–1.6)	3,586,829	27,619	17,575	40,172	321,771	9.0%	5485	2934	8188	1.7%	20% (7% - 32%)
Italy (4.4%; 1.6–7.3)	51,336,889	1,581,176	574,973	2,623,315	4,118,015	8.0%	78,501	52,730	101,393	1.9%	5% (1% - 9%)
Latvia (2.4%; 1.7–3.3)	1,731,509	29,089	20,605	39,998	271,468	15.7%	6532	2168	9209	2.4%	22% (8% - 37%)
Liechtenstein (0.9%; 0.7–1.5)	31,142	196	153	327	14,672	47.1%	172	82	223	1.2%	88% (35% - >100%)[f]

Table 1 Demographic data and CHC epidemiology in the general population and among migrants in EU/EEA countries *(Continued)*

Country (anti-HCV prevalence; range)	General Adult Population				Migrants from endemic countries						
	Total Population[a]	Estimated no. of CHC cases			Number	Proportion (of the total population)	Estimated number of CHC cases			CHC prevalence	Relative contribution (and range) to burden of CHC
		Central estimate	Lower estimate	Upper estimate			Central Estimate	Lower Estimate	Upper Estimate		
Lithuania (2.9%; 0.7–3.0)	2,535,329 [e]	51,467	12,423	53,242	127,711	5.0%	2795	1046	4142	2.2%	5% (2%- 9%)
Luxembourg (0.9%; 0.6–0.9)	417,377[d]	2629	1753	2629	104,495	25.0%	1682	659	2710	1.6%	64% (24% - >100%)[f]
Malta (0.9%; 0.7–1.5)	355,704[b]	2241	1743	3735	17,833	5.0%	295	182	438	1.7%	13% (5% - 21%)
Netherlands (0.2%; 0.1–0.4)	13,901,653	19,462	9731	38,925	978,698	7.0%	13,262	7278	18,376	1.4%	68% (10% - >100%)[f]
Norway (0.7%; (0.6–0.9)	4,122,334	20,199	17,314	25,971	357,877	8.7%	4822	2601	6907	1.3%	24% (12% - 36%)
Poland (1.1%; 0.6–1.9)	32,736,685	252,072	137,494	435,398	453,723	1.4%	9633	3080	12,877	2.1%	4% (1% - 7%)
Portugal (1.8%; 0.5–2.9)	8989,849[b]	113,272	31,464	182,494	642,212	7.1%	13,505	7474	24,179	2.1%	12% (1% - 23%)
Romania (3.2%; 2.9–3.6)	16,880,465	378,122	342,673	425,388	102,854	0.6%	2090	912	2923	2.0%	1% (0% - 1%)
Slovakia (1.4%; 0.9–2.0)	4,580,260	44,887	28,856	64,124	31,460	0.7%	588	281	782	1.9%	1% (0% - 2%)
Slovenia (1.3%; 1.1–1.6)	1,760,726	16,023	13,558	19,720	208,026	11.8%	2030	1607	2563	1.0%	13% (9% - 17%)
Spain (1.7%; 0.4–2.6)	39,637,891	471,691	110,986	721,410	3,748,924	9.5%	55,164	31,440	75,323	1.5%	12% (3% - 21%)
Sweden (0.6%; 0.5–0.7)	7,944,034	33,365	27,804	38,926	773,085	9.7%	10,579	5352	14,452	1.4%	32% (17% - 46%)
United Kingdom (0.6%; (0.4–1.2)	52,082,285[b]	218,746	145,830	437,491	4,706,765	9.0%	76,535	45,555	118,608	1.6%	35% (6% -64%)
EU/EEA (1.4%; 0.5–1.5)	429,501,677	4,222,026	1,999,421	6,621,241	36,155,438	8.4%	578,663	312,539	859,941	1.6%	14% (4% - 24%)

[a]Source is EUROSTAT 2013 unless indicated by the following letter
[b]ESS 2011 Census
[c]OECD 2012/EUROSTAT 2013 age distribution
[d]OECD 2010/EUROSTAT age distribution
[e]http://www.euras.lt (Lithuanian National Statistics Agency)/EUROSTAT 2013 age distribution
[f]The Delta method does not give a reliable confidence interval around the relative contribution as the relative contribution is close to 100% and the distribution of cases in the general population is extremely skewed

Google Scholar were searched in January 2015 for reviews, systematic reviews and meta-analyses in English about the prevalence of hepatitis C in the general population at country level. The search (described in full in Annex 1 of the Additional file 1) used a combination of disease-related (hepatitis C), outcome-related (prevalence), population-related (general population, worldwide) and study design-related (reviews) terms. Note that the search also included terms related to hepatitis B since we conducted a similar analysis for chronic hepatitis B among migrants from endemic countries (to be published in this journal). Since the aim was to identify recent reviews, the search was restricted to papers published after 2009 to the date of the search. The titles and abstracts, then the full text, of retrieved citations were assessed for relevancy by one reviewer (AF). Key exclusion criteria included studies focused on: hepatitis other than type C; natural history, clinical features or complications of hepatitis; medical treatment; other high risk groups e.g. people who inject drugs (PWID); and single case studies and cost effectiveness analyses. High quality systematic reviews/meta-analyses were selected given the recent publication of robust systematic reviews/meta-analyses of national level prevalence estimates globally.

Country-level anti-HCV prevalence estimates and uncertainty ranges/confidence intervals (CIs) were extracted from the included reviews and entered into a Microsoft Excel database of all countries. Where a country-specific estimate was unavailable, the relevant Global Burden of Disease region estimate was used. If a meta-analysis reported a statistically significant time trend, the estimate from the most recent period was selected. Where multiple estimates for a country were available from different reviews, the most robust was selected based on the assessed risk of selection bias. Risk of selection bias was assessed based on: sampling method (random favoured over convenience); sampling population (the general population was favoured over more specifically defined (risk) groups); geographical coverage (national favoured over regional; regional favoured over local); sample size (larger studies preferred over smaller one); and data collection timeframe (favouring recency). Decisions were made jointly by two reviewers (AF and IV) based on these criteria (rather than a pre-defined algorithm) with a detailed rationale recorded for each selected estimate. This rationale, together with search strategy, the inclusion/exclusion criteria and a PRISMA flowchart are available in the online supplement.

Estimating the CHC burden among migrants from endemic countries

Anti-HCV prevalence was multiplied by the number of migrants from the top 50 countries of birth of migrants in each EU/EEA country. The countries of birth were then sorted in descending order of magnitude by anti-HCV prevalence to identify all endemic (≥1% anti-HCV prevalence) countries. The total number of migrants born in anti-HCV endemic countries was used to determine both the total and proportional contribution of migrants from these countries to the overall number of migrants residing in each of the 31 EU/EEA countries. To estimate the proportion of CHC (viraemic) cases among the anti-HCV positive migrant population, the worldwide average viraemic proportion of 70% found in a recent global meta-analysis was applied [1].

Relative contribution

For each EU/EEA country, the estimated number of infected cases among migrants from endemic countries was divided by the total number of infected persons (based on the general population CHC prevalence estimate and the total population) to estimate the relative contribution of migrants from endemic countries to the overall number of people infected with CHC. Given uncertainty in both the size of the migrant population and CHC prevalence estimates in countries of birth, a range in the relative contribution (a lower limit and a higher limit) was also calculated using the Delta method [21].

Part 2: Anti-HCV prevalence in migrant populations in Europe

The online databases Medline, Embase, the Cochrane library, Web of Science, Scopus, PubMed publisher and Google Scholar were searched in November 2014 for studies in English that estimate the prevalence of hepatitis C in migrants in any of the 31 EU/EEA countries. The search used a combination of disease-related (hepatitis C), outcome-related (prevalence), population-related (migrants) and geographical area (EU/EEA countries) terms and was limited to studies published between 2000 and 2014. We expected a limited retrieval from this search and therefore included only selection bias (how representative the study population was of the general population) as a key parameter in the risk of bias assessment. This operationalised through the exclusion of studies sampled from higher risk migrant groups such as refugees/asylum seeker and higher risk (general) populations such as STI clinic attendees, outpatient clinics, international health centres etc. The full search strategy, inclusion/exclusion criteria and PRISMA flowchart are available in the online supplement.

Data from the included studies were entered into Microsoft Excel. Pooled estimates for countries of birth were produced by combining the numbers tested and the number of cases. A 95% CI was re-calculated using the Fisher's exact method. Prevalence estimates pooled from multiple studies or extracted from large single studies (>25 subjects from a single country) were compared with the in-country estimates to determine whether in-country estimates reflect the prevalence found among migrants. When the point prevalence from a study in migrants (Part 2) fell within the CI/uncertainty range of the in-country estimate (from Part 1), this estimate was considered to be comparable; when it fell below the lower CI/uncertainty range, it was considered to be lower than the in-country prevalence; and when it was higher than the upper CI/uncertainty range, it was considered to be higher.

Results

Estimated CHC prevalence and number of infected cases in 31 EU/EEA countries (Table 1)

The anti-HCV prevalence in the general population in the EU/EEA is estimated at 1.4% (range of 0.7–2.2%). However, prevalence estimates range from 0.2% in the Netherlands to 4.4% in Italy and 14 EU/EEA countries are considered endemic by the definition adopted in our study (≥1% anti-HCV prevalence). Table 1 lists the estimated number and range of CHC cases among adults in EU/EEA countries. An estimated 4.2 million (range 2.0–6.6 million) adults in the EU/EEA have CHC infection. Italy has the highest absolute number, with an estimated 1.6 million CHC cases. Other EU/EEA countries with a high absolute number of CHC cases among adults are Romania, with 380,000, and Spain, with 470,000.

The distribution of migrants in the EU/EEA based on HCV endemicity in country of birth

The top 50 migrant populations in each EU/EEA country included in the analysis make up at least 95% of the total migrant population in 19 countries and at least 90% in all but three EU/EEA countries (Denmark, Sweden and the United Kingdom, where the proportion is at least 85%). These migrant populations account for approximately 10.7% of the total adult population in the EU/EEA although the proportion in each country varies, ranging from 0.7% in Romania, 1.1% in Bulgaria and 1.7% in Poland to 42.0% in Luxembourg and 65.2% in Liechtenstein (Fig. 2).

Nearly 80% of the total migrant population were born in HCV endemic countries. Other than in Slovakia, where 23% of the total migrant population are from endemic countries, over half of all migrants in the other 30 EU/EEA countries were born in countries where the anti-HCV prevalence is ≥1%. In Croatia, Estonia, Latvia, Lithuania, Romania and Slovenia, more than 90% of all migrants are from endemic countries (Fig. 2). The number and proportion of all migrants that from endemic countries, at country level and in the EU/EEA as a whole are shown in Table 2.

Country-specific anti-HCV prevalence estimates

The most comprehensive review with country-specific estimates of anti-HCV prevalence identified by the search was published in 2014 by Gower et al. [1]. This review includes studies published after the year 2000 and provides estimates for 87 countries and for each of the 21 Global Burden of Disease regions. The country-level estimates from Gower do not have 95% CIs but a lower and upper uncertainty range; the lower range is based on studies among populations considered representative of 'healthy adults' (such as blood donors), but the methodology applied to derive the upper limit is unclear. For nine countries, Gower's regional or in-country estimate was replaced with estimates from other systematic reviews deemed more robust according to the criteria described in the methods [2, 22–26]. The 224

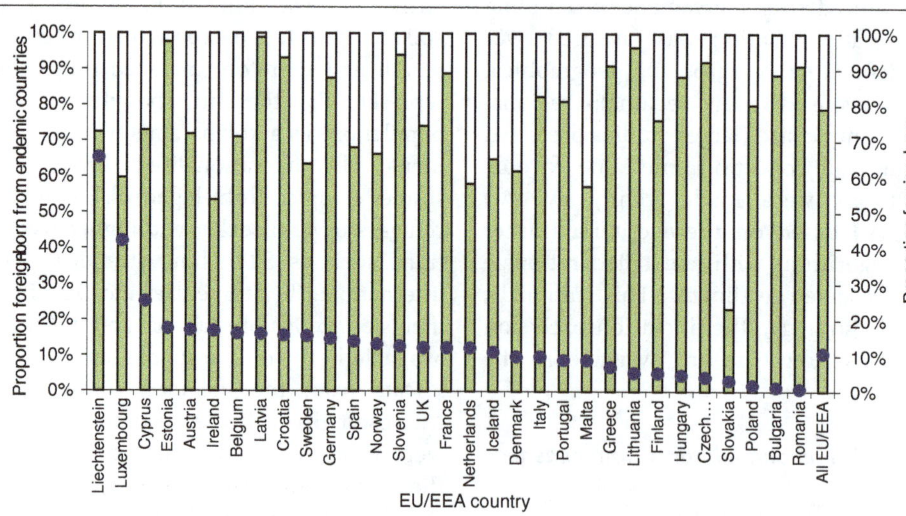

Fig. 2 Total (%) migrant population in each EU/EEA country and the proportion born in endemic countries

Table 2 The ten migrant groups (from endemic countries) accounting for the highest number of CHC cases

Migrant country of birth	Total adult migrant population	Anti-HCV prevalence	Number (rounded) of CHC cases	Host countries (first 6 with largest populations)[a]
Romania	2,646,392	3.2	59,000	Italy, Spain, Germany, Hungary, UK, Austria
Russia	1,713,636	4.1	49,000	Germany, Latvia, Estonia, Italy, Lithuania, Spain
Italy	1,114,683	4.4	34,000	France, Germany, UK, Belgium, Spain, The Netherlands
Poland	4,103,409	1.1	32,000	Germany, UK, Italy, France, Ireland, The Netherlands
Morocco	2,418,072	1.6	27,000	France, Spain, Italy, Belgium, The Netherlands, Germany
Pakistan	756,170	5.0	27,000	UK, Italy, Spain, Germany, Greece, France
Ukraine	993,459	3.6	25,000	Poland, Germany, Italy, Czech Republic, Spain, Latvia
Egypt	194,852	15.7	21,000	Italy, UK, France, The Netherlands, Austria, Greece
Kazakhstan	807,781	3.3	19,000	Germany, Latvia, Czech Republic, Poland, Lithuania, Estonia
Nigeria	313,212	8.4	18,000	UK, Italy, Spain, Ireland, Austria, The Netherlands

[a]if migrant population is at least 1000

country-level prevalence estimates and the source, together with an overview of decision rationale where an estimate other than Gower was available, are listed in the online supplement.

Estimated prevalence and number of CHC infections among migrants

Across the EU/EEA, the overall anti-HCV prevalence among migrants from endemic countries is estimated at 2.3%, which corresponds to a CHC prevalence of 1.6% and an estimated 580,000 CHC infections (Table 2). The estimated prevalence of CHC infection among migrants from endemic countries ranges from 0.9% in Croatia to 2.4% in Estonia. Table 2 lists the ten migrant populations with the highest estimated number of CHC cases and the host EU/EEA countries with the largest populations of migrants born in these countries. Based on cumulative analysis of the CHC burden among the different migrant populations from endemic countries to or within the EU, migrants from Romania, Russia, Italy and Poland contribute most, in descending order, to the overall number of CHC cases. An estimated 50,000–60,000 CHC cases are found among migrants from Romania and from Russia.

Some countries of birth of migrants are common across EU/EEA countries. Adult migrants from Russia, a high CHC prevalence country (2.9%), are represented among the top ten migrant populations in 25 of 31 EU/EEA countries. Migrants from Romania and Italy are among the top ten migrant groups in 20 EU/EEA countries. Although small in number, migrants from Egypt are among the top ten CHC-infected migrant populations in 16 of 31 EU/EEA countries due the very high anti-HCV prevalence (15.7%) in Egypt. In Estonia, Lithuania and Latvia, the top ten migrant populations with the highest number of infected cases are all from countries of the former Soviet Union. This is also the case in five to six of the top ten migrant populations with the highest number of infected cases in Bulgaria, the Czech Republic and Poland. People born either in Yugoslavia before 1992 or in one of the countries that emerged from the fall of Yugoslavia since 1992are represented in six of the top ten migrant populations with the largest of number of CHC cases in Croatia and Slovenia and three of the top ten in Austria. Migrants from the Algeria, Morocco and Tunisia are represented among the ten most CHC-affected migrant populations in France. EU/EEA countries with three to five African countries represented among the top ten CHC-affected migrant groups include Belgium, France, Luxembourg, Portugal and the UK. Prevalence, population size and number and range of CHC infections among, for all 50 countries of birth of migrants in each EU/EEA country can be found in the online supplement.

Relative contribution of migrants to the CHC burden in EU/EEA countries

The relative proportion (and range) of infected migrants from endemic countries within the overall CHC burden in EU/EEA countries is shown in Table 1 and Fig. 3. The relative contribution is low (<4%) in Bulgaria, Poland, Romania and Slovakia and much higher (64%–92%) in Cyprus, Liechtenstein, Luxembourg and the Netherlands.

Comparing migrant-derived anti-HCV prevalence with country of birth estimates

The literature search identified thirteen anti-HCV prevalence estimates from studies in migrants in the EU/EEA

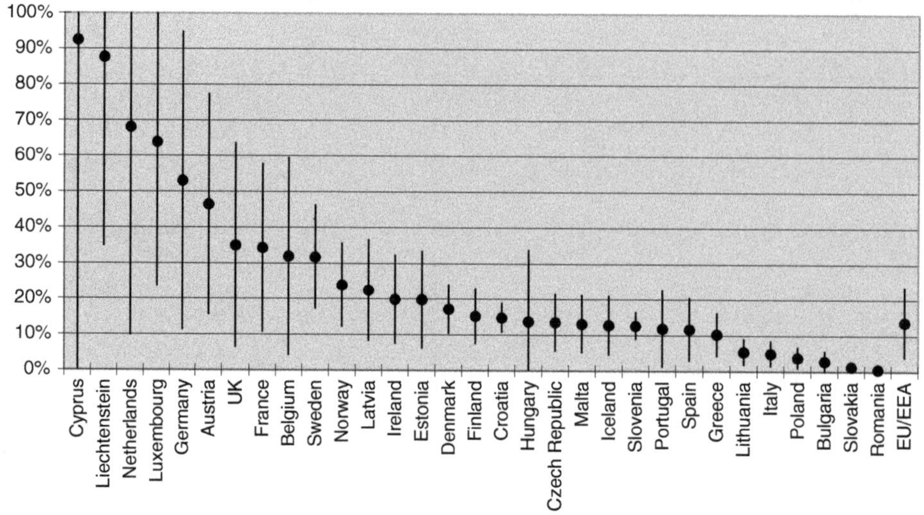

Fig. 3 Estimated relative contribution (upper/lower range) of migrants to the total number of CHC cases

for comparison with the in-country estimates derived in Part 1. Two of the thirteen estimates, from studies among migrants from the former Dutch Antilles and Suriname, were higher than the comparator regional prevalence [1]. One estimate, from a study among migrants from the former Soviet Union, could not be compared with in-country anti-HCV prevalence since this nation state is now dissolved. Of the remaining ten estimates, seven were comparable with the in-country estimate and three, among migrants from Egypt, Pakistan and Turkey, were lower than the in-country prevalence (Egypt: 2.4% in migrants vs. 15.7% in-country; Pakistan: 2.8% in migrants vs. 5.5% in-country; and Turkey: 0.2% in migrants vs. 1.0% in-country), although for Turkey the two confidence intervals overlap. See Table 3 for details.

Discussion

This is the first study we know of that attempts to systematically estimate the overall number of CHC cases among migrants, as well as the relative contribution of cases among migrants to the overall burden of CHC in EU/EEA countries. Migrants from endemic countries account for one in 12 EU/EEA adult citizens and for one in seven of all CHC cases in the EU/EEA. As the contribution of migrants to the overall burden of CHC varies between EU/EEA countries, effective approaches to secondary prevention will, therefore, also differ. Screening

Table 3 Comparing migrant study-derived prevalence to country of birth-derived prevalence

Country of birth	Migrants			In-country		Comparison
	N. tested	Prevalence (95% CI)	Reference	Prevalence (95% CI)	Reference	
Afghanistan	293	1.0 (0.2–3.0)	[32]	1.1 (0.6–1.9)	[1]	Comparable
Bangladesh	934	0.4 (0.1–1.1)	[52, 53]	1.3 (0.2–2.2)	[1]	Comparable
Dutch Antilles	38	2.6 (0.1–13.8)	[15, 45]	0.8[b] (0.2–1.3)	[1]	Higher
Egypt	465	2.4 (1.2–4.2)	[54]	15.7 (13.9–17.5)	[25]	Lower
Former USSR	65	3.1 (0.4–10.7)	[32]	3.3[a] (1.6–4.5)	[1]	Comparable
India	1334	0.4 (0.2–1.0)	[52, 53]	0.8 (0.4–1.0)	[1]	Comparable
Iran	153	0.7 (0–3.6)	[32]	0.5 (0.2 – 1[a])	[1]	Comparable
Iraq	290	0.3 (0–1.9)	[32]	3.2 (0.3–3.2[a])	[1]	Comparable
Morocco	331	0.9 (0.2–2.6)	[15, 45]	1.6 (0.6–1.9[a])	[1]	Comparable
Pakistan	3562	2.8 (2.3–3.4)	[30, 52, 53]	5.5 (4.4–5.5)	[26]	Lower
Suriname	225	2.4 (0.5–7.0)	[15, 45]	0.8[b] (0.2–1.3)	[1]	Higher
Turkey	965	0.2 (0–0.8)	[15, 45, 46]	1.0 (0.7–1.1)	[22]	Lower
Vietnam	126	1.6 (0.2–5.6)	[32]	1.0 (0.8–1.8)	[1]	Comparable

[a]Regional estimate from GBD Eastern European region
[b]Caribbean GBD Regional estimate

programmes targeting migrant populations will be most effective in EU/EEA countries such as Austria, France, Germany, the Netherlands and the UK where migrants account for a large proportion of the disease burden (32–92%, see Fig. 3) and a small proportion of the total population (7–15%, see Fig. 2).

In contrast, in countries where HCV prevalence is high in the general population and the contribution of migrants is low, it may be more cost-effective to implement population-based screening [27, 28]. Examples of such countries include Bulgaria, Poland, Romania and Slovakia where less than 4% of the CHC burden is attributable to migrants from endemic countries. The differences in general population prevalence between EU/EEA countries, together with the contribution of migrants moving within the EU/EEA from high to low prevalence countries, suggests that there may also be value in allocating EU health funding to scale up and systematise screening and treatment efforts in EU/EEA countries with a high general population prevalence, to strengthen efforts to reduce cross-border health threats and to improve overall population health in the EU. A recent modelling study estimated that only around a third of all CHC cases across Europe have been diagnosed and that there are wide differences in both the proportion diagnosed and the proportion on treatment comparing EU/EEA countries [6]. There is however no data on the estimated proportion of migrants from endemic countries that are diagnosed. The data reported, as well as the strategies and interventions suggested, in this study can contribute to increasing the proportion of cases of CHC diagnosed and on treatment.

Previous studies of hepatitis B/C screening implemented among migrant populations describe different models. These include: outreach offering awareness raising and/or on-site screening by public health teams in social, civic or cultural locations familiar to the target community [29–31]; invitation-based screening where municipal, population or patient registries are used to send postal invitations to attend screening to people born in higher prevalence countries [32, 33]; opportunistic offering of screening to patients with country of birth-related risk factors who attend health care services for other health issues [34, 35]; and adding viral hepatitis screening to an existing screening programme, such as for tuberculosis, that targets people from high prevalence countries [36]. Each of these models differs in terms of logistical and resource requirements, uptake and case yield, but few studies have compared the characteristics and effectiveness of different models [37]. The characteristics of screening programmes that have demonstrated success in uptake and yield include: involvement of the community in planning and raising awareness; provision of screening in suitable and accessible locations for the target community; provision of language support, for example, translated materials and interpreters; planning and provision for people without health insurance coverage; cultural sensitivity about and efforts to reduce or eliminate stigma; and availability of follow-up and care in the community. Retention within a follow-up care and treatment pathway is crucial to ensure that the public health benefits of screening are realised [38]. A summary of migrant-specific screening programmes, an appraisal of factors contributing to success, and a range of other scientific and practical resources are available as part of the HEPscreen Toolkit, produced by the EU-funded HEPscreen project, which focused on screening for chronic viral hepatitis among migrants [39].

In four countries, (Cyprus, Lichtenstein, Luxembourg and the Netherlands) the upper range of the estimated relative contribution of migrants as a proportion of the total number of estimated cases was found to be over 100%. This reflects unmeasured correlation between the input parameters (prevalence in countries of birth and the size of the migrant population) for the Delta method as well as the strong skew in the distribution of cases in the general population in these countries. It is also possible that the prevalence in the general population in these EU/EEA countries is under-estimated, due to unrepresentative sampling or low participation of risk populations who are harder to reach, such as PWID and ethnic minorities as well as migrants. Under-representation of migrants and ethnic minorities is a widely recognised phenomenon in clinical trial and health survey research, [40, 41] although literature specifically focused on sero-prevalence sampling and uptake is very limited [23]. In addition, it is possible that estimates based on prevalence in countries of birth results in over-estimation of the prevalence among migrants. For example, it is probable that no longer living in a high prevalence country would reduce the risk of transmission of HCV, especially since much of the transmission in higher prevalence countries is nosocomial [42] and most EU/EEA countries have successfully controlled nosocomial transmission through health care infection control procedures. Over-estimation may also be due to the characteristics of migrants to the EU/EEA, who may be younger and healthier, and so less likely to have experienced hospitalisation or serious medical intervention and more likely to have benefited from improved primary prevention in the last two decades. Migrants to the EU may also be from higher socio-economic groups in their countries of birth and able to afford better, safer health care [43]. We sought to test out this theory of over-estimation and found that, for just three of the ten countries of birth for which we retrieved estimates for, [15, 29, 30, 44–47] the prevalence in migrants was lower than the reported in-country prevalence.

Despite the systematic nature of data retrieval, there are some data limitations. Detailed demographic data was available from Eurostat for only 21 EU/EEA countries. There is also heterogeneity in the parameters and methods used by the different demographic databases and in the way that demographic data on migration is collected and reported by EU/EEA countries. From other literature, we know that countries such as Germany, France and the Netherlands require municipal registration upon arrival in a new area and collect country of birth data as part of registration. Other countries, like the UK, rely on population census data to systematically collect population size and origin [48]. However, there is very limited information in the literature on the methods used by each database or on the heterogeneity of demographic data collection methods across the EU/EEA. Despite these differences, the demographic data used in this study are derived from databases that in turn derive data from national statistical institutes. We believe it to be the best and most reputable available. These analyses do not include undocumented migrants, partly because the size and origin of this population is very dynamic, but mostly because of the imprecision and unreliability of the data [49]. The use of systematic reviews and meta-analyses for the country of birth prevalence input has reduced the reliance on less reliable single study estimates, and whilst we critically appraised the quality of the systematic reviews and meta-analyses, which all applied quality criteria to select studies, we did not directly assess the quality of the estimates included in these reviews. A further note of caution relates to the studies retrieved on prevalence in migrants, as just ten countries of birth were represented in the estimates and few studies had the specific aim of estimating the prevalence in migrants. The use of convenience sampling in many of these studies increases the chance of selection bias and, specifically, that people already diagnosed may not present for screening.

Conclusions

Advances in antiviral treatment open up the possibility of eliminating hepatitis C infection in Europe, but achieving this will require countries to scale up and better target screening, linkage to care and treatment. This study provides strategic, timely and detailed epidemiological intelligence for EU/EEA countries on the hepatitis C burden among migrant populations, a key population group affected by this infection in Europe. It also provides prevalence estimates for 224 countries and territories, which should serve as a useful resource for other countries and regions wishing to understand the relative contribution of migrants to the burden of hepatitis C. This intelligence, together with the learning from previous migrant-specific screening projects in the EU/EEA [39], can help to inform the design of screening programmes to reach migrant populations most affected by chronic hepatitis C infection. A targeted approach in higher risk populations makes more effective use of health care resources and contributes to reducing health inequalities. The World Health Organisation's Global Strategy for Viral Hepatitis [50] and the European Action Plan [51] both share the ambitious goal of elimination of viral hepatitis by 2030. If this goal is to be realised, it will be essential to dramatically increase the proportion of people who are diagnosed, aware of their infection and on treatment. Future research can contribute by focussing on improving the evidence base on effective strategies to reach and retain migrant and other risk populations in screening and treatment and on cost-effectiveness across the treatment cascade.

Additional file

Additional file 1: Annex 1. Search strategy for systematic reviews and meta-analyses of global/worldwide prevalence studies; **Annex 2.** PRISMA diagram of systematic search for global HBsAg/anti-HCV sero-prevalence; **Annex 3.** Description of the search strategy and retrievals for chronic hepatitis B/C prevalence studies among migrants; **Annex 4.** PRISMA flow diagram of systematic search for HBsAg/anti-HCV sero-prevalence in migrants in the EU/EEA; **Annex 5.** Inclusion/exclusion criteria for systematic reviews/meta analyses reporting the prevalence worldwide/in various continents/regions; **Annex 6.** Inclusion/exclusion criteria for studies retrieved by the search for articles reporting the prevalence among migrants; **Annex 7.** Comparison of anti-HCV estimates from SRs/MAs and rationale for estimate selected for analysis; **Annex 8.** Anti-HCV prevalence estimates selected from systematic reviews; **Annex 9.** Chronic Hepatitis C burden country tables: 50 largest migrant populations per EU/EEA country; **Annex 10.** Countries of birth of foreign-born migrants found amongst the ten migrant groups most affected by chronic hepatitis C in 10 or more of the 31 EU/EEA countries. (DOCX 308 kb)

Abbreviations

CHC: Chronic hepatitis c; CIs: Confidence Intervals; DAAs: Direct acting antivirals; ECDC: European centre for disease prevention and control; EU/EEA: European Union/European Economic Area; GBD: Global burden of disease; HCC: Hepatocellular carcinoma; HCV: Hepatitis C virus; OECD: Organisation for economic co-operation and development; PRISMA: Preferred reporting items for systematic reviews and meta analyses; PWID: People who inject drugs; UK: United Kingdom; WHO: World Health Organisation

Acknowledgements

Wichor Bramer (Medical Librarian, Erasmus MC) for assistance with the systematic search queries. Jelle Koopson (RIVM), Daan Nieboer (Statistician, Department of Public Health, Erasmus MC) and Dr. Luc Coffeng (Assistant Professor, Department of Public Health, Erasmus MC) for statistical advice regarding the comparison of in-country with migrant derived prevalence estimates. Dr. Jan van de Kassteele (Statistician, RIVM) for assistance with the Delta method to derive the relative contribution range.

Funding

This study was funded by the European Centre for Disease Control and Prevention (ECDC) under contract number ECD.4999. The ECDC contributed to the design of the study, the interpretation of the results and the drafting/editing of the manuscript.

Authors' contributions

AMF: study concept and design, literature search, acquisition of data, analysis and interpretation of data, drafting of the manuscript and critical revision of the manuscript for important intellectual content. AAA: study concept and design, literature search, acquisition of data, analysis and interpretation of data, drafting of the manuscript and critical revision of the manuscript for important intellectual content. ED: study concept and design, interpretation of data, critical revision of the manuscript for important intellectual content, supervised the study, and obtained funding. TN: study concept and design, interpretation of data, critical revision of the manuscript for important intellectual content, supervised the study, and obtained funding. IKV: study concept and design, literature search, analysis and interpretation of data, critical revision of the manuscript for important intellectual content, and supervised the study. All authors read and approved the final manuscript.

Consent for publication

Not applicable.

Competing interests

All authors declare that they have no competing interests.

Author details

[1]Department of Public Health, Erasmus MC, University Medical Center Rotterdam, Rotterdam, the Netherlands. [2]Division of Infectious Disease Control, Municipal Public Health Service Rotterdam-Rijnmond, PO Box 70032, 3000, LP, Rotterdam, The Netherlands. [3]Department of Health Sciences, Hamburg University of Applied Sciences, Faculty Life Sciences / Public Health Research, Ulmenliet 20, 21033 Hamburg, Germany. [4]Department of Internal Medicine, University Medical Center Hamburg-Eppendorf, Martinistr 52, 20246 Hamburg, Germany. [5]European Centre for Disease Prevention and Control, Granits väg 8, 171 65 Solna, Sweden. [6]Center for Infectious Disease Control, National Institute for Public Health and the Environment, Bilthoven, the Netherlands.

References

1. Gower E, et al. Global epidemiology and genotype distribution of the hepatitis C virus infection. J Hepatol. 2014;61(1):S45–57.
2. Mohd Hanafiah K, et al. Global epidemiology of hepatitis C virus infection: new estimates of age-specific antibody to HCV seroprevalence. Hepatology. 2013;57(4):1333–42.
3. Lozano R, et al. Global and regional mortality from 235 causes of death for 20 age groups in 1990 and 2010: a systematic analysis for the global burden of disease study 2010. Lancet. 2012;380(9859):2095–128.
4. European Association for the Study of the Liver (EASL). EASL clinical practice guidelines: management of hepatitis C virus infection. J Hepatol. 2014;60(2): 392–420.
5. Wolffram I, et al. Prevalence of elevated ALT values, HBsAg, and anti-HCV in the primary care setting and evaluation of guideline defined hepatitis risk scenarios. J Hepatol. 2015;62(6):1256–64.
6. Collaborators TE. Hepatitis C virus prevalence and level of intervention required to achieve the WHO targets for elimination in the European Union by 2030: a modelling study. Lancet Gastroenterol Hepatol. 2017;2(5):325–36.
7. European Liver Patients Association (ELPA), Report on hepatitis patient self-help in Europe. Brussels: European Liver Patients Assocation; 2010.
8. Kohli A, et al. Treatment of hepatitis C: a systematic review. JAMA. 2014; 312(6):631–40.
9. Wedemeyer H, et al. Strategies to manage hepatitis C virus (HCV) disease burden. J Viral Hepat. 2014;21(Suppl 1):60–89.
10. Razavi H, et al. The present and future disease burden of hepatitis C virus (HCV) infection with today's treatment paradigm. J Viral Hepat. 2014; 21(Suppl 1):34–59.
11. Negro F. Epidemiology of hepatitis C in Europe. Dig Liver Dis. 2014;46(Suppl 5): S158–64.
12. Deuffic-Burban S, et al. Predicted effects of treatment for HCV infection vary among European countries. Gastroenterology. 2012;143(4):974 85. e14
13. Hope VD, et al. Prevalence and estimation of hepatitis B and C infections in the WHO European region: a review of data focusing on the countries outside the European Union and the European free trade association. Epidemiol Infect. 2014;142(2):270–86.
14. Buggisch P, et al. High prevalence of chronic hepatitis C in 8009 patients with migration background living in Germany. J Hepatol. 2013;58:S325.
15. Urbanus AT, et al. Hepatitis C in the general population of various ethnic origins living in the Netherlands: should non-western migrants be screened? J Hepatol. 2011;55(6):1207–14.
16. Jafferbhoy H, et al. The effectiveness of outreach testing for hepatitis C in an immigrant Pakistani population. Epidemiol Infect. 2012;140(6):1048–53.
17. Eurostat. Immigration by five-year age group, sex and country of birth [migr_imm3ctb]. 2013 [cited 2015; Available from: http://appsso.eurostat.ec.europa.eu/nui/show.do?dataset=migr_imm3ctb&lang=en.
18. European Statistical System. EU 2011 - housing and Polulation census. 2011; Available from: https://ec.europa.eu/CensusHub2/.
19. Organisation for Economic Cooperation and Development (OECD). International migration database. 2013; Available from: http://stats.oecd.org/Index.aspx?DatasetCode=MIG.
20. Lithuanian National Statistics Service. International migration flows. 2013; Available from: http://osp.stat.gov.lt/en/temines-lenteles1.
21. Casella G, Berger RL. Statistical inference. Michigan: Thomson Learning; 2002.
22. Bruggmann P, et al. Historical epidemiology of hepatitis C virus (HCV) in selected countries. J Viral Hepat. 2014;21(Suppl 1):5–33.
23. Cornberg M, et al. A systematic review of hepatitis C virus epidemiology in Europe, Canada and Israel. Liver Int. 2011;31(Suppl. 2):30–60.
24. Godzik P, et al. Prevalence of anti-HCV antibodies among adults in Poland–results of cross-sectional study in general population. Przegl Epidemiol. 2012;66(4):575–80.
25. Lehman EM, Wilson ML. Epidemiology of hepatitis viruses among hepatocellular carcinoma cases and healthy people in Egypt: a systematic review and meta-analysis. Int J Cancer. 2009;124(3):690–7.
26. Waheed Y, et al. Hepatitis C virus in Pakistan: a systematic review of prevalence, genotypes and risk factors. World J Gastroenterol. 2009;15(45):5647–53.
27. Gane E, et al. Strategies to manage hepatitis C virus (HCV) infection disease burden - volume 2. J Viral Hepat. 2015;22(Suppl 1):46–73.
28. Brady JE, et al. Uptake of hepatitis C screening, characteristics of patients tested, and intervention costs in the BEST-C study. Hepatology. 2016;65(1):44–53.
29. Uddin G, et al. Prevalence of chronic viral hepatitis in people of south Asian ethnicity living in England: the prevalence cannot necessarily be predicted from the prevalence in the country of origin. J Viral Hepatitis. 2010;17(5):327–35.
30. O'Leary MC, et al. The prevalence of hepatitis C virus among people of south Asian origin in Glasgow - results from a community based survey and laboratory surveillance. Travel Med Infect Dis. 2013;11(5):301–9.
31. Veldhuijzen IK, et al. Identification and treatment of chronic hepatitis B in Chinese migrants: results of a project offering on-site testing in Rotterdam, the Netherlands. J Hepatol. 2012;57(6):1171–6.
32. Richter C, et al. Screening for chronic hepatitis B and C in migrants from Afghanistan, Iran, Iraq, the former soviet republics, and Vietnam in the Arnhem region, The Netherlands. Epidemiol Infect. 2014;142(10):2140–6.
33. van der Veen YJ, et al. Cultural tailoring to promote hepatitis B screening in Turkish Dutch: a randomized control study. Health Promot Int. 2014;29(4): 692–704.
34. Bottero J, et al. Current state of and needs for hepatitis B screening: results of a large screening study in a low-prevalent, metropolitan region. PLoS One. 2014;9(3).
35. Heidrich B, et al. High prevalence of hepatitis markers in immigrant populations: a prospective screening approach in a real-world setting. Eur J Gastroenterol Hepatol. 2014;26(10):1090–7.
36. Barnett ED. Infectious disease screening for refugees resettled in the United States. Clin Infect Dis. 2004;39(6):833–41.
37. Rein DB, et al. Models of community-based hepatitis B surface antigen screening programs in the U.S. and their estimated outcomes and costs. Public Health Rep. 2011;126(4):560–7.
38. Miners AH, et al. Assessing the cost-effectiveness of finding cases of hepatitis C infection in UK migrant populations and the value of further research. J Viral Hepat. 2014;21(9):616–23.
39. The HEPscreen Project. 2015; Available from: www.hepscreen.eu.
40. Murthy VH, Krumholz HM, Gross CP. Participation in cancer clinical trials: race-, sex-, and age-based disparities. JAMA. 2004;291(22):2720–6.
41. Downing NS, et al. Participation of the elderly, women, and minorities in pivotal trials supporting 2011-2013 U.S. Food and Drug Administration approvals. Trials. 2016;17:199.

42. Sievert W, et al. A systematic review of hepatitis C virus epidemiology in Asia, Australia and Egypt. Liver Int. 2011;31(Suppl. 2):61–80.
43. Rechel B, et al. Migration and health in an increasingly diverse Europe. Lancet. 2013;381(9873):1235–45.
44. McPherson S, et al. Targeted case finding for hepatitis B using dry blood spot testing in the British-Chinese and south Asian populations of the north-east of England. J Viral Hepatitis. 2013;20(9):638–44.
45. Veldhuijzen IK, et al. Viral hepatitis in a multi-ethnic neighborhood in the Netherlands: results of a community-based study in a low prevalence country. Int J Infect Dis. 2009;13(1):e9–e13.
46. Richter C, et al. Hepatitis B prevalence in the Turkish population of Arnhem: implications for national screening policy? Epidemiol Infect. 2012;140(4):724–30.
47. Zuure FR, et al. Screening for hepatitis B and C in first-generation Egyptian migrants living in the Netherlands. Liver Int. 2013;33(5):727–38.
48. Rechel B, Mladovsky P, Deville W. Monitoring migrant health in Europe: a narrative review of data collection practices. Health Policy. 2012;105(1):10–6.
49. Clandestino – Database on irregular migration. *http://irregular-migration.net//index.php?id=161*. [cited 2015.
50. World Health Organisation (WHO). Global Health sector strategy on viral hepatitis 2016–2021: towards ending viral hepatitis. Geneva: World Health Organisation; 2016.
51. World Health Organisation (WHO). Action plan for the health sector response to viral hepatitis in the WHO European region. Geneva: World Health Organisation; 2016.
52. Uddin G, et al. Prevalence of chronic viral hepatitis in people of south Asian ethnicity living in England: the prevalence cannot necessarily be predicted from the prevalence in the country of origin. J Viral Hepat. 2010;17(5):327–35.
53. McPherson S, et al. Targeted case finding for hepatitis B using dry blood spot testing in the British-Chinese and south Asian populations of the north-east of England. J Viral Hepat. 2013;20(9):638–44.
54. Zuure FR, et al. Reasons for compliance or noncompliance with advice to test for hepatitis C via an internet-mediated blood screening service: a qualitative study. BMC Public Health. 2011;11:293.

5

Novel serum biomarkers modified by the body mass index z-score for the detection of liver fibrosis and steatosis in children with chronic hepatitis C

Maria Pokorska-Śpiewak[1,2*], Barbara Kowalik-Mikołajewska[1,2], Małgorzata Aniszewska[1,2], Magdalena Pluta[1,2] and Magdalena Marczyńska[1,2]

Abstract

Background: There is a need for validation of noninvasive alternatives to liver biopsy for the evaluation of fibrosis in children with chronic hepatitis C (CHC). The aim of this study was to evaluate the diagnostic performance of serum biomarkers modified by the body mass index z-score (BMI z-score) for the detection of fibrosis and steatosis in children with CHC.

Methods: Thirty children aged 9.4 ± 3.7 years (14 males, 16 females) with CHC underwent liver biopsy. Fibrosis was scored using a 5-point METAVIR scale (≥2 = significant fibrosis). For all the children, the following noninvasive markers were calculated: The aspartate transaminase (AST)-to-platelets ratio index (APRI), the modified APRI (M-APRI: BMI z-score × APRI), the Fibrosis-4 index (FIB-4), the modified FIB-4 (M-FIB-4: BMI z-score × FIB-4), and a novel marker, B-AST (BMI z-score × AST). The area under the receiver operator characteristic curve (AUROC) was calculated to detect significant fibrosis and steatosis.

Results: In the histopathological evaluation, 22/30 (73%) patients presented with fibrosis, and 8/30 (27%) presented with steatosis. For the detection of significant fibrosis, the AUROCs for M-APRI, M-FIB-4 and B-AST were 0.842, 0.823, and 0.848, respectively. For significant steatosis, the AUROCs were more than 0.9 for all markers that included the BMI z-score. B-AST, with a cut-off of 92.8, showed 71% sensitivity and 95% specificity for detecting significant fibrosis. For predicting severe steatosis, B-AST had 100% sensitivity and 92% specificity. Negative values of all three markers that included BMI z-scores excluded all patients with both significant fibrosis and significant steatosis.

Conclusions: Including the BMI z-score in serum biomarker formulas enhances their diagnostic ability to detect significant fibrosis and steatosis. B-AST may thus act as an effective alternative to liver biopsy.

Keywords: Hepatitis C, Liver biopsy, Liver fibrosis, Liver steatosis

Background

Liver biopsy has been considered a standard method for evaluating liver fibrosis and steatosis in children with chronic hepatitis C (CHC) [1–3]. However, it has several limitations: it is invasive and painful, has inter- and intraobserver variability, and is prone to sampling errors [1, 3]. Therefore, efforts have been made to develop alternative, noninvasive methods to liver biopsy, including imaging studies (elastography) and serum biomarkers [3, 4]. According to the recent recommendations of the European Association for the Study of the Liver (EASL), noninvasive methods can be used instead of liver biopsy to assess liver disease severity prior to antiretroviral therapy, and liver biopsy should be reserved only for cases with potential additional comorbidities or any uncertainty [2]. Many of these noninvasive methods have been evaluated in adults with CHC for their ability to determine fibrosis [5]. However, data on the accuracy of

* Correspondence: mpspiewak@gmail.com
[1]Department of Children's Infectious Diseases, Medical University of Warsaw, ul. Wolska 37, 01-201 Warsaw, Poland
[2]Hospital of Infectious Diseases, ul. Wolska 37, 01-201 Warsaw, Poland

noninvasive tests in pediatric patients with HCV are limited, and none of these methods has been fully validated in children to date [3, 4].

The serum biomarkers include both direct and indirect markers. Direct markers (e.g., glycoproteins, collagens, collagenases, and metalloproteases) reflect the removal or deposition of extracellular matrix in the liver [5]. Indirect markers can be identified in routine blood tests and indicate alterations in liver function [5]. Such markers include the aspartate transaminase-to-platelets ratio index (APRI) and the Fibrosis-4 index (FIB-4), which have been validated to predict significant fibrosis and cirrhosis in adult patients with chronic HCV infection [5–7]. Simple serum biomarkers are widely available, inexpensive, and easy to calculate and therefore provide a desirable alternative to liver biopsy [8].

In our recent studies, we have shown that in children with CHC, both fibrosis and steatosis were positively associated with the body mass index z-score (BMI z-score) [9, 10]. Thus, the aim of the present study was to analyze the diagnostic performance of APRI and FIB-4 to determine liver fibrosis and steatosis in children with CHC. Additionally, the diagnostic performance of these biomarkers when modified by including the BMI z-score in the formulas was established, and B-AST, a novel simple marker based on the BMI z-score and aspartate aminotransferase (AST) only, was proposed, and its diagnostic performance was analyzed.

Methods

Patients

This prospective clinicopathological study comprised consecutive treatment-naïve patients chronically infected with HCV who underwent a liver biopsy in our tertiary health care department between 2010 and 2014. Noninvasive serum biomarker analysis was performed simultaneously with liver biopsy as part of the qualification procedure for the antiviral treatment, according to the current European recommendations [2]. In addition, liver biopsy was required by the National Health Found for every patient prior to inclusion to the therapeutic program. The CHC diagnosis was established in patients with at least a 6-month history of hepatitis based on elevated alanine and aspartate aminotransferase (ALT and AST) serum levels and positive anti-HCV testing and was confirmed with nucleic acid testing/positive HCV RNA real-time polymerase chain reaction analysis (RT-PCR method; Amplicor, Roche; Cobas TaqMan, Roche). Both biochemical and serological testing were performed using commercially available laboratory kits (Vitros 5600, Ortho-Clinical Diagnostics, Johnson & Johnson). The upper limits of normal (ULN) for ALT and AST were established as 40 IU/l. The most likely route and time of infection were established using available medical records. The putative duration of infection was calculated from the beginning of the risk exposure.

Patients with hepatitis B virus, human immunodeficiency virus infection, autoimmune hepatitis, nonalcoholic fatty liver disease, Wilson's disease, or alpha 1-antitrypsin deficiency were excluded from this study. The patients' weights and heights were recorded on the day of the biomarker examination. BMI z-scores were calculated using the World Health Organization (WHO) Child Growth Standards and Growth Reference data with the WHO anthropometric calculator, AnthroPlus v.1.0.4.

Biomarker evaluation

The biomarker determinations were performed using commercially available laboratory kits (XT-1800i, Sysmex for platelets; Vitros 5600, Ortho-Clinical Diagnostics, Johnson & Johnson for biochemical parameters). The noninvasive serum biomarker analysis included APRI and FIB-4, which were calculated according to the published analytic recommendations [6, 7], as follows:

$$\begin{aligned}\text{APRI} &= [\text{AST(IU/L)}/\text{AST ULN(IU/L)}/\text{platelet count}(10^9/\text{L})] \\ &\quad \times 100; \\ \text{FIB-4} &= [\text{age(years)} \times \text{AST(IU/L)}]/[\text{platelet count}(10^9/\text{L}) \\ &\quad \times \sqrt{\text{ALT(IU/L)}}]\end{aligned}$$

Additionally, modified APRI (M-APRI) and modified FIB-4 (M-FIB-4) were calculated by including BMI z-scores in both formulas, as follows:

$$\begin{aligned}\text{M-APRI} &= \text{BMI z-score} \times \text{APRI}; \text{M-FIB-4} \\ &= \text{BMI z-score} \times \text{FIB-4}.\end{aligned}$$

A novel simple biomarker, B-AST = BMI z-score × AST (IU/L), was also proposed and calculated.

Histopathological evaluation

Liver biopsy was performed percutaneously using a Menghini needle (Hepafix kit 1.4 or 1.6 mm, Braun). An experienced pathologist who was unaware of the clinical data performed the histopathological evaluation. Fibrosis staging was evaluated using the METAVIR scoring system on a 5-point scale (F0 – no fibrosis; F1 – portal fibrosis without septa; F2 – portal fibrosis with few septa; F3 – numerous septa without cirrhosis; and F4 – cirrhosis) [11]. Fibrosis was considered significant if the METAVIR F score was ≥2. Liver steatosis was determined semi-quantitatively according to the percentage of hepatocytes containing fat droplets and was staged as follows: 0 – no steatosis; 1 – minimal (≤ 5% hepatocytes affected); 2 – mild (6–33%); 3 – moderate (34–66%); and 4 – severe (> 66%). Steatosis was considered significant if more than 33% of the hepatocytes were affected (steatosis score > 2).

Statistical analysis

Continuous variables were tested for normal distribution using the Kolmogorov-Smirnov test and are expressed as the mean ± standard deviations (SD) or as medians with interquartile ranges (IQR), as required. To analyze associations between the results of the five serum biomarkers and fibrosis and steatosis stages, Spearman correlation coefficients were obtained. A two-sided *p*-value <0.05 was considered significant.

Receiver operating characteristic (ROC) curves and areas under the ROC curve (AUROC) calculations were performed to assess the diagnostic performances of the noninvasive tests for identifying patients with any or significant liver fibrosis and steatosis, using liver biopsy as a reference standard. An analyzed method is considered perfect when the AUROC is 100%, excellent when the AUROC is over 90%, and good when the AUROC is over 80% [3, 5]. Optimal cutoffs, sensitivity, specificity, and positive and negative predictive values were also calculated for each noninvasive test.

All statistical analyses were performed using the licensed MedCalc Statistical Software, ver. 17.2 (MedCalc, Mariakerke, Belgium).

Ethical statement

The investigation was concordant with the principles outlined in the Declaration of Helsinki and its amendments. Written informed consent was collected from all the patients and/or their parents/guardians before their inclusion in the study.

Results

Patient characteristics

Thirty children (14 male and 16 female) aged 9.4 ± 3.7 years with a mean HCV infection duration of 8.2 ± 3.1 years were included in this study. Most of the children (73%) were infected vertically by an infected mother. The predominant HCV genotype in this group was 1b. In 2/30 (7%) cases, the BMI z-score indicated obesity (> 2 SD). The clinical and laboratory characteristics of the study group are presented in Table 1.

Table 1 Clinical and laboratory characteristics of the study group

Characteristics		Data
Number		30
Sex	Male (%)/female (%)	14 (47)/16 (53)
Age at liver biopsy (years)	Mean ± SD	9.4 ± 3.7
Duration of infection (years)	Mean ± SD	8.2 ± 3.1
BMI z-score	Mean ± SD	0.39 ± 1.04
Mode of infection	Vertical (%)	22 (73)
	Nosocomial (%)	7 (23)
HCV genotype (%)	1a	2 (7)
	1b	19 (63)
	3	5 (17)
	4	4 (13)
Viral load (IU/ml)	HCV median (IQR)	5.95×10^5 (2.25×10^5–1.53×10^6)
Laboratory findings Mean ± SD/median (IQR)	ALT (IU/l)	60.5 (36–79)
	AST (IU/l)	50 (37–68)
	Platelets (× 10^9/l)	308.2 ± 90.5
METAVIR F	0	8 (27)
	1	15 (50)
	2	7 (23)
	3–4	0
Steatosis	Any (%)	8 (27)
	Significant (%)	4 (13)
APRI	Mean ± SD	0.48 ± 0.26
FIB-4	Mean ± SD	0.22 ± 0.13
M-APRI	Mean ± SD	0.28 ± 0.69
M-FIB-4	Mean ± SD	0.09 ± 0.28
B-AST	Mean ± SD	31.71 ± 69.87

ALT alanine aminotransferase, *AST* aspartate aminotransferase, *BMI* body mass index, *APRI* aspartate-to-platelet Ratio Index, *FIB-4* Fibrosis-4 test, *M-APRI* modified aspartate-to-platelet ratio index (BMI z-score x APRI); *M-FIB-4* modified Fibrosis-4 index (BMI z-score x FIB-4), *B-AST* BMI z-score x AST

Histopathological evaluation

Histopathological evaluation of the liver biopsy specimens revealed a mild stage of fibrosis in most cases: 22/30 (73%) patients presented with some stage of fibrosis, and in 7/30 (23%) patients, the fibrosis was significant (METAVIR F score ≥ 2 points). No cirrhosis cases were observed. Liver steatosis was detected in 8/30 (27%) patients, and in 4/30 (13%) patients, the steatosis was significant (> 33% of hepatocytes affected, Table 1).

Noninvasive evaluation

Five noninvasive serum biomarkers were calculated according to the formulas described above, and the mean values for each test are presented in Table 1. The APRI exceeded 0.7 in 6/30 (20%) cases, and in 3/30 (10%) patients, the APRI was greater than 1.0. The maximal FIB-4 value was 0.57, and it did not exceed 1.0 in any case.

Relationship between noninvasive and histopathological evaluations

Positive associations between the fibrosis stages determined by the histopathological evaluation and the M-APRI and B-AST scores were revealed ($p = 0.01$ and $p = 0.001$, respectively, Table 2). A trend toward such an association was observed for APRI and M-FIB-4 ($p = 0.06$ and $p = 0.05$, respectively, Table 2). Steatosis stages were positively associated with the APRI, M-APRI, and M-FIB-4 scores ($p = 0.02$ for all evaluations), and they trended toward an association with the B-AST score ($p = 0.08$, Table 2).

Table 2 Association between the five biomarkers and the stage of fibrosis (METAVIR F score) and between the biomarkers and the presence of steatosis

Marker	METAVIR F	Steatosis
APRI	0.34 (−0.03–0.63), p = 0.06	0.42 (0.08–0.68), p = 0.02
M-APRI	0.44 (0.08–0.69), p = 0.01	0.40 (0.05–0.67), p = 0.02
FIB-4	0.18 (−0.20–0.51), p = 0.35	0.09 (−0.27–0.44), p = 0.61
M-FIB-4	0.36 (−0.01–0.64), p = 0.05	0.40 (0.04–0.66), p = 0.02
B-AST	0.56 (0.24–0.77), p = 0.001	0.32 (−0.05–0.61), p = 0.08

Data are presented as correlation coefficients (95% confidence intervals) and p-values

Figure 1 shows the diagnostic performance (ROC curves) of the five analyzed noninvasive tests for all fibrosis diagnoses (Fig. 1a) and for significant fibrosis diagnoses (METAVIR F ≥ 2 points, Fig. 1b). For the diagnosis of any fibrosis stage, the corresponding AUROCs were below 0.8 for all tests, and the highest AUROC value was observed for APRI: 0.719 (0.526–0.867) (Fig. 1a). In the significant fibrosis cases, the AUROCs for all three tests that included BMI z-scores exceeded 0.8 (0.842, 0.823, and 0.848 for the M-APRI, M-FIB-4, and B-AST, respectively), whereas the AUROCs for the APRI and FIB-4 were below 0.8 (Table 3). The novel marker, B-AST, predicted significant fibrosis with a cut-off of 92.8 with 71.4% sensitivity and 95.7% specificity.

The diagnostic performances of the five noninvasive tests for determining steatosis are presented in Fig. 2 and Table 4. For the detection of any steatosis stage, the AUROC was highest for the APRI (0.768). The AUROCs for the other tests did not exceed 0.7 (Fig. 2a). The diagnostic value of the tests for detecting significant steatosis was excellent (AUROC >0.9) for all three tests that included the BMI z-scores (0.923, 0.942, and 0.942 for M-APRI, M-FIB-4, and B-AST, respectively). For the APRI, the AUROC was good (0.837); however, for the FIB-4, the AUROC was insufficient (0.683). B-AST, with a cut-off of 92.8, predicted significant steatosis with 100% sensitivity and 92.3% specificity (Table 4).

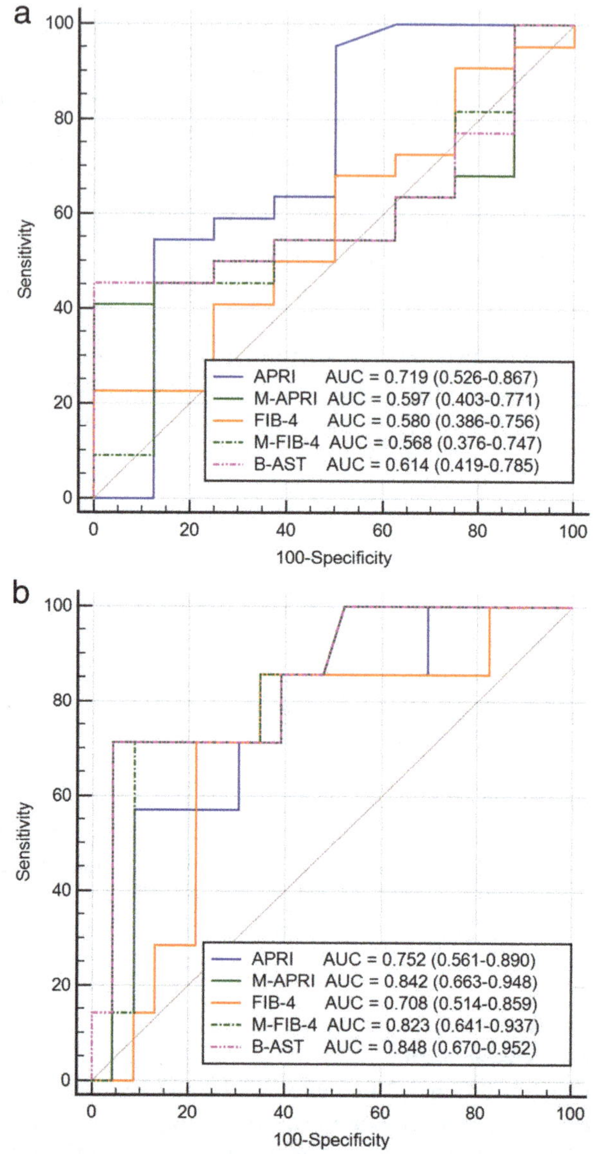

Fig. 1 Receiver operating characteristic (ROC) curves of the five noninvasive liver fibrosis tests for detecting fibrosis. **a** for fibrosis at any stage (METAVIR F score > 0 points). **b** for significant fibrosis (METAVIR F score ≥ 2 points)

Discussion

In the era of direct-acting antivirals (DAAs), successful treatment of CHC is achievable for nearly all infected patients, and DAAs are recommended for all adults with chronic HCV infection [2, 12]. The availability of DAAs for pediatric patients with CHC is expected within the coming months. According to the current recommendations, histopathological evaluation of liver disease may not be necessary for all patients prior to therapy. However, the majority of patients require testing to determine the stage of fibrosis, which is vital for determining the urgency of treatment, the duration of treatment in some instances, and the need for more intensive clinical monitoring [12].

Several noninvasive markers of liver fibrosis based on a combination of different biochemical parameters have been developed recently and analyzed in adult patients with CHC [5, 7, 8, 13]. A meta-analysis of 40 studies revealed that an APRI score greater than 1.0 had a sensitivity of 76% and specificity of 72% for predicting cirrhosis. Additionally, APRI scores greater than 0.7 had a sensitivity of 77% and specificity of 72% for predicting significant hepatic fibrosis [13]. In a study by Sterling et al., FIB-4 scores <1.45 had a negative predictive value of

Table 3 Diagnostic performance of five non-invasive tests for determining significant fibrosis (METAVIR F ≥ 2)

Significant fibrosis (METAVIR F ≥ 2)					
Test	APRI	M-APRI	FIB-4	M-FIB-4	B-AST
AUROC (95% CI)	0.752 (0.561–0.890)	0.842 (0.663–0.948)	0.708 (0.514–0.859)	0.823 (0.641–0.937)	0.848 (0.670–0.952)
Cut-off	0.656	0.577	0.180	0.179	92.82
Sensitivity (95% CI)	57.1 (18.4–90.1)	71.4 (29.0–96.3)	85.7 (42.1–99.6)	71.4 (0.29–96.3)	71.4 (0.29–96.3)
Specificity (95% CI)	91.3 (72.0–98.9)	95.6 (78.1–99.9)	65.2 (42.7–83.6)	91.30 (72.0–98.9)	95.7 (78.1–99.0)
+ PV	66.7 (31.5–89.7)	83.3 (41.0–97.3)	42.9 (28.4–58.6)	71.4 (38.0–91.1)	83.3 (41.0–97.3)
- PV	87.5 (74.7–94.3)	91.7 (77.3–97.3)	93.7 (70.5–99.0)	91.3 (76.4–97.2)	91.7 (77.3–97.3)

APRI aspartate-to-platelet ratio index, *FIB-4* Fibrosis-4 index, *M-APRI* modified aspartate-to-platelet ratio index (BMI z-score x APRI), *M-FIB-4* modified Fibrosis-4 index (BMI z-score x FIB-4), *B-AST* BMI z-score x AST, *AUROC* area under the receiver operating characteristic, *95% CI* 95% confidence interval, + *PV* positive predictive value, − *PV* negative predictive value

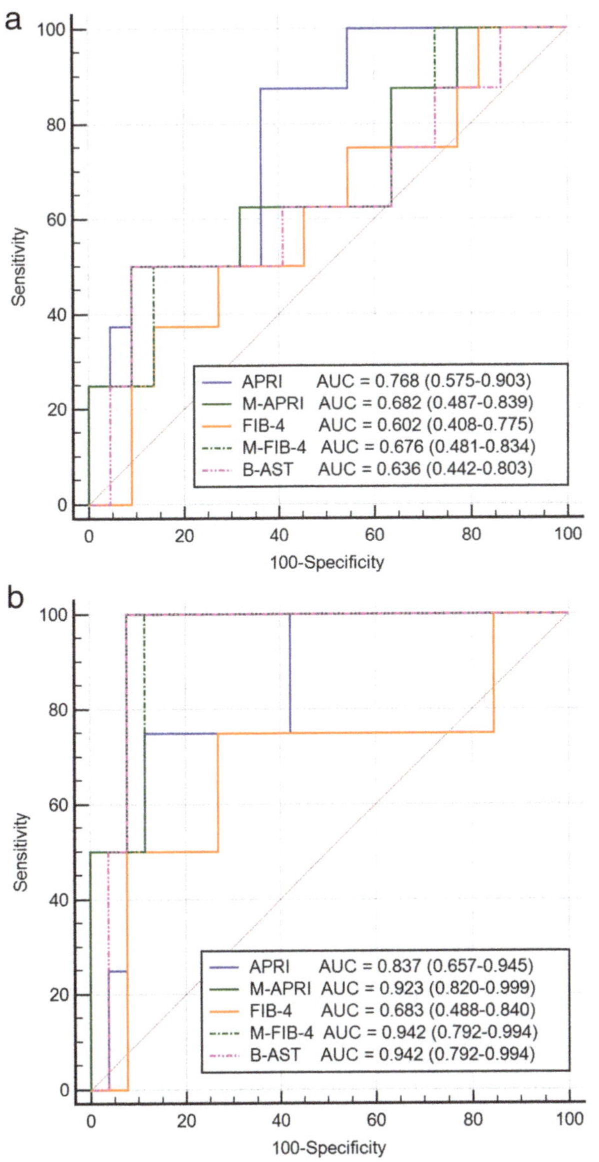

Fig. 2 Receiver operating characteristic (ROC) curves of the five noninvasive liver fibrosis tests for detecting steatosis. **a** for any steatosis. **b** for significant steatosis (> 33% of hepatocytes affected)

90% for advanced fibrosis, and FIB-4 scores >3.25 had a 97% specificity and a positive predictive value of 65% for advanced fibrosis [6].

There are only limited published data on the use of these noninvasive methods in children, and, to our knowledge, none of these serum biomarkers have been fully validated in children with CHC to date. De Ledinghen et al. prospectively analyzed the feasibility of a liver stiffness measurement using FibroScan (elastography method) in 116 children with chronic liver diseases and compared the results with those of FibroTest (a commercial biomarker), the APRI and liver biopsy [4]. All three noninvasive methods correlated significantly with the METAVIR fibrosis score. The AUROCs for cirrhosis diagnoses were 0.88 for FibroScan, 0.73 for FibroTest, and 0.73 for the APRI. However, the cohort of patients in this study was heterogenic and included children with liver diseases of different etiologies.

In a study conducted in children and adolescents with chronic hepatitis B and C, the AUROC was 0.71 for identifying patients with fibrosis and 0.52 for identifying those with liver cirrhosis [14]. For children infected with HCV, the AUROC was 0.75; it was more effective for vertically infected patients than for those infected via blood transfusion (1.00 vs. 0.53). The authors concluded that a validated noninvasive marker of fibrosis is needed for pediatric patients; however, the results of their study indicated that the APRI is not such a marker [14].

Our recent observations suggest that liver fibrosis in children with CHC is positively associated with the BMI z-score. In both univariate and multivariate analyses, the BMI z-score was found to be an independent predictor of fibrosis among our 42 pediatric patients with CHC (p = 0.03) [9]. Therefore, we proposed including the BMI z-score in the formulas of previously used biomarkers. The obtained results indicate that these modified tests perform better than the APRI and FIB-4 for predicting severe fibrosis. Additionally, we proposed a new simple biomarker, B-AST, that can easily detect liver fibrosis based on very simple parameters. B-AST,

Table 4 Diagnostic performance of five non-invasive tests for determining significant steatosis (> 33% of hepatocytes)

Significant steatosis (> 33% of hepatocytes)					
Test	APRI	M-APRI	FIB-4	M-FIB-4	B-AST
AUROC (95% CI)	0.837 (0.657–0.945)	0.923 (0.820–0.999)	0.683 (0.488–0.840)	0.942 (0.792–0.994)	0.942 (0.792–0.994)
Cut-off	0.656	0.577	0.216	0.179	92.82
Sensitivity (95% CI)	75 (19.4–99.4)	100 (39.8–100)	75 (19.4–99.4)	100 (39.8–100)	100 (39.8–100)
Specificity (95% CI)	88.46 (69.8–97.6)	92.3 (74.9–99.1)	73.1 (52.2–88.4)	88.46 (69.8–97.6)	92.3 (74.9–99.1)
+ PV	50.0 (23.1–76.9)	66.7 (34.6–88.3)	30.0 (15.5–50.0)	57.1 (31.5–79.4)	66.7 (34.6–88.3)
- PV	95.8 (80.7–99.2)	100	95.0 (77.4–99.1)	100	100

APRI aspartate-to-platelet ratio index, *FIB-4* Fibrosis-4 index, *M-APRI* modified aspartate-to-platelet ratio index (BMI z-score x APRI), *M-FIB-4* modified Fibrosis-4 index (BMI z-score x FIB-4), *B-AST* BMI z-score x AST, *AUROC* area under the receiver operating characteristic, *95% CI* 95% confidence interval, + *PV* positive predictive value, − *PV* negative predictive value

with a cut-off of 92.8, showed 71% sensitivity and 95% specificity for detecting significant fibrosis.

Several studies have demonstrated that liver steatosis in patients with CHC may have prognostic and metabolic implications [15–17]. In our recent study, moderate to severe steatosis was independently associated with the BMI z-score in a group of 48 patients with CHC ($p = 0.02$) [10]. In addition, it was found to be a predictor of advanced fibrosis in children with HCV infection; this was a unique finding because unlike in adults, no correlation between liver steatosis and fibrosis had previously been confirmed in pediatric patients with CHC [10]. Noninvasive markers of steatosis have been studied in patients with nonalcoholic fatty liver disease (NAFLD) but not in patients with CHC [18]. The results of our study suggest that biomarkers that include the BMI z-score perform excellently for diagnosing significant steatosis in children with CHC. B-AST had a very high sensitivity (100%) and specificity (92%) for predicting severe steatosis with a cut-off of 92.8. Considering that negative B-AST values excluded all patients with both significant fibrosis and significant steatosis, one may speculate that liver biopsy could be avoided in children with B-AST <0. In this study, 11/30 (37%) of children had B-AST <0 and consequently would not require the liver biopsy.

Despite the novel and unique findings presented in this study, several issues should be considered as limitations. First, the small number of patients in the study group should be acknowledged, and the obtained results should be confirmed with other, larger cohorts of children. However, currently, liver biopsy is rarely performed in children; thus, the opportunity to compare noninvasive methods with histopathological assessment as a reference standard is lacking. Another important issue arose from the relatively mild liver disease observed in the histopathological evaluations: a low number of children presented with significant fibrosis, and no children presented with cirrhosis, which could lead to a spectrum bias. However, children with CHC usually present with mild liver disease, and cirrhosis is rarely observed [9]. Therefore, in most cases, distinguishing no or mild fibrosis from significant fibrosis would be most desirable for therapeutic decision-making.

Conclusions

In conclusion, the results of this study indicate that noninvasive biomarkers that include BMI z-scores in their formulas have a good to excellent performance for detecting significant liver disease. The novel simple B-AST serum test may be an inexpensive and widely available alternative to liver biopsy due to its high sensitivity and specificity for detecting significant liver fibrosis and steatosis. Continued research in this area in pediatric populations is needed to fully validate these noninvasive diagnostic tools for children with chronic liver diseases of different etiologies.

Abbreviations

ALT: Alanine aminotransferase; APRI: Aspartate aminotransferase-to-platelet ratio index; AST: Aspartate aminotransferase; AUROC: Area under the receiver operating characteristic; BMI z-score: Body mass index z-score; CHC: Chronic hepatitis C; CI: Confidence interval; HCV: Hepatitis C virus; IQR: Interquartile ranges; PV: Predictive value; ROC: Receiver operating characteristic; SD: Standard deviation; ULN: Upper limit of normal

Acknowledgements

Not applicable.

Funding

Not applicable.

Authors' contributions

MPS performed the research, designed the research study, conducted the statistical analysis, and drafted the manuscript; MPS, BKM, MA, and MP collected and analyzed the data; MM contributed to the study design; BKM, MA, MP, and MM contributed to the interpretation of the data, and critically revised the manuscript; all authors read and approved the final manuscript.

Competing interests

The authors declare that they have no competing interests.

Consent for publication

Not applicable.

References

1. Dezsofi A, Baumann U, Dhawan A, Durmaz O, Fischler B, Hadzic N, Hierro L, Lacaille F, McLin VA, Nobili V, et al. Liver biopsy in children: position paper of the ESPGHAN Hepatology committee. J Pediatr Gastroenterol Nutr. 2015;60(3):408–20.
2. European Association for the Study of the Liver. EASL recommendations on treatment of hepatitis C 2016. J Hepatol. 2017;66(1):153–94.
3. Pokorska-Śpiewak M, Kowalik-Mikołajewska B, Aniszewska M, Pluta M, Marczyńska M. Is liver biopsy still needed in children with chronic viral hepatitis? World J Gastroenterol. 2015;21(42):12141–9.
4. de Ledinghen V, Le Bail B, Rebouissoux L, Fournier C, Foucher J, Miette V, Castera L, Sandrin L, Merrouche W, Lavrand F, et al. Liver stiffness measurement in children using FibroScan: feasibility study and comparison with Fibrotest, aspartate transaminase to platelets ratio index, and liver biopsy. J Pediatr Gastroenterol Nutr. 2007;45(4):443–50.
5. Castera L. Noninvasive methods to assess liver disease in patients with hepatitis B or C. Gastroenterology. 2012;142(6):1293–1302.e1294.
6. Sterling RK, Lissen E, Clumeck N, Sola R, Correa MC, Montaner J, S Sulkowski M, Torriani FJ, Dieterich DT, Thomas DL et al: Development of a simple noninvasive index to predict significant fibrosis in patients with HIV/HCV coinfection. Hepatology 2006, 43(6):1317–1325.
7. Wai CT, Greenson JK, Fontana RJ, Kalbfleisch JD, Marrero JA, Conjeevaram HS, Lok AS. A simple noninvasive index can predict both significant fibrosis and cirrhosis in patients with chronic hepatitis C. Hepatology. 2003;38(2):518–26.
8. Zeng DW, Dong J, Liu YR, Jiang JJ, Zhu YY. Noninvasive models for assessment of liver fibrosis in patients with chronic hepatitis B virus infection. World J Gastroenterol. 2016;22(29):6663–72.
9. Pokorska-Śpiewak M, Kowalik-Mikołajewska B, Aniszewska M, Pluta M, Walewska-Zielecka B, Marczyńska M. Determinants of liver disease progression in children with chronic hepatitis C virus infection. Pol J Pathol. 2015;66(4):368–75.
10. Pokorska-Śpiewak M, Kowalik-Mikołajewska B, Aniszewska M, Pluta M, Walewska-Zielecka B, Marczyńska M. Liver steatosis in children with chronic hepatitis B and C: prevalence, predictors, and impact on disease progression. Medicine (Baltimore). 2017;96(3):e5832.
11. Bedossa P, Poynard T. An algorithm for the grading of activity in chronic hepatitis C. The METAVIR Cooperative Study Group. Hepatology. 1996;24(2):289–93.
12. Panel AIHG. Hepatitis C guidance: AASLD-IDSA recommendations for testing, managing, and treating adults infected with hepatitis C virus. Hepatology. 2015;62(3):932–54.
13. Lin ZH, Xin YN, Dong QJ, Wang Q, Jiang XJ, Zhan SH, Sun Y, Xuan SY. Performance of the aspartate aminotransferase-to-platelet ratio index for the staging of hepatitis C-related fibrosis: an updated meta-analysis. Hepatology. 2011;53(3):726–36.
14. McGoogan KE, Smith PB, Choi SS, Berman W, Jhaveri R. Performance of the AST-to-platelet ratio index as a noninvasive marker of fibrosis in pediatric patients with chronic viral hepatitis. J Pediatr Gastroenterol Nutr. 2010;50(3):344–6.
15. Adinolfi LE, Gambardella M, Andreana A, Tripodi MF, Utili R, Ruggiero G. Steatosis accelerates the progression of liver damage of chronic hepatitis C patients and correlates with specific HCV genotype and visceral obesity. Hepatology. 2001;33(6):1358–64.
16. Bjornsson E, Angulo P. Hepatitis C and steatosis. Arch Med Res. 2007;38(6):621–7.
17. Guido M, Bortolotti F, Jara P, Giacomelli L, Fassan M, Hierro L, Nebbia G, Zancan L, Rugge M. Liver steatosis in children with chronic hepatitis C. Am J Gastroenterol. 2006;101(11):2611–5.
18. Papagianni M, Sofogianni A, Tziomalos K. Non-invasive methods for the diagnosis of nonalcoholic fatty liver disease. World J Hepatol. 2015;7(4):638–48.

6

Hepatitis C seropositivity among newly incarcerated prisoners in Estonia: data analysis of electronic health records from 2014 to 2015

Kristel Kivimets[1*], Anneli Uusküla[2], Jeffrey V. Lazarus[3,4] and Kristi Ott[5]

Abstract

Background: Hepatitis C virus (HCV) infection is a widespread problem in prisons. The present study aimed to assess the prevalence of HCV seropositivity, HCV genotypes, factors associated with HCV seropositivity in newly incarcerated prisoners and to report experiences of treatment with pegylated interferon/ribavirin for HCV-positive inmates.

Methods: Patient data were extracted from the Estonian prison medical information system (*Vanglate meditsiiniline infosüsteem*) databases.

Results: Among 1845 prisoners newly incarcerated from January 2014 to January 2015, the overall prevalence of HCV was 56.3% (95% CI: 54 to 59), and 25.5% (95% CI: 23.5 to 27.6%) had HIV (39.0% had neither). The all-inclusive HCV testing strategy identified 37.7% more HCV infected prisoners than the risk-based (drug use history, HIV status) case finding. Factors associated with HCV seropositivity included history of drug use (aOR 6.51 95%CI 5.12–8.28), HIV co-infection (aOR 2.56 95%CI 1.92–3.43), previous incarceration (aOR 3.61 95%CI 2.48–4.04), and increasing age. The main HCV genotypes were 3a ($n = 172$, 44.4%) and 1b ($n = 135$, 35.2%). Twenty-five prisoners received HCV treatment: 60% ($n = 15$) were cured, 16% ($n = 4$) relapsed (3 with genotype 3a, one with 1b), and 12% ($n = 3$) were unresponsive (all with genotype 3a).

Conclusions: HCV seropositivity rate is high and HCV tretment rate is very low in Estonian prisons. Optimizing case finding and scaling up treatment is critical to addressing the health needs of prisoners and meeting public health goals.

Keywords: Prison health, Viral hepatitis, Hepatitis C, HIV, Case finding, Estonia

Background

Hepatitis C virus (HCV) infection is an escalating global health issue and prisoners are emerging as an important high-risk group. HCV prevalence in this subpopulation ranges from 3 to 38% [1, 2]. Although this high burden of HCV is gaining notoriety and modern treatment can provide noticeable improvements in the health statuses of most patients, many countries still lack HCV prevalence data for high-risk groups. Epidemic patterns of HCV infection related to injection drug use persist in Europe. Understanding the risk factors for HCV infection among prisoners may inform HCV prevention and treatment intervention measures [2–5].

HCV prevalence is higher among prisoners than in the general population [2]. Intravenous drug use (IDU) is one of the major risk factors for HCV infection. The prevalence of IDU in prisons is ranging from 2 to 38% in Europe while the relevant percentage in the general population is estimated at 0.3% in the European Union and 0.2% in Australia. [6]. A metaanalysis showed that people who inject drugs (PWID) were about 24 times more likely to be infected with HCV than individuals in the general population in Europe [7]. IDU [8] and tattooing [9, 10] are the main risk behaviours for acquiring HCV infection in prisons.

* Correspondence: kristel.kivimets@tai.ee
[1]National Institute for Health Development, 42, 11619 Tallinn, Hiiu, Estonia
Full list of author information is available at the end of the article

Prisoners with human immunodeficiency virus (HIV) are more likely to be infected with HCV probably because of the similarity in the routes of transmission of these blood-borne infections [1, 3]. According to recent studies in Italian and US prisons, the HCV prevalence was more than four times higher among HCV-HIV coinfected patients than among those not infected with HIV (65.5–89.6% vs. 15.5–27.5%, respectively) [3, 11].

Another risk factor related to HCV infection is repeated incarceration [12, 13], an association that may be confounded by low socioeconomic status, poor access to health care, high-risk sexual behaviors and injection drug use [14].

In some studies HCV infection was observed more frequently in female inmates than in males. [1]. In part that may have been because the number of women in prison has grown and women prisoners are more likely than their male counterparts to have been incarcerated for drug offences [15] and to have serious drug-related health problems [16], including infectious diseases [17].

Direct-acting antivirals (DAAs) are relatively new and expensive, but cost-effective when well utilised as interventions for chronic hepatitis C, and preliminary results suggest that DAAs may eradicate HCV from the blood (sustained virological response). The effect of long-term treatment with DAA (hepatitis C morbidity and mortality) is yet to be convincingly demonstrated [18]. Still, ribavirin has been an integral component of treatment for hepatitis C virus (HCV) infection, and the safety profile of ribavirin is improved when co-administered with all-oral DAA combinations in the absence of interferon [19]. Several studies have shown that prisoners can be effectively treated for HCV infection [20–22], although treatment is administered less frequently to prisoners because of the cost of treatment, treatment often exceeding average prison stay combined with a lack of continuity of care, and unawareness of the HCV infected status of the prisoners [1].

Most HCV infected people are unaware of their condition [23]. Prisons may be a good venue to detect many of those cases. Although exact data are not available, each year, up to one million people with undiagnosed HCV infection may come into contact with the correctional system in the United States [24]. Strategies of case finding should be developed that are based on current infections rates and feasibility.

The situation in Estonian prisons

The prison population in Estonia has stabilised at nearly 3000 individuals in recent years but the incarceration rate, with 222 prisoners per 100,000 population, still remains very high. According to the Council of Europe's annual penal statistics, the highest incarceration rates in Europe are recorded in the former Soviet Union countries (439 per 100,000 population in the Russian Federation, 277 per 100,000 in Lithania, 274 per 100,000 in Georgia, 248 per 100,00 in Azerbaijan and 223 per 100,000 in Latvia) [25].

Needle and syringe exchange programmes (NSP) in Estonia were launched in 1997. In addition to NSP, condom distribution, different counselling services incl. social, health, psychological, legal, experience counselling), basic humanitarian aid, primary hygiene possibilities [26], naloxone take-home program training (since 2013), and motivation and referral to treatment/rehabilitation are offered under harm reduction services in Estonia. From 2015, naloxone is available also in prisons [27]. In all Estonian prisons, opioid substitution therapy (OST) in the form of methadone treatment is provided. NSP are not operating in Estonian prisons [28].

According to the Estonian Ministry of Justice, there were 3580 prisoners in Estonia's four prisons during the period between 1 January 2014 and 1 January 2015 (personal communication with Asko Oruste, the information systems manager with Estonian IT Support System). A study conducted in Estonia in 2012–2013 found that, of all prisoners, one-third had a history of drug use, 15.6% were infected with HIV and, of those that were HIV-positive, 54.1% were receiving antiretroviral therapy (ART) [28].

The implementation of the project "Improvement of Prevention and Treatment of Infectious Diseases in Estonian prisons" [29] targeting testing, treatment and infrastructure buildings was a milestone in the diagnosis and care of HCV in prisons [30]. Before that, HCV testing targeted only prisoners considered at high risk for HCV (identified by their drug use history or HIV status; "the old testing strategy") (personal communication with Maret Miljan from the rehabilitation department of the Estonian prison department,). Since the launch of the project in January 2014, HCV tests have been offered for all newly incarcerated prisoners ("the new testing strategy").

The aim of this study was to assess the prevalence of HCV seropositivity and its related factors among newly incarcerated prisoners and to describe the effects of treatment of HCV infection in Estonian prisons.

Methods

This study was carried out from 1 January 2014 to 1 January 2015. The term 'newly incarcerated prisoner' is used for all people, including adults and juveniles, detained during the investigation of a crime, while awaiting trial, after conviction, before sentencing and after sentencing, and incarcerated in one of the four Estonian prisons.

Data and data sources

For this study we relied on the secondary data available in the administrative and health databases of the Estonian prison medical information system.

Prison electronic patient database

The prison electronic patient database is designed for prison healthcare and contains electronic health records. For those tested for HCV, the following data were extracted from prisoners' health records: (i) HCV test result, (ii) HCV genotype, (iii) age, (iv) gender, (v) HIV serostatus, (vi) history of drug use (based on the International Classification of Diseases codes F11-F16 or F18-F19), and (vii) HCV treatment results. HCV in prisons is treated by prison infectious diseases physicians who also make HCV-genotype testing decisions.

For all samples collected in the prison medical information system over the study period, HIV testing (VironostikaHIV Uniform II Ag/Ab, BioMerieux method), anti-HCV antibodies testing (Siemens, A HCV200T KIT), and HCV genotyping (The VERSANT® HCV Genotype 2.0 Assay) were performed at Synlab Estonia (an accredited laboratory following the requirements of ISO 15189 Medical Laboratories).

Database of prisoners, detained persons, persons in custody and probationers

Data on tattoos and previous incarceration were extracted from the databases of prisoners, detained persons, persons in custody and probationers (hereinafter referred to as the *prisoners' register*). The prisoners' register is an electronic database containing selected information on the details of prison sentence as well as personal data. Information on tattoos included in the register is based on inspection of prisoners' skin at prison entry.

Statistical analysis

Descriptive statistics are presented for categorical variables (absolute number (n) and relative frequencies (%)) and continuous variables (mean, standard deviation and range). A chi-squared test was used to explore differences in categorical variables and the Wilcoxon rank sum test for age comparisons between the HCV infected and non-infected groups. Associations between antibodies to HCV (the outcome of interest) and covariables were explored bivariably and multivariably (by including all independent variables in the model) by logistic regression analyses. Odds ratios (OR) and adjusted OR (AOR) together with 95% confidence intervals (CI) are presented. Associations between covariables were also tested to assess the reliability of the multivariate models (according to the possibility of multicollinearity). The statistical software program SPSS version 16.0 (Chicago, Illinois, USA) was used.

Results

HCV and HIV diagnosis

Between 1 January 2014 and 1 January 2015, 1957 new prisoners were admitted to the Estonian prison system. Of those, 603 were already infected with HCV (based on data from previous testing in prison). As per the new testing strategy, the rest of the newly imprisoned individuals (n = 1242) were tested for HCV with the exception of 112 prisoners (26 prisoners declined testing and the reason for not testing was unknown for the other 86).

The final sample consisted of 1845 newly incarcerated prisoners with known HCV status. They had an average age of 35 years (SD = 11.54, range 15–78). Of these prisoners, 94.4% were male (n = 1742), 58.1% had previously used illicit drugs (n = 1034), 28.1% were tattooed (n = 519), and 68.9% had been previously incarcerated (n = 1272). The prevalence of HCV seropositivity was 56.3% (n = 1038, 603 + 435) and the prevalence of HIV 25.5% (95% CI 23.5–27.6%) (n = 469). One fifth (n = 379; 20.5, 95% CI 19.8–23.6%) of the newly incarcerated prisoners had HCV-HIV co-infections. The majority (80.8, 95% CI 77.2–84.4%) of the HIV-positive prisoners were also infected with HCV (Table 1).

The old testing strategy – high-risk based case finding - would have identified only 37.7% (164/435) of the HCV infected newly incarcerated prisoners.While comparing HCV infected and non-infected newly incarcerated prisoners, we found that HCV-infected prisoners tended to be slightly older, and were more likely to have a tattoo (63.8% vs 36.2%, $p < 0.001$), to have a history of drug use (76.6% vs 23.4%; $p < 0.001$), to be HIV-infected (80% vs 19.2%, $p < 0.001$), and to have previously been incarcerated (65.1% vs 4.9%, $p < 0.001$). There were no gender differences in HCV seropositivity (Table 2).

After adjustment, history of drug use emerged as the factor most strongly associated with HCV seropositivity (AOR 6.51 95% CI 5.12–8.28). The risk of HCV seropositivity was also significantly higher among those who were HIV-positive (AOR 2.56 95% CI 1.92–3.43) and those previously incarcerated (AOR 3.16 95% CI 2.48–4.04). The risk of HCV positivity increased with age. While tattooing was associated with the HCV rates in the bivariable analysis, this association was not found in the multivariable analysis.

HCV genotypes

Of the 1038 prisoners who tested positive for HCV, 383 (36.9%) underwent HCV genotype testing. The main genotypes identified were 3a (44.4%, n = 172) and 1b (35.2%, n = 135). A further 17% (n = 65) had genotype 1a, and 2.6% prisoners (n = 10) had genotype 2. Only one prisoner had HCV genotype 4.

HCV treatment

Between 1 January 2014 and 1 January 2015, all HCV cases, 25 prisoners (24 male and 1 female), received HCV treatment (pegylated interferon (PEG-INF) and ribavirin). The decision to treat was reached after an in-depth, individualized process including informed consent and considering

Table 1 Factors associated with hepatitis C infection among newly incarcerated prisoners in Estonia, 2014 to 2015 ($n = 1845$)

Variable	All $N = 1845$	HCV +[b] (n; %)	HCV-[c] (n; %)	p-value (HCV + vs HCV-)
Age (mean; SD)	34.1; 10.92	35.66; 11.49	34.11; 11.56	$p < 0.001$
Gender (male: n; %)	1742; 94.4%	978; 56.1%	764; 43.9%	$p = 0.675$
Age group				
15–20	107	36; 33.6%	71; 66.4%	
21–30	620	330; 53.2%	290; 46.8%	
31–40	494	304; 61.5%	190; 38.5%	
41–50	304	177; 58.2%	127; 41.8%	
51–60	183	103; 56.3%	80; 43.7%	
61–70	30	25; 83.3%	5; 16.7%	
71–78	4	3; 75%	1; 25%	
Tattoo (yes: n; %)	519; 28.1%	331; 63.8%	188; 36.2%	$p < 0.001$
Drug use history (yes: n; %)	1034; 56.2%	819; 76.6%	250; 23.4%	$p < 0.001$
HIV[a] infected (n; %)	469; 25.5%	379; 80.8%	90; 19.2%	$p < 0.001$
Previous incarceration (yes: n; %)	1271; 68.9%	827; 65.1%	444; 34.9%	$p < 0.001$

[a]HIV: human immunodeficiency virus
[b]HCV+: Hepatitis C virus positive
[c]HCV-: Hepatitis C virus negative

other factors such as co-morbid addiction and mental illnesses. For patients with a history of drug use, a program-based addiction treatment [31] was required to initiate HCV treatment. Inmates who had a history of depression or another psychiatric disorder were referred to an on-site psychiatrist for evaluation. Prisoners with HCV genotype 1b or with HIV infection were treated for 48 weeks, and those with genotypes 2 or 3 were treated for 24 weeks [32]. Individual treatment decisions were made by prison infectious disease physicians based on whether the expected length of stay was long enough to allow for the completion of a treatment course (24 to 48 weeks). Clinical indicators for treatment and funds available for the medications were also taken into consideration. Of those who received HCV treatment, 21 (84%) had a history of drug use (11 opiate users, 5 stimulant users and 5 users of multiple drugs including opiates), 5 (20%) were HIV infected, none was hepatitis B infected, 24 (96%) had received hepatitis B vaccination before treatment.

None of the patients had previous experience with interferon and ribavirin. The average age of treated patients was 35.5 years (range 29–45). Fifteen of 25 (60%) treated patients underwent ultrasound-guided liver biopsies. The Metavir scoring system was used to classify fibrosis levels [33]. 11 (91.7%) of those biopsied had no to mild fibrosis, 1 person had moderate (9%) and 3 (27.3%) had severe fibrosis of the liver. Of all the patients treated, 15 (60%) were cured based on a negative HCV RNA test at the end of the treatment and 6 months after the treatment; 4 (16%) relapsed based on a negative HCV RNA at the end of the treatment and positive HCV RNA test 6 months after the treatment (3 patients with genotype 3a, one with 1b); 3 (12%) were unresponsive to treatment based on an HCV RNA test at 24 weeks of treatment (all with genotype 3a); 1 person (4%) stopped treatment; and treatment outcome data were missing for 2 (8%) of the patients as they had been released from prison.

Table 2 Factors associated with hepatitis C infection among newly admitted prisoners in Estonia, 2014 to 2015, univariate and multivariable logistic regression analyses ($n = 1845$)

Variable	Bivariable analysis		Multivariable analysis	
	OR[c]	CI[b] (95%)	Adjusted OR	CI (95%)
Age	1.01	1.00–1.02***	1.01	1.00–1.02***
Gender (female)	1.09	0.73–1.63	1.30	0.79–2.15
Tattoo (yes)	1.54	1.25–1.90***	0.81	0.62–1.04
Drug use history (yes)	8.49	6.87–10.49***	6.51	5.12–8.28***
HIV[a] infected (yes)	4.62	3.59–5.96***	2.56	1.92–3.43***
Previous incarceration (yes)	3.2	2.61–3.93***	3.16	2.48–4.04***

*** p-value < 0.01

Discussion

To our knowledge, this is the first study focusing on HCV prevalence and HCV treatment outcomes in the entire prison population of a European country. The studies that do exist are often restricted to individual prisons or subgroups of prisoners [2].

We found high HCV seropositivity rates (56%) among newly imprisoned individuals in Estonia. HCV seropositivity among newly incarcerated and tested prisoners (with either unknown HCV status or previous negative HCV test) was 35%. These prevalence figures are consistent with those from Italy (38%) [34] and Scotland (19%) [35], where available data suggest that HCV is highly prevalent among prisoners.

The risk factors for HCV seropositivity we observed (drug use, previous incarceration, HIVstatus, age) are in accordance with previous research [1, 2, 8, 14, 36]. According to previous studies in other countries, the main risk factor associated with HCV infection in prison populations is IDU [1, 2, 8, 37]. In our study, the odds for being HCV-positive were about three times higher among HIV-positive than HIV-negative prisoners. HIV and HCV share common routes of transmission, and are therefore expected to some extent co-infect the same individuals.

Previous incarceration has been significantly associated with HCV infection in studies from Australia, England, and Wales [36–38]. Multiple incarcerations were also found to be a risk factor for HCV seropositivity in our study. The contribution of HCV transmission in prison to the overall disease burden among PWID is difficult to document owing to uncertainties regarding precise date of infection and risk behaviours in the community (both prior to and post-incarceration). The role of prisons as a risk environment for the reinforcement, concentration and amplification of infections such as HIV and HCV has been suggested [39].

In our study, the seropositivity of HCV was higher among those with tattoos. However, this association was lost while adjusting for potential confounders. It is known that tattooing is common in prisons and jails [10] and prisoners who acquired their tattoos in prisons are more likely to be HCV-infected [1, 12, 34]. The risks and benefits of legal tattooing in prison should be discussed. Evidence from studies on the relationship between tattooing and HCV transmission in prisons appears to be mixed. Some studies report significant correlations [10, 36, 40] while others do not [41].

We found the presence of hepatitis C antibodies in 12 individuals (0.6%) who were HIV negative and had no records indicative of drug use. While we do not have data on other HCV risk factors (such as history of blood transfusion, high risk sexual behviour), all of the 12 prisoners had tattoos. Eight of them had acquired their tattoos while in prison during the Soviet era (personal communication with prisoners). One might speculate that the traditions of tattooing in prisons have changed (there appear to be fewer tattoos among more recent prison populations and drug using individuals).

Data on the relationship between HCV and gender in prison populations is also conflicting. In some studies, HCV infection was observed more frequently in incarcerated women than in incarcerated men. [1, 3]. Other studies did not find the same result [42]. In our study, after accounting for other risk factors, gender did not emerge to be associated with HCV seropositivity.

Screening strategies based on risk factors have traditionally failed to identify all patients at risk of infection, leaving a sizable proportion of patients unaware of their infection. We observed that a screening system for HCV case finding relying only on known risk factors misses a sizeable proportion of newly incarcerated individuals with HCV infection. The all-inclusive HCV testing strategy identified 37.7% more HCV infection cases among the newly incarcerated than would have been detected on the basis of known risk factors (drug use history, HIV infected status) screening.

In our study, the main HCV genotypes were 3a ($n = 172$, 44%) and 1b ($n = 135$, 35.2%). HCV genotypes have geographically distinct distributions. HCV genotype 1 and 3 infections are globally more prevalent than all other genotypes. Those genotypes, more commonly found in lower-income countries, account for a significant proportion of HCV cases worldwide [43]. Meyer et al. found that genotype 3 prevailed in prisoners from the independent states of the former Soviet Union [44]. Tyczyno et al. compared the HCV genotyping performed on Polish prisoners and hospital patients, and found that HCV genotype 3 prevailed in the prisoners (60.1%) and genotype 1 in patients at large (79.6%). This distinction is most probably due to the fact that genotype 3 is more frequent in PWID [45]. In Estonia, the following distribution of genotypes was documented among hospital patients: genotype 1b was found in 32% of the patients, 3a was found in 20%, 2a in 12%, and 1a/b (double infection) in 28% [46]. Among the Estonian prisoners tested for HCV genotypes nearly two decades later, we were unable to replicate the finding of 1a/b double infection occurrence.

The response to antiviral treatment in prisoners is similar to that of the general population [1]. Our study observed a 60% sustained viral response among treated prisoners. Importantly, this result does not differ from the treatment response reported from the community (in a hospital setting in Estonia) where a 60.3% sustained treatment response was achieved [47]. This suggests that acceptable HCV treatment outcomes can be achieved in prisons. There are clear advantages to HCV treatment in prison settings. In-prison, treatment provides the opportunity to access population groups for whom treatment options may be limited after release. Treatment in prisons occurs in controlled, directly observed settings, potentially achieving increased compliance and monitoring for side effects and complications [48, 49].

Our study has some strengths and limitations. A key feature of our study is the all-inclusive testing strategy and national coverage of the data collection. This is different from other, similar studies [11, 12, 14] conducted in the region because testing was offered and data were collected from all new prisoners entering all Estonian prisons. However, given the nature of the data used, we were unable to determine the frequency or duration of drug injection and, particularly importantly, distinguish between injecting and other types of drug use. Thus, some of the important details might have been lost. Importantly, we were unable to assess the impact of other potential HCV risk factors (such as sexual behaviour and previous blood transfusions, or surgery).

Conclusions

Case finding for HCV infection in prisons, HCV treatment and educational programmes to discourage high-risk behaviours might help curtail the rise in HCV infection in prison populations. Our study suggests that HCV treatment in infected inmates is feasible and the results (sustained viral response achievement) do not differ from that in the community.

Reducing HCV prevalence among prisoners has the potential to reduce the burden of disease in the general public in the community. When developing HCV screening strategies in prisons, policy-makers should consider the risk factors that we have highlighted in our study.

Our findings have several implications: they show that (i) universal HCV testing at prisonentry has the potential to increase the number of people who are aware of their infection, (ii) there is a need to scale up comprehensive HCV care to those infected. We believe that the results of this study might be applicable to other countries in the region that have witnessed injection drug use and related HIV epidemics in the late 1990s and early 2000s.

Abbreviations

AOR: Adjusted odds ratio; ART: Antiretroviral therapy; CI: Confidence interval; DAA: Direct-acting antivirals; HCV: Hepatitis C virus; HIV: Human immunodeficiency virus; IDU: Injection drug use; NSP: Needle and syringe exchange programmes; OR: Odds ratio; OST: Opioid substitution therapy; PWID: People who inject drugs

Authors' contributions

Authors KK, AU were involved in the design of the study. KK abstracted the data from databases and conducted data analysis. JL and KO participated in manuscript writing and revision. All authors revised and approved the manuscript.

Ethics approval and consent to participate

The study procedures were in accordance with local data protection regulations, and the study was approved by the Tartu University Research Ethics Committee. The analysis was based on preexisting records containing pseudo identification codes which allows tracking care provided to this person but not personal identification. Informed consent was deemed unnecessary according to national regulations.

Consent for publication

Not applicable.

Competing interests

The authors declare that they have no competing interests.

Author details

[1]National Institute for Health Development, 42, 11619 Tallinn, Hiiu, Estonia. [2]Department of Family Medicine and Public Health, University of Tartu, Ravila 19, 50411 Tartu, Estonia. [3]Barcelona Institute for Global Health (ISGlobal), Hospital Clínic, University of Barcelona, Carrer de Casanova, 143, 08036 Barcelona, Spain. [4]CHIP, Rigshospitalet, University of Copenhagen, Blegdamsvej 9, DK-2100 Copenhagen, Denmark. [5]West Tallinn Central Hospital, Infectious Diseases Clinic, Paldiski maantee 68, 10617 Tallinn, Estonia.

References

1. Zampino R, Coppola N, Sagnelli C, Di Caprio G, Sagnelli E. Hepatitis C virus infection and prisoners: epidemiology, outcome and treatment. World J Hepatol. 2015;7(21):2323–30.
2. Dolan K, Wirtz AL, Moazen B, Ndeff o-mbah M, Galvani A, Kinner SA, et al. Global burden of HIV, viral hepatitis, and tuberculosis in prisoners and detainees. Lancet. 2016;388:1089–102.
3. Solomon L, Flynn C, Muck K, Vertefeuille J. Prevalence of HIV, syphilis, hepatitis B, and hepatitis C among entrants to Maryland correctional facilities. J Urban Health. 2004;81:25.
4. Macalino GE, Vlahov D, Sanford-Colby S, Patel S, Sabin K, Salas C, et al. Prevalence and incidence of HIV, hepatitis B virus, and hepatitis C virus infections among males in Rhode Island prisons. Am J Public Health. 2004; 94(7):1218–23.
5. Fox RK, Currie SL, Evans J, Wright TL, Tobler L, Phelps T, et al. Hepatitis C virus infection among prisoners in the California state correctional system. Clin Infect Dis. 2005;41(2):177–86.
6. European Monitoring Centre for Drugs and Drug Addiction. Prisons and drugs in Europe: the problem and responses. Luxembourg: Publications Office of the European Union; 2012. Accessed 1 Sept 2015
7. Vescio MF, Longo B, Babudieri S, Starnini G, Carbonara S, Rezza G, et al. Correlates of hepatitis C virus seropositivity in prison inmates: a meta-analysis. J Epidemiol Community Health. 2008;62(4):305–13.
8. UNAIDS. UNAIDS report on the AIDS global epidemic 2013 (appendix). Geneva: Joint United Nations Programme on HIV/AIDS; 2013.
9. Tohme RA, Holmberg SD. Transmission of hepatitis C virus infection through tattooing and piercing: a critical review. Clin Infect Dis. 2012; 54:1167–78.
10. Hellard ME, Aitken CK, Hocking JS. Tattooing in prisons—not such a pretty picture. Am J Infect Control. 2007;35:477–80.
11. Brandolini M, Novati S, De Silvestri A, Tinelli C, Patruno SF, Ranieri R, et al. Prevalence and epidemiological correlates and treatment outcome of HCV infection in an Italian prison setting. BMC Public Health. 2013;13:981.
12. Pourahmad M, Javady AA, Karimi I, Ataei B, Kassaian N. Seroprevalence of and risk factors associated with hepatitis B, hepatitis C, and human immunodeficiency virus among prisoners in Iran. Infect Dis Clin Pract. 2007;15:368–72.
13. Briggs ME, Baker C, Hall R, Gaziano JM, Gagnon D, Bzowej N, et al. Prevalence and risk factors for hepatitis C virus infection at an urban veterans' administration medical center. Hepatology. 2001;34:1200–5.
14. Nokhodian Z, Ataei B, Kassaian N, Yaran M, Hassannejad R, Adibi P. Seroprevalence and risk factors of hepatitis C virus among juveniles in correctional center in Isfahan, Iran. J Prev Med. 2012;3(Suppl1):S113–7.

15. Borrill, J., Maden, A., Martin, A., Weaver, T., Stimson, G., Farrell, M. and Barnes, T. Differential substance misuse treatment needs of women, ethnic minorities and young offenders in prison: prevalence of substance misuse and treatment needs (2003). (Available online).
16. Fazel S, Bains P, Doll H. Substance abuse and dependence in prisoners: a systematic review. Addiction. 2006;101:181–91.
17. UNODC (2008), Drug dependence treatment: interventions for drug users in prison, United Nations Office on drugs and Crime, Vienna (available online).
18. Jakobsen JC, Nielsen EE, Feinberg J, Katakam KK, Fobian K, Hauser G, et al. Direct-acting antivirals for chronic hepatitis C. Cochrane Database Syst Rev. 2017;6:CD012143. https://doi.org/10.1002/14651858.CD012143.pub2.
19. Feld JJ, Jacobson IM, Sulkowski MS, Poordad F, Tatsch F, Pawlotsky JM. Ribavirin revisited in the era of direct-acting antiviral therapy for hepatitis C virus infection. Liver Int. 2017;37:5–18.
20. Allen SA, Spaulding AC, Osei AM, et al. Treatment of chronic hepatitis C in a state correctional facility. Ann Intern Med. 2003;138:187–90.
21. Farley J, Vasdev S, Fischer B, et al. Feasibility and outcome of HCV treatment in a Canadian federal prison population. Am J Public Health. 2005;95:1737–9.
22. Sterling RK, Hofmann CM, Luketic VA, et al. Treatment of chronic hepatitis C virus in the Virginia Department of Corrections: can compliance overcome racial differences to response? Am J Gastroenterol. 2004;99:866–72.
23. Arain A, Robaeys G, Stöver H. Hepatitis C in European prisons: a call for an evidence-informed response. BMC Infect Dis. 2014;14(Suppl 6):S17. https://doi.org/10.1186/1471-2334-14-S6-S17.
24. Spaulding AC, Thomas DL. Screening for HCV infection in jails. JAMA. 2012; 307(12):1259–60. https://doi.org/10.1001/jama.2012.374.
25. Council of Europe Annual Penal Statistics. Available from: http://wp.unil.ch/space/space-i/prison-stock-on-1st-january/prison-stock-on-01-jan-2015-2016/. Accessed: 10 Nov 2017.
26. Uusküla A, Des Jarlais DC, Raag M, Pinkerton SD, Feelemyer J. Combination prevention for persons who inject drugs in the HIV epidemic in a transitional country: the case of Tallinn, Estonia. AIDS Care. 2015;27(1):105–11. https://doi.org/10.1080/09540121.2014.940271.
27. European Monitoring Centre for Drugs and Drug Addiction. Preventing fatal overdoses: a systematic review of the effectiveness of take-home naloxone, EMCDDA Papers. Luxembourg: Publications Office of the European Union; 2015.
28. Kivimets K, Uusküla A. HIV testing and counselling in Estonian prisons, 2012 to 2013: aims, processes and impacts. Euro Surveill. 2014;19(47):20970.
29. Foreign support. Projects funded from European economic area and Norway grants. Tallinn: Estonian Ministry of Justice. Available from: http://www.just.ee/en/foreign-support. Accessed: 10 Nov 2015.
30. Vanglateenistus. [Prison Service]. Uimastiseire. [Drug Monitoring Report 2014]. Tallinn: Estonian Ministry of Justice; 2014.
31. Social Rehabilitation Programmes for Offenders. Prison Service. Prisons Department of Ministry of Justice. Tallinn: Estonian Ministry of Justice. http://www.vangla.ee/en/socialwork/social-rehabilitation-programmes-offenders. Accessed 24 Jan 2015.
32. Kroonilise C- hepatiidi ravijuhend. (National Guidelines on treatment of HCV). Tallinn: Estonian Society of Gastroenterology and the Estonian Society for Infectious Diseases in 2006 and updated in 2007 and 2010. http://www.esid.ee/cms/tl_files/failid/failid/Kroonilise%20C-hepatiidi%20%20ravijuhend%202010.pdf.
33. Bedossa P, Poynard T. An algorithm for the grading of activity in chronic hepatitis C. The METAVIR Cooperative Study Group. Hepatology. 1996;24:289–93.
34. Babudieri S, Longo B, Sarmati L, Starnini G, Dori L, Suligoi B, et al. Correlates of HIV, HBV and HCV infections in a prison inmate population: results from a multicenter study Italy. J Med Virol. 2005;76(3):311–7. https://doi.org/10.1002/jmv.20375.
35. Taylor A, Munro A, Allen E, Dunleavy K, Cameron S, Miller L, Hickman M. Low incidence of hepatitis C virus among prisoners in Scotland. Addiction. 2013;108:1296–304.
36. Hellard ME, Hocking JS, Crofts N. The prevalence and the risk behaviours associated with the transmission of hepatitis C virus in Australian correctional facilities. Epidemiol Infect. 2004;132:409–15.
37. Butler T, Boonwat L, Hailstone S, Falconer T, Lems P, Ginley T, et al. The 2004 Australian prison entrants' blood-borne virus and risk behaviour survey. Aust N Z J Public Health. 2007;31:44–50.
38. Weild AR, Gill ON, Bennett D, Livingstone SJ, Parry JV, Curran L. Prevalence of HIV, hepatitis B, and hepatitis C antibodies in prisoners in England and Wales: a national survey. Commun Dis Public Health. 2000;3:121–6.
39. Altice FL, Azbel L, Stone J, et al. The perfect storm: incarceration and the high-risk environment perpetuating transmission of HIV, hepatitis C virus, and tuberculosis in Eastern Europe and Central Asia. Lancet (London, England). 2016;388(10050):1228–48. https://doi.org/10.1016/S0140-6736(16)30856-X.
40. Jafari S, Copes R, Baharlou S, Etminan M, Buxton J. Tattooing and the risk of transmission of hepatitis C: a systematic review and meta-analysis. Int J Infect Dis 2010;14(11):e928–40. https://doi.org/10.1016/j.ijid.2010.03.019.
41. Miller ER, Bi P, Ryan P. Hepatitis C virus infection in south Australian prisoners: seroprevalence, seroconversion, and risk factors. Int J Infect Dis. 2009;13(2):201–8. https://doi.org/10.1016/j.ijid.2008.06.011.
42. MAM P, Bandeira LM, Pompilio MA, Croda J, GRd R, LFP D, et al. Prevalence and Incidence of HCV Infection among Prisoners in Central Brazil. PLoS ONE. 2017;12(1):e0169195.
43. Messina JP, Humphreys I, Flaxman A, et al. Global distribution and prevalence of hepatitis C virus genotypes. Hepatology. 2015;61(1):77–87. https://doi.org/10.1002/hep.27259.
44. Meyer MF, Wedemeyer H, Monazahian M, Dreesman J, Manns MP, Lehmann M. Prevalence of hepatitis C in a German prison for young men in relation to country of birth. Epidemiol Infect. 2007;135:274–80.
45. Tyczyno M, Halota W, Nowak W, Pawlowska M. Distribution of HCV genotypes in the populations of inmates in polish prison potulice and patients hospitalized in Bydgoszcz. Hepat Mon. 2014;14:e14559.
46. Tallo T, Lappalainen M, Tefanova V, Priimagi I. Distribution of hepatitis C virus genotypes in patients with chronic hepatitis C in northern Estonia. Acta Virol. 2000;44:175–8.
47. Brjalin V, Salupere R, Tallo T, Kuznetsova T, Priimägi L, Tefanova V. Efficacy of peginterferon alpha-2A and ribavirin combination therapy in treatment-naive Estonian patients with chronic hepatitis C. Cent Eur J Public Health. 2012;20(2):150–5.
48. Negro F. Epidemiology of hepatitis C in Europe. Dig Liver Dis. 2014; 46(Suppl. 5):S158e64.
49. Stone J, Martin NK, Hickman M, et al. Modelling the impact of incarceration and prison-based hepatitis C virus (HCV) treatment on HCV transmission among people who inject drugs in Scotland. Addiction (Abingdon, England). 2017;112(7):1302-14. https://doi.org/10.1111/add.13783.

7

The rs738409 polymorphism of the PNPLA3 gene is associated with hepatic steatosis and fibrosis in Brazilian patients with chronic hepatitis C

Caroline Manchiero[1], Arielle Karen da Silva Nunes[1], Mariana Carvalheiro Magri[1], Bianca Peixoto Dantas[1], Celso Carmo Mazza[2], Antonio Alci Barone[1,2] and Fátima Mitiko Tengan[1,2*]

Abstract

Background: Prospective studies have shown that 80% of acute hepatitis C virus (HCV) cases progress to chronic infection; approximately 10-20% of patients with these conditions will develop liver cirrhosis within 2 to 3 decades, and 1-5% will develop liver cancer. Some studies have indicated that the rs738409 polymorphism of the PNPLA3 gene is associated with steatosis and the progression of advanced fibrosis. This study assessed the contribution of the PNPLA3 rs738409 polymorphism with regard to the steatosis and degree of liver fibrosis in Brazilian patients diagnosed with chronic hepatitis C.

Methods: A total of 290 patients were evaluated at the Clinics Hospital of the School of Medicine, University of São Paulo, between 2010 and 2015. The inclusion criteria were age ≥ 18 years and positive anti-HCV antibody and HCV RNA tests. The participants were evaluated based on medical consultation, blood tests, and liver biopsies conducted before specific antiviral therapies were applied. The associations between the rs738409 PNPLA3 gene polymorphism and steatosis and advanced fibrosis were tested under a recessive inheritance model using logistic regression analysis, including age, gender, BMI, ethnicity/color, HOMA-IR, alcohol intake, HCV genotype 3, and the rs58542926 TM6SF2 gene polymorphism as covariates.

Results: The mean age of the patients was 54.9 years old (range, 28 to 82 years), and 124 (42.8%) patients were male; 226 (77.9%) were white, 43 (14.8%) were *pardo,* and 21 (7.2%) were black Brazilians. Of the patients included in this study, 133 (45.9%) presented with the CC genotype, 63 (21.7%) with the CG genotype, and 94 (32.4%) with the GG genotype of the PNPLA3 gene I148M variant. We observed that the associations between PNPLA3 rs738409 GG genotype and steatosis was significant (OR: 2.16; 95% CI 1.26-3.72). The same genotype was associated to advanced fibrosis too (OR:2.64; 95% CI 1.26-5.53).

Conclusions: Associations between the rs738409 polymorphism of the PNPLA3 gene genotype GG and hepatic steatosis and advanced fibrosis were observed. Studies are still needed to clarify the influence of these polymorphisms on hepatic steatosis and degree of fibrosis among individuals diagnosed with chronic hepatitis C.

Keywords: Hepatitis C, PNPLA3, Steatosis, Fibrosis, Polymorphism rs738409, TM6SF2, Polymorphism rs58542926, Brazil

* Correspondence: fatima.tengan@uol.com.br
[1]Medical Research Laboratory for Virus (Laboratório de Investigação Médica por Vírus - LIM47) of the Clinics Hospital, School of Medicine, University of São Paulo (Universidade de São Paulo - USP), São Paulo, Brazil
[2]Department of Infectious and Parasitic Diseases, School of Medicine, University of São Paulo, São Paulo, Brazil

Background

The hepatitis C virus (HCV) has a worldwide distribution, occurring among individuals of all ages and ethnicities and across various regions of the world. HCV infection affects 2.2-3.0% of all people in the world (130-170 million people), with greater rates in Africa and Asia [1]. The estimated prevalence in Brazil is 1.4%, with 2,609,670 people infected [1]. Prospective studies have shown that 80% of acute hepatitis C cases progress to chronic infection. Approximately 10-20% of these cases develop complications of chronic liver disease, such as liver cirrhosis within 2 to 3 decades, and 1-5% will develop liver cancer [2, 3].

Clinical factors (e.g., advanced age, male gender, elevated body mass index [BMI], and alcohol consumption [> 30-50 g/day]), histological factors (e.g., steatosis), viral factors (primarily genotype 3), and HCV-human immunodeficiency virus (HIV) coinfection are associated with a greater risk of fibrosis progression. However, even when considered together, these factors have a predictive value of less than 30% [4].

The genetic factors that influence the evolution of hepatitis C are being studied, including the rs738409 polymorphism of the patatin-like phospholipase domain containing 3 (PNPLA3) gene. This polymorphism, located on chromosome 22, is characterized by the replacement of isoleucine with methionine at position 148 (I148M) due to exchange of a C nucleotide by a G (C>G) and has been strongly associated with liver fat content and high levels of serum alanine aminotransferase and aspartate aminotransferase [5]. Studies of Caucasian patients suggest that the rs738409 polymorphism is associated with steatosis and the progression of advanced fibrosis [6–8].

More recently, a single-nucleotide polymorphism encoding the E167K variant of the transmembrane six superfamily member 2 gene (TM6SF2) was determined to be independently associated with liver steatosis [9, 10] and necroinflammation [10] in chronic hepatitis C patients.

The aim of this study was to evaluate the contribution of the PNPLA3 rs738409 genetic variant to steatosis and the degree of liver fibrosis in Brazilian patients diagnosed with chronic hepatitis C. The secondary objective was to evaluate the role of the gene TM6SF2 E167K variant in the occurrence of the same outcomes.

Methods

Patient selection

A total of 290 patients were evaluated at the outpatient clinic of infectious diseases in the Clinics Hospital of the School of Medicine, University of São Paulo (Hospital das Clínicas da Faculdade de Medicina da Universidade de São Paulo; HCFMUSP). The inclusion criteria were age ≥ 18 years and positive anti-HCV antibody (3rd generation ELISA) and HCVRNA tests (Cobas Amplicor HCV Monitor Test, Roche Diagnostics, Branchburg, New Jersey, USA). Patients co-infected with hepatitis B virus (HBV) or HIV or who had received previous HCV treatment were excluded.

In the period from 01/01/2010 to 31/12/2015, 452 patients with anti-HCV positive tests were attended at the outpatient clinic of infectious diseases in the Clinics Hospital of the HCFMUSP. Of these, 413 were positive for HCV RNA, and 39 were negative for HCV RNA (Fig. 1). Of the 413 positive for HCV RNA, 21 patients were anti-HIV antibody-positive, and 9 were HBsAg-positive. Of the remaining 383 patients, 93 reported previous treatment for hepatitis C. Therefore, 290 patients with chronic hepatitis C were included in the study. The participants were evaluated based on medical consultation, blood tests, and liver biopsies conducted before specific antiviral therapies were applied. The ethics committee of HCFMUSP approved this study and all study participants provided written consent.

Data collection

The epidemiological factors collected included gender, age, ethnicity/color, alcohol consumption, and body mass index (BMI). Alcohol consumption was divided into two categories: ≤ 20 g/day or > 20 g/day. BMI was calculated as the ratio between weight in kg and height (meters squared). Insulin resistance was estimated using the HOMA-IR (homeostasis model assessment) value and was defined by the equation fasting insulin (μU/mL) x fasting glucose (mmol/L)/22.5.

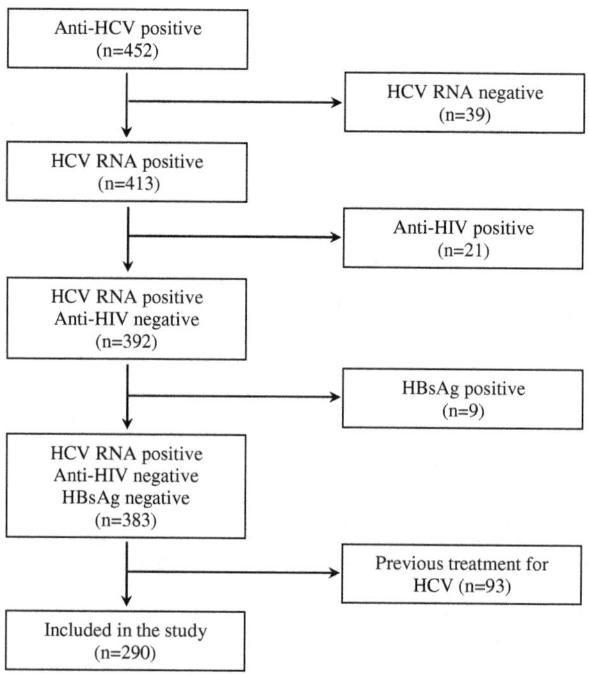

Fig. 1 Patient selection flowchart for the present study

In the present study, Brazilians were classified according to their own self-identification of ethnicity/color: African Brazilians, self-identified as "black"; European Brazilians, self-identified as "white"; a mixture of one or more ethnicities, self-identified as "*pardo*"; Brazilian Asian, self-identified as "yellow"; and indigenous Brazilian, self-identified as "indigenous." In Brazil, the term most used to define multiracial people is *pardo* (brown), which is the result of a mixture of various ethnicities [11]. The term has been officially adopted by the Instituto Brasileiro de Geografia e Estatística (BGE - Brazilian Institute of Geography and Statistics), which conducts the Brazilian demographic census [11].

Histological abnormalities were scored using the Metavir system. Liver fibrosis was rated using a 5-point scale, where F0 = no fibrosis, F1 = portal fibrosis without septa, F2 = rare septa, F3 = numerous septa without cirrhosis, and F4 = cirrhosis. Necroinflammatory activity was rated using a 4-point scale, where A = no histological activity, A1 = mild activity, A2 = moderate activity, and A3 = severe activity [12]. Steatosis was evaluated based on the percentage of hepatocytes containing fat droplets and was classified as 0 (<5%), 1 (5-33%), 2 (34-66%), or 3 (> 66%).

Genotyping was conducted using the Versant ® HCV Genotype 2.0 (LiPA) test (Imunogenetics, Ghent, Belgium) according to the manufacturer's instructions.

PNPLA3 and TM6SF2 genotyping

The extraction and purification of genomic DNA from the serum were conducted using a PureLink Genomic DNA Mini kit (Invitrogen/Life Technologies, Carlsbad, California, USA) according to the manufacturer's instructions.

After DNA extraction, the samples were subjected to a PCR-RFLP reaction to analyze the rs738409 polymorphism of the PNPLA3 gene where the dominant homozygous genotype is CC, the heterozygous genotype is CG and the recessive / mutated homozygote is GG. The following primers were used: F: 5'-TGGGCC TGAAGTCCGAGGGT-3' and R: 5'-CCGACACCAGTG CCCTGCAG-3'. To determine the rs738409 (C>G) polymorphism genotype, the restriction endonuclease BtsCI (BtsCI, 20,000 U/ml, New England BioLabs, Massachusetts, USA) was used based on the descriptions of Dutta [13]. The products of the restriction enzyme digestion were subjected to electrophoresis in a 2% agarose gel with 6 μL of *Diamond*™ Nucleic Acid Dye (Promega, Fitchburg, Wisconsin, USA) in a horizontal electrophoretic tank containing TBE buffer (0.5X concentration) with a constant current of 110 V for 1 hour and 15 minutes. The resulting bands were visualized under ultraviolet (UV) light using a UVIdoc HD2 gel documentation system (Uvitec Cambridge, Cambridge, UK). The images were recorded to digital files.

Regarding the rs58542926 polymorphism (C>T) of the TM6SF2 gene, samples were subjected to a real-time PCR using the system "TaqMan genotyping assay", dbSNP rs58542926 assay C_89463510_10, #4351379 (Applied Biosystems, Foster City, CA, USA) on a StepOnePlus™ (96-well) Real-Time PCR System (Applied Biosystems, Foster City, CA, USA). The assay was standardized in a final volume of 25 μL: 12.5 μL of TaqMan MasterMix (Applied Biosystems, Foster City, CA, USA), 0.63 μL of Genotyping Assay 40X (Applied Biosystems, Foster City, CA, USA), 0.63 μL of ultrapure water (Promega, Fitchburg, Wisconsin, USA), and 11.25 μL of genomic DNA. The cycling was as follows: 95°C for 10 minutes, followed by 50 cycles of 95°C for 15 seconds and 60°C for 1 minute, and finally, 60°C for 1 minute. The interpretation of genotypes was given by CC, CT, and TT, where T is the mutated allele.

Genetic inheritance model

The role of the polymorphism rs738409 of the PNPLA3 gene on steatosis and fibrosis was investigated using the recessive genetic inheritance model, comparing patients with the homozygous G allele (GG genotype) with patients with one or no copy of the G allele (CG or CC). The model of recessive genetic inheritance was chosen, based on previous results of studies on the association between genotypes of polymorphism rs738409 PNPLA3 and fibrosis in patients with nonalcoholic fatty liver disease (NAFLD) and Hepatitis C performed by other authors [7, 14].

In addition, in order to better understand the risk associated with the rs738409 polymorphism of the PNPLA3 gene, we compared, as an additional analysis, patients with the G allele (CG+GG) and patients with the genotype CC (dominant model) and patients with GG genotype and patients with genotype CC (additive model).

Finally, as a secondary objective, we evaluated the role of the gene TM6SF2 E167K variant in the occurrence of the same outcomes.

Statistical analyses

As a primary objective we assessed the effect of PNPLA3 on steatosis and degree of liver fibrosis in Brazilian patients diagnosed with chronic hepatitis C using a recessive (genotype CG+CC vs GG.) inheritance genetic model and as an additional analysis we evaluate the same effects under a dominant (genotype CC vs. CG+GG) and additive (genotype CC vs. GG) genetic model. As a secondary objective, we evaluated the role of the TM6SF2 gene E167K variant in the occurrence of the same outcomes.

The associations between the rs738409 PNPLA3 gene polymorphism and steatosis and advanced fibrosis were tested using logistic regression analysis, including age, gender, BMI, ethnicity/color, HOMA-IR, alcohol intake,

HCV genotype 3, and the rs58542926 TM6SF2 gene polymorphism as covariates. The effect on advanced fibrosis was evaluated by comparing patients with no fibrosis, mild fibrosis, or moderate fibrosis (F0-F1-F2) with those with severe fibrosis or cirrhosis (F3-F4). The presence of steatosis was studied as a qualitative variable (< 5% versus ≥ 5%). To perform the analyses, the software IBM-SPSS for Windows version 20.0 was used; for data tabulation, the software Microsoft Excel 2003 was used. The tests were performed with a significance level of 5%.

Results

The characteristics of the patients with chronic hepatitis C included in the study are shown in Table 1. The mean age of the patients was 54.9 years old (range, 28 to 82 years), and 124 (42.8%) patients were male. Of the 290 patients included in the study, 226 (77.9%) were white, 43 (14.8%) were *pardo,* and 21 (7.2%) were black Brazilians. The mean BMI was 27 kg/m^2; 107 (36.9%) and 66 (22.8%) of these patients were classified as overweight (25.0-29.9 kg/m^2) and obese (≥30 kg/m^2), respectively. Of the 290 patients, 133 (45.9%) presented with the CC genotype, 63 (21.7%) presented with the CG genotype, and 94 (32.4%) presented with the GG genotype of PNPLA3 polymorphism. For the TM6SF2, 29 (10.0%) presented with CT genotype, and 261 (90.0%) presented with the CC genotype.

The most frequent GG genotype of the PNPLA3 gene was found in white Brazilians (35.4%), followed by *pardo* (23.3%) and black (19.1%) Brazilians. Thus, the highest frequency of the PNPLA3 allele G was found in white Brazilians (45.6%), followed by black (35.7%) and *pardo* (34.9%) Brazilians; details of the clinical characteristics stratified by ethnicity and genotype polymorphism at rs738409 PNPLA3 are shown in Additional file 1.

After adjusting for age, gender, BMI, HOMA-IR, ethnicity/color, alcohol use, HCV genotype 3, and TM6SF2 genotypes, the association between PNPLA3 rs738409 GG genotype and steatosis remained significant in the recessive (p=0.01) model (Table 2).

After adjusting for age, gender, BMI, HOMA-IR, ethnicity/color, alcohol use, HCV genotype 3, and TM6SF2 genotypes, the association between PNPLA3 rs738409 GG genotype and advanced fibrosis remained significant in the recessive model (p=0.01) (Table 2). The gene TM6SF2 E167K variant (genotype CT) was also associated advanced fibrosis (p=0.00).

When analyzing the data, using the dominant and additive genetic inheritance model, we observed that patients with the GG genotype presented a higher risk of steatosis than patients with the CC genotype (p= 0.03, additive model) (Additional file 2). Patients with G allele presented higher risk of advanced fibrosis than those with the CC genotype (p=0.02, dominant model). However, patients carrying the GG genotype presented no greater risk of advanced fibrosis than those with the CC genotype (p=0.08, additive model) (Additional file 2). Regarding the TM6SF2 gene polymorphism, we observed that T-allele carriers presented a higher risk of fibrosis than patients with CC genotype (p = 0.01; dominant model).

Table 1 Baseline characteristics of patients included in the study

Characteristics	Total
N	290
Age (mean±SD)	54.9±12.1
Male gender	124 (42.8%)
Ethnicity/color	
White	226 (77.9%)
Pardo	43 (14.8%)
Black	21 (7.2%)
Alcohol > 20 g/day	55(19.3%)
BMI (mean±SD)	27.1±6.1
Glucose (mean±SD)	93.1±49.4
Insulin (mean±SD)	15.2±32.2
ALT (mean±SD)	62.3±49.4
AST (mean±SD)	49.8±38.1
Total cholesterol (mean±SD)	173.9±39.8
LDL-C (mean±SD)	95.5±32.8
HDL-C (mean±SD)	55.3±18.5
VLDL-C (mean±SD)	23.9±20.9
Triglycerides (mean±SD)	109.3±66.8
Hepatic steatosis ≥ 5%	143 (49.3%)
Liver fibrosis (Metavir ≥ F3)	58 (20%)
HCV genotype 3	45 (15.7%)
PNPLA3 rs738409	
CC	133 (45.9%)
CG	63 (21.7%)
GG	94 (32.4%)
TM6F2 rs58542926	
CC	261 (90%)
CT	29 (10%)

Abbreviations: *BMI* body mass index, *ALT* alanine aminotransferase, *AST* aspartate aminotransferase, *LDL-C* low-density lipoprotein-cholesterol, *HDL-C* high-density lipoprotein-cholesterol, *VLDL* very-low-density lipoprotein-cholesterol

Discussion

This study assessed the influence of the rs738409 polymorphism of the PNPLA3 gene on hepatic steatosis and the degree of fibrosis among individuals diagnosed with chronic hepatitis C and observed that the prevalence rates of genotypes CC, CG, and GG of the PNPLA3

Table 2 Analysis of the association between genotype polymorphism at rs738409 PNPLA3 and steatosis and advanced liver fibrosis in patients with HCV infection according to the univariate and multivariate analysis in the recessive model

Variables	n[a]/N[b] (%)	n[a]/N[b] (%)	Univariate analysis			Multivariate analysis		
	No steatosis	Steatosis	OR[c]	95% CI	*P*	OR	95% CI	*P*
PNPLA3 genotype								
CC/CG	108/147 (74.1)	88/143 (61.5)	1.00			1.00		
GG	38/147 (25.9)	55/143 (38.5)	1.73	(1.05 – 2.84)	0.03	2.16	(1.26 – 3.72)	0.01
Age (years)	52.2±11.7	57.6±11.8	0.03	(0.01 – 0.06)	0.00	1.04	(1.02 – 1.06)	0.00
Sex								
Female	78/147 (53.1)	88/143 (61.5)	1.00			1.00		
Male	69/147 (46.9)	55/143(38.6)	1.41	(0.88 – 2.25)	0.14	0.62	(0.35 – 1.08)	0.09
BMI (kg/m2)	26±3.8	28.1±7.6	0.07	(0.03 – 0.13)	0.00	1.10	(1.04 – 1.18)	0.00
Ethnicity/color								
White	108/147 (73.5)	118/143 (82.5)	1.00			1.00		
Pardo	28/147 (19.0)	15/143(10.5)	0.64	(0.33 – 1.24)	0.19	0.77	(0.36 – 1.66)	0.50
Black	11/147 (7.5)	10/143 (7.0)	1.34	(0.53 – 3.23)	0.55	0.71	(0.25 – 2.05)	0.53
HOMA-IR	3.1±8.2	3.8±3.7	0.02	(0.01 – 0.07)	0.38	0.99	(0.95 – 1.03)	0.72
Alcohol								
<20 g/day	113/147 (76.9)	117/143 (81.8)	1.00			1.00		
>20 g/day	31/147 (21.1)	24/143(16.8)	0.75	(0.41 – 1.36)	0.35	1.38	(0.77 – 2.48)	0.29
HCV genotype								
Non 3	130/147 (88.4)	111/143 (77.6)	1.00			1.00		
3	15/147 (10.2)	29/143(20.3)	2.34	(1.19 – 4.57)	0.01	2.15	(1.02 – 4.53)	0.04
TM6SF2 (genotype								
CC	135/147 (91.8)	126/143 (88.1)	1.00			1.00		
CT	12/147 (8.2)	17/143(11.9)	0.95	(0.44 – 2.05)	0.90	2.28	(0.93 – 5.61)	0.07
	Mild fibrosis (F0-F1-F2)	Advanced Fibrosis (F3-F4)						
PNPLA3 genotype								
CC/CG	162/232 (69.8)	34/58 (58.6)	1.00			1.00		
GG	70/232 (30.2)	24/58(41.4)	1.63	(1.15 – 2.95)	0.01	2.64	(1.26 – 5.53)	0.01
Age (years)	53.4±13.3	60.7±9.2(84.5)	0.05	(0.02 – 0.08)	0.00	1.08	(1.04 – 1.11)	0.00
Sex								
Female	145/232 (62.5)	21/58 (36.2)	1.00			1.00		
Male	87/232 (37.5)	37/58(63.8)	2.93	(1.61 – 5.33)	0.00	1.06	(1.03 – 1.09)	0.00
BMI (kg/m2)	27.1±6.4	26.8±4.8	1.00	(0.95 – 1.05)	0.71	1.03	(0.97 – 1.09)	0.37
Ethnicity/color								
White	183/232 (78.9)	43/58 (74.1)	1.00			1.00		
Pardo	16/232 (6.9)	10/58(17.3)	1.36	(0.62 – 2.99)	0.43	2.46	(0.93 – 6.48)	0.07
Black	33/232 (14.2)	5/58(8.6)	2.25	(0.85 – 5.94)	0.10	1.76	(0.45 – 6.93)	0.42
HOMA-IR	3.2±6.7	4.6±4.5	0.02	(0.01 – 1.02)	0.21	1.03	(0.99 – 1.08)	0.15
Alcohol								
<20 g/day	187/232 (80.6)	43/58 (74.1)	1.00			1.00		
>20 g/day	40/232 (17.2)	15/58(25.9)	0.59	(0.30 – 1.17)	0.13	0.91	(0.39 – 2.12)	0.82
HCV genotype								
Non 3	196/232 (84.5)	45/58 (77.6)	1.00			1.00		
3	32/232 (13.8)	13/58(22.4)	1.76	(0.86 – 3.64)	0.12	1.43	(0.59 – 3.45)	0.43

Table 2 Analysis of the association between genotype polymorphism at rs738409 PNPLA3 and steatosis and advanced liver fibrosis in patients with HCV infection according to the univariate and multivariate analysis in the recessive model *(Continued)*

Variables	n[a]/N[b] (%)	n[a]/N[b] (%)	Univariate analysis			Multivariate analysis		
	No steatosis	Steatosis	OR[c]	95% CI	*P*	OR	95% CI	*P*
TM6SF2 (genotype								
CC	215/232 (92.7)	46/58 (79.3)	1.00			1.00		
CT	17/232 (7.3)	12/58(20.7)	3.51	(1.18 – 10.47)	0.02	4.81	(1.67 – 13.87)	0.00

Abbreviations: *BMI* Body mass index, *HOMA-IR* homeostatic model assessment of insulin resistance
[a]Number of patients with the characteristic; [b]Total number of patients with the outcome (no steatosis, steatosis, no advanced fibrosis or advanced fibrosis); [c]In the case of continuous variables (age, BMI and HOMA-IR) means OR in one unit increase

polymorphism were 45.9%, 21.7%, and 32.4%, respectively. We also observed that the GG genotype of the same polymorphism was associated with steatosis and advanced fibrosis. We also found an association between TM6SF2 polymorphism and advanced fibrosis. Our additional analysis reinforced the finding that the carriers of the rs847309 polymorphism genotype GG of the PNPLA3 gene are at increased risk of developing hepatic steatosis.

The influence of the rs738409 polymorphism on liver fat deposition was initially demonstrated in patients with NAFLD [5, 15, 16]. Sookoian et al. [16] also described the association between the polymorphism and fibrosis intensity, including nonalcoholic steatohepatitis. Later, this polymorphism was revealed to play a similar role in individuals with other liver diseases [17–19]. Regarding hepatitis C, several authors [7, 8, 20] have observed that the GG genotype is associated with a greater risk of steatosis and advanced fibrosis, whereas a study in Taiwan [21] observed that the G allele (CG + GG) was associated with the same events (i.e., the presence of steatosis and a greater degree of fibrosis). Our finding is in accordance with the data described above, as we also found that the G allele was an independent determinant of hepatic steatosis and advanced fibrosis.

PNPLA3, also referred to as adiponutrin, encodes a 481-amino-acid protein that contains a highly conserved patatin-like domain at the N terminus; in human tissues, its expression is highest in the liver, followed by skin and adipose tissue [22]. *In vitro* assays using recombinant PNPLA3 confirmed that the wild-type enzyme hydrolyzes emulsified TG and that the I148M substitution abolishes this activity. Expression of PNPLA3-I148M, but not wild-type PNPLA3, in cultured hepatocytes or in the livers of mice increased cellular TG contents [23]. The exact mechanism by which variation in PNPLA3 affects liver TG content is not known.

Related to the association between PNPLA3 and hepatic fibrosis, Pirazzi et al. [24] presented evidence of the mechanism involved in the association between PNPLA3 activity and hepatic fibrosis, regardless of the presence of steatosis. In that study, the authors demonstrated that PNPLA3 is highly expressed in human hepatic stellate cells (HSCs) suggesting a potential link between HSCs, retinoid metabolism, and PNPLA3 in determining the susceptibility to hepatic fibrosis.

Another finding of our study is that the E167K variant is an independent determinant of severity of fibrosis, as other researchers have also observed in NAFLD [25, 26] and hepatitis C [10]. In vivo [27, 28] and in vitro [27–29] studies suggest that TM6SF2 controls hepatic lipid efflux. Deletion or mutation of TM6SF2 results in reduced lipoprotein secretion (very-low-density lipoprotein [VLDL], TG, and apolipoprotein B [APOB]), which coincides with increased hepatocellular lipid droplet size and TG accumulation. The mechanism by which the E167K variant influences the severity of fibrosis is not known. In our study, rs58542926 TM6SF2 polymorphism was associated with advanced fibrosis independent of factors known to be associated with fibrosis, including the rs738409 PNPLA3 polymorphism.

The highest frequency of the PNPLA3 allele G was found in white Brazilians (45.6%), followed by black (35.7%) and *pardo* (34.9%) Brazilians. The prevalence of the GG genotype found in the study (32.4%) was higher than those found in European (2.2% to 12%) [7, 30–32] and Japanese studies (17.7% to 21.2%) [33–36]. However, the frequency of the G allele in white Brazilians was similar to that reported by Romeo et al. in American Hispanics (49.8%) [5]. Patients who considered themselves to be black had a higher prevalence of the G allele than the African Americans, according to Romeo et al [5].

According to the Brazilian census of 2010 [11] and to an autosomal DNA study [37], most Brazilians come from three large ancestral populations: European, African, and Brazilian Amerindians, in various combinations and varying degrees. Many Brazilians who define themselves as white may present African or Amerindian ancestors [38, 39], since in Brazil, individuals define themselves as white, black, or *pardo* based on skin color rather than on ancestry [11, 38, 39]. The mixture of ethnicities, even in patients who are considered white or black, could explain, at least in part, the different prevalence rates of the G allele of the rs738409 PNPLA3 gene polymorphism found in our study, although we could not locate the ethnic source of that difference.

Our study has limitations. The participants were recruited from a single tertiary care center linked to the university, limiting the number of participants in the study. Our results cannot be generalized to all patients with hepatitis C, although our case sample did not have a high proportion of patients with advanced liver disease (20.0%). In addition, the interpretation of our findings is also limited by the lack of a comparison group (e.g., patients with chronic liver disease of other etiologies or healthy volunteers) to help contextualize the events and characteristics present in patients with HCV.

Finally, despite these limitations, the data obtained should be added to the extant evidence regarding the roles that the rs738409 polymorphism of the PNPLA3 gene and the rs58542926 polymorphism of the TM6SF2 gene play in hepatic steatosis and advanced fibrosis among individuals with chronic hepatitis C. In addition, this study examined Brazilian patients, who (to the best of our knowledge) have not yet been studied from this perspective.

Conclusions

Associations between the rs738409 polymorphism PNPLA3 gene genotype GG and hepatic steatosis and advanced fibrosis were observed among Brazilian patients with chronic HCV. In addition, we found that the rs58542926 polymorphism of the TM6SF2 gene is associated with advanced liver fibrosis independent of rs738409 polymorphism of the PNPLA3 gene.

Further studies are needed with comparison groups and larger numbers of patients to clarify the influence of the rs738409 polymorphism of the PNPLA3 gene and the rs58542926 polymorphism of the TM6SF2 gene (genotype CT) on hepatic steatosis and degree of fibrosis among individuals diagnosed with chronic hepatitis C.

Abbreviations

γ-GT: Gamma-glutamyltransferase; ALT: Alanine aminotransferase; AST: Aspartate aminotransferase; BMI: Body mass index; CI: Confidence interval; DNA: Desoxyribunucleic acid; ELISA: Enzyme-linked immunosorbent assay; HBV: Hepatitis B virus; HCFMUSP: Hospital das Clínicas da Faculdade de Medicina da Universidade de São Paulo; HCV: Hepatitis C virus; HDL-C: High-density lipoprotein-cholesterol; HIV: Human immunodeficiency virus; HOMA-IR: Homeostatic model assessment; LDL-C: Low-density lipoprotein-cholesterol; OR: Odds ratio; PCR: Polymerase chain reaction; PNPLA3: Patatin-like phospholipase domain-containing 3 protein; RFLP: Restriction fragment length polymorphism; RNA: ribonucleic acid; SD: Standard deviation; SNP: Single-nucleotide polymorphism; SPSS: Statistical Software for the Social Sciences; TBE: Tris-Borate; TG: Triglycerides; TM6SF2: Transmembrane six superfamily member 2; VLDL-C: Very-low-density lipoprotein-cholesterol

Acknowledgments

Not Applicable.

Funding

No specific funding was obtained for this study.

Authors' contributions

CM conceived the study design, performed data collection, and drafted the manuscript. AKSN performed data collection and helped to draft the manuscript. CM, AKSN, MCM, and BPD performed the experiments. CCM and AAB participated in the collection of clinical data. FM conceived the study design and was in charge of the critical revision of the manuscript content. All authors read and approved the final manuscript.

Consent for publication

Not applicable for this study.

Competing interests

The authors declare that they have no competing interest.

References

1. Lavanchy D. Evolving epidemiology of hepatitis C virus. Clin Microbiol Infect. 2011;17:107–15.
2. Seeff LB. Natural history of chronic hepatitis C. Hepatology. 2002;36:S35–46.
3. Davis GL, Alter MJ, El-Serag H, Poynard T, Jennings LW. Aging of hepatitis C virus (HCV)-infected persons in the United States: a multiple cohort model of HCV prevalence and disease progression. Gastroenterology. 2010;138 513–21, 521.e1
4. Wright M, Goldin R, Fabre A, Lloyd J, Thomas H, Trepo C, et al. Measurement and determinants of the natural history of liver fibrosis in hepatitis C virus infection: a cross sectional and longitudinal study. Gut. 2003;52:574–9.
5. Romeo S, Kozlitina J, Xing C, Pertsemlidis A, Cox D, Pennacchio LA, et al. Genetic variation in PNPLA3 confers susceptibility to nonalcoholic fatty liver disease. Nat Genet. 2008;40:1461–5.
6. Stättermayer AF, Rutter K, Beinhardt S, Scherzer TM, Stadlmayr A, Hofer H, et al. Association of the IL28B genotype with insulin resistance in patients with chronic hepatitis C. J Hepatol. 2012;57:492–8.
7. Trépo E, Pradat P, Potthoff A, Momozawa Y, Quertinmont E, Gustot T, et al. Impact of patatin-like phospholipase-3 (RS738409 C>G) polymorphism on fibrosis progression and steatosis in chronic hepatitis C. Hepatology. 2011;54:60–9.
8. Valenti L, Aghemo A, Stättermayer AF, Maggioni P, De Nicola S, Motta BM, et al. Implications of PNPLA3 polymorphism in chronic hepatitis C patients receiving peginterferon plus ribavirin. Aliment Pharmacol Ther. 2012;35:1434–42.
9. Coppola N, Rosa Z, Cirillo G, Stanzione M, Macera M, Boemio A, et al. TM6SF2 E167K variant is associated with severe steatosis in chronic hepatitis C, regardless of PNPLA3 polymorphism. Liver Int. 2015;35:1959–63.
10. Milano M, Aghemo A, Mancina RM, Fischer J, Dongiovann P, Nicola S, et al. Transmembrane 6 superfamily member 2 gene E167K variant impacts on steatosis and liver damage in chronic hepatitis C patients. Hepatology. 2015;62:111–7.
11. Instituto Brasileiro de Geografia e Estatistica. Ethno-Racial Characteristics of the population. https://biblioteca.ibge.gov.br/index.php/biblioteca-catalogo?id=263405&view=detalhes. Accessed 12 Dec 2017.
12. The French METAVIR Cooperative Study Group. Intraobserver and interobserver variations in liver biopsy interpretation in patients with chronic hepatitis C. The French METAVIR Cooperative Study Group. Hepatology. 1994;20:15–20.
13. Dutta AK. A new PCR-RFLP method for diagnosing PNPLA3 RS738409 polymorphism. Webmedcentral Genet. 2012;3:WMC002928.
14. Valenti L, Al-Serri A, Daly AK, Galmozzi E, Rametta R, Dongiovanni P, et al. Homozygosity for the PNPLA3 / adiponutrin I148M polymorphism influences liver fibrosis in patients with nonalcoholic fatty liver disease. Hepatology. 2010;51:1209–17.
15. Kotronen A, Johansson LE, Johansson LM, Roos C, Westerbacka J, Hamsten A, et al. A common variant in PNPLA3, which encodes adiponutrin, is associated with liver fat content in humans. Diabetologia. 2009;52:1056–60.
16. Sookoian S, Castaño GO, Burgueño AL, Gianotti TF, Rosselli MS, Pirola CJA. nonsynonymous gene variant in the adiponutrin gene is associated with nonalcoholic fatty liver disease severity. J Lipid Res. 2009;50:2111–6.
17. Buch S, Stickel F, Trépo E, Way M, Herrmann A, Nischalke HD, et al. A genome-wide association study confirms PNPLA3 and identifies

TM6SF2 and MBOAT7 as risk loci for alcohol-related cirrhosis. Nat Genet. 2015;47:1443–8.
18. Vigano M, Valenti L, Lampertico P, Facchetti F, Motta BM, D'Ambrosio R, et al. Patatin-like phospholipase domain-containing 3 affects liver steatosis in patients with chronic hepatitis B. Hepatology. 2013;58:1245–52.
19. Zampino R, Coppola N, Cirillo G, Boemio A, Grandone A, Stanzione M, et al. Patatin-like phospholipase domain-containing 3 I148M variant is associated with liver steatosis and fat distribution in chronic hepatitis B. Dig Dis Sci. 2015;60:3005–10.
20. Stättermayer AF, Rutter K, Beinhardt S, Wrba F, Scherzer TM, Strasser M, et al. Role of FDFT1 polymorphism for fibrosis progression in patients with chronic hepatitis C. Liver Int. 2014;34:388–95.
21. Huang CF, Dai CY, Yeh ML, Huang CI, Tai CM, Hsieh MH, et al. Association of diabetes and PNPLA3 genetic variants with disease severity of patients with chronic hepatitis C virus infection. J Hepatol. 2015;62:512–8.
22. Huang Y, He S, Li JZ, Seo YK, Osborne TF, Cohen JC, et al. A feed-forward loop amplifies nutritional regulation of PNPLA3. Proc Natl Acad Sci U S A. 2010;107:7892–7.
23. He S, McPhaul C, Li JZ, Garuti R, Kinch L, Grishin NV, et al. A sequence variation (I148M) in PNPLA3 associated with nonalcoholic fatty liver disease disrupts triglyceride hydrolysis. J Biol Chem. 2010;285:6706–15.
24. Pirazzi C, Valenti L, Motta BM, Pingitore P, Hedfalk K, Mancina RM, et al. PNPLA3 has retinyl-palmitate lipase activity in human hepatic stellate cells. Hum Mol Genet. 2014;23:4077–85.
25. Liu YL, Reeves HL, Burt AD, Tiniakos D, McPherson S, Leathart JBS, et al. TM6SF2 rs58542926 influences hepatic fibrosis progression in patients with non-alcoholic fatty liver disease. Nat Commun. 2014;5:4309.
26. Wang X, Liu Z, Wang K, Wang Z, Sun X, Zhong L, et al. Additive effects of the risk alleles of PNPLA3 and TM6SF2 on non-alcoholic fatty liver disease (NAFLD) in a Chinese population. Front Genet. 2016;7:140. https://doi.org/10.3389/fgene.2016.00140.
27. Kozlitina J, Smagris E, Stender S, Nordestgaard BG, Zhou HH, Tybjærg-Hansen A, et al. Exome-wide association study identifies a TM6SF2 variant that confers susceptibility to nonalcoholic fatty liver disease. Nat Genet. 2014;46:352–6.
28. Holmen OL, Zhang H, Fan Y, Hovelson DH, Schmidt EM, Zhou W, et al. Systematic evaluation of coding variation identifies a candidate causal variant in TM6SF2 influencing total cholesterol and myocardial infarction risk. Nat Genet. 2014;46:345–51.
29. Mahdessian H, Taxiarchis A, Popov S, Silveira A, Franco-Cereceda A, Hamsten A, et al. TM6SF2 is a regulator of liver fat metabolism influencing triglyceride secretion and hepatic lipid droplet content. Proc Natl Acad Sci U S A. 2014;111:8913–8.
30. Valenti L, Rumi M, Galmozzi E, Aghemo A, Del Menico B, De Nicola S, et al. Patatin-like phospholipase domain-containing 3 polymorphism, steatosis, and liver damage in chronic hepatitis C. Hepatology. 2011;53:791–9.
31. Zampino R, Coppola N, Cirillo G, Boemio A, Pisaturo M, Marrone A, et al. Abdominal fat interacts with PNPLA3 I148M, but not with the APOC3 variant in the pathogenesis of liver steatosis in chronic hepatitis C. J Viral Hepat. 2013;20:517–23.
32. Ampuero J, Del Campo JA, Rojas L, García-Lozano JR, Solá R, Andrade R, et al. PNPLA3 RS738409 causes steatosis according to viral & IL28B genotypes in hepatitis C. Ann Hepatol. 2014;13:356–63.
33. Nakamura M, Kanda T, Nakamoto S, Miyamura T, Jiang X, Wu S, et al. No correlation between PNPLA3 RS738409 genotype and fatty liver and hepatic cirrhosis in Japanese patients with HCV. PLOS One. 2013;8:e81312.
34. Yasui K, Kawaguchi T, Shima T, Mitsuyoshi H, Seki K, Sendo R, et al. Effect of PNPLA3 rs738409 variant (I148 M) on hepatic steatosis, necroinflammation, and fibrosis in Japanese patients with chronic hepatitis C. J Gastroenterol. 2015;50:887–93.
35. Nakaoka K, Hashimoto S, Kawabe N, Nitta Y, Murao M, Nakano T, et al. PNPLA3 I148M associations with liver carcinogenesis in Japanese chronic hepatitis C patients. Springerplus. 2015;4:83.
36. Tamaki N, Kurosaki M, Higuchi M, Takada H, Nakakuki N, Yasui Y, et al. Genetic polymorphisms of IL28B and PNPLA3 are predictive for HCV related rapid fibrosis progression and identify patients who require urgent antiviral treatment with new regimens. PLOS One. 2015;10:e0137351.
37. Lins TC, Vieira RG, Abreu BS, Grattapaglia D, Pereira RW. Genetic composition of Brazilian population samples based on a set of twenty-eight ancestry informative SNPs. Am J Hum Biol. 2010;22:187–92. https://doi.org/10.1002/ajhb.20976.
38. Ferreira LB, Mendes-Junior CT, Wiezel CE, Luizon MR, Simões AL. Genomic ancestry of a sample population from the state of São Paulo, Brazil. Am J Hum Biol. 2006;18:702–5.
39. Probst CM, Bompeixe EP, Pereira NF. de O Dalalio MM, Visentainer JE, Tsuneto LT, et al. HLA polymorphism and evaluation of European, African, and Amerindian contribution to the white and mulatto populations from Paraná, Brazil. Hum Biol. 2000;72:597–617.

8

Glomerular filtration rate change during chronic hepatitis C treatment with Sofosbuvir/Ledipasvir in HCV/HIV Coinfected patients treated with Tenofovir and a boosted protease inhibitor

Cristina Aurora São Pedro Soeiro*, Celina Andreia Melo Gonçalves, Marta Sofia Correia Marques, Maria Josefina Vazquez Méndez, Ana Paula Ribeiro Almeida Tavares, Ana Maria Lacerda Morgado Fernandes de Carvalho de Aboim Horta and Rui Manuel do Rosário Sarmento-Castro

Abstract

Introduction: Concomitant use of ledipasvir and boosted protease inhibitors (PIs) may increase the risk of tenofovir (TDF) nephrotoxicity, since both these drugs increase TDF levels. Our aim was to evaluate glomerular filtration rate (eGFR) evolution during HCV treatment with sofosbuvir/ledipasvir (SOF/LDV) in HCV/HIV coinfected patients, according to their antiretroviral treatment (ARV).

Methods: Observational prospective study of HCV/HIV coinfected patients treated with SOF/LDV. eGFR evolution was evaluated during and 12 weeks after HCV treatment. Patients were categorized in three groups based on ARV regimen: non TDF, non-boosted TDF and TDF + boosted PI.

Results: We included 273 patients: 145 were receiving a non-TDF regimen, 78 a non-boosted TDF scheme and 50 were receiving TDF + boosted PI. We observed a statistically significant decrease in eGFR during treatment in all groups (non TDF $p = 0.03$, 95%CI [0.23–3.86], non-boosted TDF $p < 0.01$, 95%CI [3.36–7.44], TDF + PI $p = 0.01$, 95%CI [1.09–7.53]). The decrease was more pronounced in those receiving unboosted TDF (– 5.40 ml/min/1.73m^2), but differences in eGFR decrease between the three groups were small and not statistically different ($p = 0.06$). eGFR decrease was greater in patients treated for 24 weeks ($p = 0.009$) and in cirrhotic patients ($p = 0.036$). At the end of follow up a recovery of eGFR was observed in all groups.

Conclusion: We observed a significant decrease in eGFR during treatment in all study groups, that was small and reversible after SOF/LDV discontinuation. TDF was not associated with an increase in renal toxicity.

Keywords: Co-infection HIV/HCV, HCV treatment, Sofosbuvir/ledipasvir, Renal toxicity, Tenofovir, Protease inhibitor, Drug-drug interactions

* Correspondence: cristinaaspsoeiro@hotmail.com
Infectious Diseases Department, Centro Hospitalar do Porto, Largo do Prof. Abel Salazar, 4099-001 Porto, Portugal

Background

According to the World Health Organization (WHO), 2–15% of the people infected by the human immunodeficiency virus (HIV) are coinfected with hepatitis C virus (HCV), and this percentage goes up to 90% in those who acquired the infection through intravenous drug use [1]. Liver disease is currently one of the leading causes of morbidity and mortality in HIV infected people [2, 3] and HIV coinfected patients seem to have a faster progression to cirrhosis, a higher rate of liver decompensation and liver death and a lower response to HCV therapy [4–6] . However, HCV treatment has been shown to decrease the risk of negative outcomes even in co-infected patients [7].

With the advent of direct acting antivirals (DAAs), the sustained virologic response (SVR) rates in mono and HIV co-infected patients are similar. With these agents, high cure rates are achieved in the co-infected population, with excellent tolerability and convenient posology [8, 9]. HIV specialists have always been aware of the importance of surveilling and managing drug-drug interactions (DDIs) between antiretroviral medication (ARV) and other co-medication. DDIs are currently one of the problems in the use of DAAs in co-infected patients [8–10]. Clinicians are advised to check possible DDIs between the HCV DAAs and other chronic medication, using up to date resources such as the one found at http://www.hep-druginteractions.org [8].

The association in a single tablet of sofosbuvir (SOF), a nucleotide NS5B polymerase inhibitor, and ledipasvir (LDV), an inhibitor of nonstructural protein 5A (NS5A), is one of the possible treatment options for HCV genotypes 1 and 4, and has shown impressive results in co-infected patients both in clinical trials [11] and in real life cohorts [12]. This combination has few interactions with ARV and can be used with nonnucleoside reverse transcriptase inhibitors (NNRTIs), integrase inhibitors or ritonavir-boosted HIV protease inhibitors (PIs), excluding tipranavir [8, 10].

However, recent studies have raised concerns regarding the interaction between LDV and tenofovir (TDF). Although the mechanism is not completely understood, it is thought that LDV increases TDF levels through the inhibition of P-glycoprotein (P-gp) and breast cancer resistance protein (BCRP) [13]. Moreover, it has been shown that TDF exposure is even greater (30–60%) when SOF/LDV was co-administered with a boosted PI [14]. As administration of TDF with a boosted PI already increases TDF by 20–30%, most authors and guidelines recommend changing ARV or DAA therapy; if, however, this triple combination must be used, renal function should be closely monitored [13, 15–17]. In those with a glomerular filtration rate < 60 mL/min, these drugs should be avoided [13, 15–17].

The aim of our study was to evaluate the effect of the combination SOF/LDV in the eGFR in HCV/HIV patients who were receiving TDF as part of their antiretroviral therapy, and to analyze the added risk of the concomitant use of a boosted PI.

Methods

This was a single center observational prospective study regarding all HCV/HIV patients treated with DAAs in our department. Data on baseline characteristics, co-morbidities, medication and evolution during HCV treatment was collected in a database that was previously approved by the hospital's ethical commission, as well as by the National Data Protection Commission. Informed consent was obtained for all patients.

We analyzed the data of those patients who were treated with SOF/LDV for HCV and who had completed at least 12 weeks of follow up after treatment, from February 2015 to July 2017; patients who did not complete 12 weeks of follow up after treatment were excluded (death or abandonment) as well as patients with incomplete records. Patients were categorized in three groups according to their ARV regimen: (1) non TDF containing regimen (non TDF), (2) TDF without a boosted PI (non-boosted TDF) or (3) TDF with a ritonavir boosted PI (boosted TDF). Evolution of estimated glomerular filtration rate (eGFR) during and after HCV treatment was compared amongst the three groups. eGFR was calculated using the Chronic Kidney Disease Epidemiology Collaboration (CKD-EPI) formula.

Statistical analysis was performed using Statistical Package for the Social Sciences (SPSS®) software, version 23. Paired t- test was used for comparing baseline and end of treatment (EOT) mean eGFR evolution in each group, likelihood ratio was used for categorical variable analysis, ANOVA for analysis of mean difference within the 3 groups and Wilcoxon signed-rank test to evaluate the impact of cirrhosis in the eGFR. P-value < 0.05 was defined as statistically significant.

All patients in our cohort were evaluated for liver fibrosis using transient hepatic elastography (Fibroscan®) and, in some cases, liver biopsy. Patients with an hepatic elastrography value ≥12.5 KPa were considered cirrhotic.

Results

From February 2015 until July 2017, 333 HCV/HIV coinfected patients were treated for chronic HCV infection in our department. Of these, 273 (81.9%) were prescribed the combination SOF/LDV for 12–24 weeks and completed 12 weeks of follow up. We excluded 19 patients from our analysis (three died during HCV treatment, three were lost to follow up and 13 had incomplete records).

All the 273 HCV/HIV patients were receiving antiretroviral medication: 53.1% ($n = 145$) received a non-TDF regimen, 28.6% ($n = 78$) used an unboosted TDF scheme and TDF plus boosted PI was administered in 18.3% ($n = 50$). Efavirenz was the most used third agent in both the non-TDF and unboosted-TDF groups ($n = 50$, 34,5% and $n = 52$, 66,7%, respectively); other drugs less used included rilpivirine ($n = 2$, 1,4% and $n = 6$, 7,7% respectively) and dolutegravir ($n = 10$, 6,9% and $n = 1$, 1,3%, respectively). Regarding the TDF + PI group, the most frequently used boosted PI was darunavir ($n = 27$, 54%), followed by atazanavir ($n = 14$, 28%) and finally lopinavir ($n = 9$, 18%); ritonavir was the booster used in all cases.

The baseline characteristics of the three groups (non-TDF, non-boosted TDF and with TDF + PI) are shown in Table 1. Almost all patients had undetectable HIV RNA ($n = 258$, 94.5%) and the mean CD4 cell count was 650/mm^3 (±338/mm^3).

The mean baseline eGFR was 100.9 ml/min/1.73m^2 (±16.3) in the non TDF group, 104.1 ml/min/1.73m^2 (±11.3) in non-boosted TDF and 98.2 ml/min/1.73m^2 (± 11.8) in the TDF + boosted PI group. In all groups, we observed a decrease in eGFR during treatment, as is shown in Fig. 1.

The decrease of eGFR between the baseline and the end of treatment (EOT) was statistically significant in all groups (non TDF $p = 0.03$, 95%CI [0.23–3.86], non-boosted TDF $p < 0.01$, 95%CI [3.36–7.44], TDF + PI $p = 0.01$, 95%CI [1.09–7.53]). The decrease was more pronounced in those receiving unboosted TDF (mean difference 5.40 ml/min/1.73m^2; 95%CI [(− 7.44) -(− 3.37)]), than in those receiving either TDF + boosted PI (mean difference 4.31 ml/min/1.73m^2; 95%CI [(− 7.53) -(− 1.09)] or non TDF regimens (mean difference 2.02 ml/min/1.73m^2; 95%CI [(− 3.84) -(− 0.02)]). Differences in eGFR decrease between the three groups were small and were not statistically different ($p = 0.06$). (Table 2).

At the end of follow up a recovery of eGFR was observed in all groups (Fig. 1).

The evolution of eGFR was similar between those who were treated for 12 weeks ($n = 188$) to those treated for 24 weeks ($n = 85$). However, there was a steeper decrease in eGFR in those who receiving a longer treatment course: mean change was − 2.1 95%CI [(− 3.43) -(− 7.96)] in those treated for 12 weeks and − 6.3 ml/min/1.73m^2 95%CI [(− 9.08) -(− 3.47)] in those treated for 24 weeks ($p = 0.009$). There was a statistical significant difference in mean eGFR decrease amongst the three ARV groups in those treated for 24 weeks ($p = 0.026$), but not in those who were treated for 12 weeks ($p = 0.89$). Of note, there was a higher proportion of cirrhotic patients in those treated for 24 weeks (81.2% of patients treated for this duration, $n = 69$) than in those treated for 12 weeks (13.3% of patients treated for 12 weeks, $n = 25$).

A separate analysis of the 94 cirrhotic patients included showed a similar evolution. There were no differences amongst the three groups ($p = 0.833$). However, cirrhosis was associated with a decrease in eGFR ($p = 0.036$): mean eGFR decrease for cirrhotic patients was − 5.57 ml/min/1.73m^2 (95%CI [(− 8.16) -(− 2.98)]) vs − 2.28 ml/min/1.73 m^2 (95%CI [(− 3.64) -(− 0.91)] for non-cirrhotic patients.

Table 1 Baseline characteristics of patients according to ARV regimen

Baseline characteristics	Non TDF $n = 145$	Non-boosted TDF $n = 78$	TDF + Boosted PI $n = 50$	p
Male, *n*, (%)	127 (87.6)	67 (85.9)	45 (90.0)	0.78
Mean age ± SD (years)	47 ± 6	47 ± 6	45 ± 6	0.79
Baseline mean creatinine ± SD (mg/dL)	0.84 ± 0.19	0.8 ± 0.13	0.9 ± 0.14	0.05
Baseline mean eGFR ± SD (ml/min/1.73m^2)	100.9 ± 16.3	104.1 ± 11.3	98.2 ± 11.8	0.06
Body mass index ± SD (Kg/m^2)	23.3 ± 3.9	22.3 ± 4.3	22.8 ± 3.8	0.24
Diabetes, *n* (%)	5 (3.4)	4 (5.1)	1 (2.0)	0.63
Hypertension, *n* (%)	21 (14.5)	10 (12.8)	4 (8.0)	0.47
Median CD4$^+$ cell count ± IQ (/mm^3)	618 (457–868)	611 (443–762)	506 (279–807)	0.12
VL HIV < 20 cp/mL, *n* (%)	138 (95.2)	76 (97.4)	44 (88)	0.09
Median stiffness ± IQ (kPa)	9.4 (6.4–15.4)	9.5 (6.9–12.3)	10.5 (7.4–18.2)	0.74
Cirrhosis, *n* (%)	53 (36.6)	19 (24.4)	22 (44.0)	0.051
Median MELD ± IQ	7 (6–8)	7 (6–7)	7 (7–9)	0.07
Child-Pugh A, *n* (%)	33 (62.2)	8 (42.1)	9 (40.9)	0.10
SOF/LDV 24 weeks, *n* (%)	42 (27.2)	24 (30.0)	19 (38.0)	0.50
Ribavirin use, *n* (%)	28 (18.4)	14 (17.5)	9 (18.0)	0.96

TDF tenofovir, *PI* protease inhibitor, *Non TDF* regimens without TDF, *Non-boosted TDF* regimens with TDF without boosted PI, *TDF* Boosted PI – regimens with TDF and boosted PI, *SD* standard deviation, *IQ* interquartile range, *VL* viral load, *MELD* Model for End-Stage Liver Disease score, *SOF* sofosbuvir, *LDV* ledipasvir

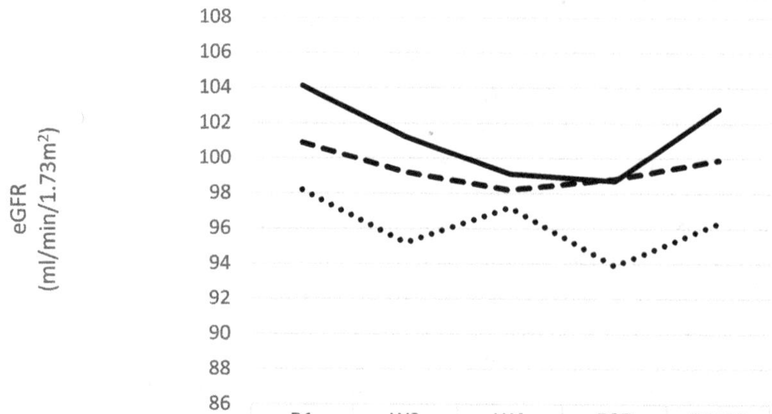

	D1	W2	W4	EOT	SVR12
Non TDF (n=145)	100.9	99.2	98.2	98.8	99.9
Non-Boosted TDF (n=78)	104.1	101.2	99.1	98.7	102.8
TDF + Boosted PI (n=50)	98.2	95.2	97.2	93.9	96.3

Fig. 1 Evolution of the eGFR during treatment and at SVR12 according to ARV regimen. (eGFR – estimated glomerular filtration rate; D1 – day 1, beginning of treatment; W2 – week 2 of treatment; W4 – week 4 of treatment; EOT – end of treatment; SVR12 – end of follow up; TDF – tenofovir; PI – protease inhibitor; Non TDF – regimens without TDF; Non-boosted TDF – regimens with TDF without boosted PI; TDF + Boosted PI – regimens with TDF and boosted PI)

There were six patients whose eGFR decreased to less than 60 ml/min/1.73m^2 during HCV treatment, but, except for one patient in the non-TDF group, these decreases were transient and were not sustained in the following assessments. The evolution of these patients is shown in Table 3.

No patient needed to interrupt HCV treatment due to renal dysfunction and no patient changed ARV during HCV treatment. The SVR12 was 98.6, 98.7 and 100% for the non-TDF, the unboosted TDF and boosted TDF group, respectively.

Discussion

The SOF/LDV combination pill is an option for the treatment of HCV genotypes 1 and 4, due to its simple posology, good tolerability and few DDIs. However, international guidelines recommend caution (and frequent renal monitoring) when using these drugs in HIV coinfected patients receiving TDF and a booster (either ritonavir or cobicistat) as part of their ARV regimen due to the increased risk of TDF exposure and renal toxicity [15, 16].

In our cohort of SOF/LDV treated HCV/HIV co-infected patients, receiving multiple of ARV therapeutic schemes which included regimens without TDF, with TDF and TDF combined with a ritonavir boosted PI, we observed a significant decrease in eGFR during treatment in all study groups. The eGFR decrease was more pronounced in those patients receiving TDF in comparison with patients receiving either TDF with a boosted PI or non-TDF containing regimens, but the changes were small in all groups and had little clinical impact. Moreover, we found no statistical differences amongst the three groups regarding comorbidities. We found no explanation for the grater decrease in eGFR in the unboosted TDF group. Treatment duration had an impact in eGFR decrease, with longer treatment courses being associated with greater eGFR decrease. However, the proportion of cirrhotic patients was much higher in the group of patients treated for 24 weeks (81.2%) and cirrhosis was also associated with a decrease in eGFR ($p = 0.036$).

Despite this overall decrease, after treatment completion eGFR returned to almost baseline values in all

Table 2 Global Mean eGFR decrease between the baseline and end-of-treatment

Global Mean eGFR Decrease between the baseline and EOT		p	Confidence Interval
Non TDF $n = 152$	5.40 ml/min/1.73m^2	0.03	95%CI [(−7.44) -(−3.37)]
Non-boosted TDF $n = 80$	4.31 ml/min/1.73m^2	< 0.01	95%CI [(−7.53) -(− 1.09)]
TDF + Boosted PI $n = 50$	2.02 ml/min/1.73m^2	0.01	95%CI [(− 3.84) -(− 0.02)]

TDF tenofovir, *PI* protease inhibitor, *Non TDF* regimens without TDF, *Non-boosted TDF* regimens with TDF without boosted PI, *TDF* Boosted PI – regimens with TDF and boosted PI, *EOT* end of treatment

Table 3 Evolution of the eGFR in patients with eGFR below 60 ml/min/1.73m^2 during treatment

	Group	Gender, Age	Cirrhosis	HCV Treatment Duration	eGFR at baseline (ml/min/m^2)	eGFR at W4 (ml/min/m^2)	eGFR at EOT (ml/min/m^2)	eGFR at SVR12 (ml/min/m^2)
1	Non-TDF	Male, 66 yo	Yes	12w	59	45.3	56.9	63.9
2	Non-TDF	Male, 48 yo	Yes	24w	60	62.8	54.3	57.5
3	Non-TDF	Male, 49 yo	Yes	24w	65.9	57.1	37.8	32
4	Non-TDF	Male, 55 yo	Yes	12w	67.7	62	59.8	57.7
5	Non-boosted TDF	Male, 55 yo	Yes	24w	72.8	57.7	60.9	71.2
6	TDF+ Boosted PI	Male, 45 yo	Yes	24w	80.6	64.1	57.7	83.4

eGFR estimated glomerular filtration rate, *W2* week 2 of treatment, *W4*, week 4 of treatment, *EOT* end of treatment, *SVR12* end of follow up, *TDF* tenofovir, *PI* protease inhibitor, *Non-TDF* regimens without TDF, *Non-boosted TDF* regimens with TDF without boosted PI, *TDF* Boosted PI – regimens with TDF and boosted PI, *yo* years old, *w* week

groups. We observed the same occurrence in those who had a longer course of treatment and in cirrhotic patients. No patient needed to interrupt HCV treatment due to renal dysfunction and there were no ARV alterations; the SVR12 was above 98% in all groups.

Our results are consistent with the already published literature. Bhattacharya and colleagues analysed a cohort of 996 HCV genotype 1 and HIV co-infected patients, of which 895 were treated with SOF/LDV ± RBV; these authors did not find any difference in creatinine change during SOF/LDV treatment in those receiving either TDF containing ARV schemes (with or without PI) or those not receiving TDF [18]. Moreover, in line with our results, the median creatinine change was small (0.15 mg/dL in those without TDF, 0.18 mg/dL with TDF and 0.17 mg/dL in those with TDF + PI) and not different between the three groups ($p = 0.30$) [18].

Taramasso et al. evaluated the renal tolerability of the SOF/LDV in patients participating in the SCOLTA project (Surveillance Cohort Long-Term Toxicity Antiretrovirals), which included 79 HCV/HIV co-infected patients: 47 taking TDF, 34 a ritonavir boosted PI and 17 TDF + boosted PI [19]. The authors found no statistically significant variation of eGFR in patients receiving a boosted PI either in combination with TDF or not [19]. Moreover, they observed that patients receiving unboosted TDF experienced the highest percentage of filtration loss (– 5.3 mL/min (SD 15.8)) and that the frequency of eGFR loss > 5% was more frequent in this group but similarly to our results, there was no difference between those who took a boosted PI and those who did not [19].

Despite these reassuring results, Bunnell and colleagues published a case of acute tubular necrosis and acute interstitial nephritis in a HCV/HIV co-infected patient taking efavirenz/tenofovir/emtricitabine and receiving HCV treatment with SOF/LDV, that resolved after discontinuation of TDF and SOF/LDV [20]. Of note, the patient was also taking other medications that could contribute to renal injury [20].

The main limitations of our study are its observational nature and the lack of analysis of other parameters of renal lesion, namely urine analysis, proteinuria, albuminuria, as well as serum and urinary measurements of calcium and phosphate. Moreover, we did not evaluate the impact of other possible causes of nephrotoxicity. Additionally, data regarding HIV and HCV history is lacking, due to the lack of informatic records in our hospital.

The ongoing clinical trial NCT02588287 (Effects of Sofosbuvir/Ledipasvir Treatment on the Pharmacokinetics and Renal Safety of Tenofovir), promoted by the University of Colorado, is likely to shed some more light on the safety of this combination [21].

Conclusion

We observed a decrease in the mean GFR in all patients treated with SOF/LDV. This decrease was higher in those receiving TDF, but the differences amongst the three groups were small and not statistically significant. Moreover, the eGFR decrease seems to be reversible after termination of HCV treatment. Our data, along with that of other authors [18, 19], reassures clinicians on the safety of SOF/LDV in combination with TDF containing regimens, regardless of the concomitant use of a boosted PI. However, from the authors point of view and as recommended in guidelines, if TDF is used in patients who are receiving SOF/LDV, signs of nephrotoxicity should be carefully monitored [15, 16], especially in cirrhotic patients.

Abbreviations

ARV: Antiretroviral medication; DAA: Direct acting antiviral; DDIs: Drug-drug interactions; eGFR: estimated Glomerular filtration rate; EOT: End of treatment; HCV: Hepatitis C virus; HIV: Human immunodeficiency virus; LDV: Ledipasvir; NNRTI: Nonnucleoside reverse transcriptase inhibitor; PI: Protease inhibitor; SOF: Sofosbuvir; SVR: Sustained virologic response; TDF: Tenofovir; WHO: World Health Organization

Acknowledgements

The authors thank Dr. J. Seabra, Dr. O. Vasconcelos, Dr. M. Abreu, Dr. M. Gonçalves and Enf. M. Santos.

Authors' contributions

CS – Manuscript writing and preparation, data collection, data analysis and interpretation. CG – Manuscript writing and preparation, data collection, data analysis and interpretation. MM - Data collection and analysis. JM – Manuscript preparation, data analysis and interpretation. APT - Data collection and analysis. AH - Data collection and analysis. RSC - Manuscript preparation, data analysis and interpretation. All authors have read and approved the manuscript.

Consent for publication

All authors agreed with the final manuscript and consented publication. Participants consented publication.

Competing interests

The authors declare that they have no competing interests.

References

1. World Health Organization. http://www.who.int/hiv/topics/hepatitis. Accessed July 2017.
2. Smith CJ, Ryom L, Weber R, Morlat P, Pradier C, Reiss P, et al. Trends in underlying causes of death in people with HIV from 1999 to 2011 (D:a:D): a multicohort collaboration. Lancet. 2014;384:241–8.
3. Weber R, Ruppik M, Rickenbach M, Spoerri A, Furrer H, Battegay M, et al. Decreasing mortality and changing patterns of causes of death in the Swiss HIV cohort study. HIV Med. 2013;14:195–207.
4. Re LR, Kallan MJ, Tate JP, Localio AR, Lim JK, Goetz MB, et al. Hepatic decompensation in antiretroviral-treated HIV/hepatitis C-Coinfected compared to hepatitis C-Monoinfected patients: a cohort study. Ann Intern Med. 2014;160(6):369–7.9.
5. Graham CS, Baden LR, Yu E, Mrus JM, Carnie J, Heeren T, et al. Influence of human immunodeficiency virus infection on the course of hepatitis C virus infection: a meta-analysis. Clin Infect Dis. 2001;33(4):562–9.
6. Chen JY, Feeney ER, Chung RT. HCV and HIV co-infection: mechanisms and management. Nat Rev Gastroenterol Hepatol. 2014;11:362–71.
7. Mira JA, Rivero-Juárez A, López-Cortés LF, Girón-González JA, Téllez F, de los Santos-Gil I, et al. Benefits from sustained virologic response to pegylated interferon plus ribavirin in HIV/hepatitis C virus-coinfected patients with compensated cirrhosis. Clin Infect Dis. 2013;56:1646–53.
8. Arends JE, Lieveld FI, Boeijen LL, Kanter CTMM, Erpecum KJ, Salmon D, et al. Natural history and treatment of HCV/HIV coinfection: is it time to change paradigms? J Hepatol. 2015;63:1254–62.
9. Cachay E, Soriano V. Is HIV still a special population for the treatment of hepatitis C? AIDS. 2016;30(12):2001–3.
10. Langness J, Larson B, Bayer J, Rogers M, Kiser J. Readying HIV/HCV coinfected patients for HCV treatment: occurrence and management of antiviral interactions. In: 16th International Workshop on Clinical Pharmacology of HIV and Hepatitis Therapy. 2015, Washington. Abstract 18. http://regist2.virology-education.com/2015/16HIVHEP/34_Langness.pdf. Accessed Dec 2016.
11. Naggie S, Cooper C, Saag M, Workowski K, Ruane P, Towner WJ, et al. Ledipasvir and Sofosbuvir for HCV in patients Coinfected with HIV-1. N Engl J Med. 2015;373:705–13.
12. Butt AA, Yan P, Shaikh OS, Chung RT, Sherman KE. Sofosbuvir-based regimens in clinical practice achieve SVR rates closer to clinical trials: results from ERCHIVES. Liver Intent. 2016;36:651–8.
13. El-Sherif O, Khoo S, Solas C. Key drug-drug interactions with direct-acting antiviral in HIV-HCV coinfection. Curr Opin HIV AIDS. 2015;10:348–54.
14. German P, Garrison K, Pang PS, Stamm LM, Ray AS, Shen G, et al. Drug-Drug Interactions Between Anti-HCV Regimen Ledipasvir/Sofosbuvir and Antiretrovirals. In: Conference on Retroviruses and Opportunistic Infections. 2015, Seattle. Abstract 82. http://www.croiconference.org/sessions/drug-drug-interactions-between-anti-hcv-regimen-ledipasvirsofosbuvir-and-antiretrovirals. Accessed Dec 2016.
15. European Association for the Study of the Liver. EASL recommendations on treatment of hepatitis C 2016. J Hepatol. 2017;66:153–94.
16. AASLD/IDSA HCV Guidance Panel. AASLD-IDSA recommendations for testing, managing, and treating adults infected with hepatitis C virus. http://www.hcvguidelines.org. Accessed July 2017.
17. Kaur K, Gandhi MA, Slish J. Drug-Drug Interactions Among Hepatitis C Virus (HCV) and Human Immunodeficiency Virus (HIV) Medications. Infect Dis Ther. 2015;4:159–72.
18. Bhattacharya D, Belperio PS, Shahoumian TA, Loomis TP, Goetz MB, Mole LA, et al. Effectiveness of All-Oral Antiviral Regimens in 996 Human Immunodeficiency Virus/Hepatitis C Virus Genotype 1-Coinfected Patients Treated in Routine Practice. Clin Infect Dis. 2017;64(12):1711–20.
19. Taramasso L, Ricci E, Celesia BM, Bonfanti P, Quirino T, Squillace N, et al. Co-administration of tenofovir plus protease inhibitor based antiretroviral therapy during sofosbuvir/ledipasvir treatment for HCV infection: much ado about nothing? Clin Res Hepatol Gastroenterol. 2017;S2210-7401(17):30085–2.
20. Bunnell KL, Vibhakar S, Glowacki RC, Gallagher MA, Osei AM, Huhn G. Nephrotoxicity associated with concomitant use of Ledipasvir-Sofosbuvir and Tenofovir in a patient with hepatitis C virus and human immunodeficiency virus coinfection. Pharmacotherapy. 2016;36(9):e148–53.
21. ClinicalTrials.gov. Effects of Sofosbuvir/Ledipasvir Treatment on the Pharmacokinetics and Renal Safety of Tenofovir. https://clinicaltrials.gov/ct2/show/NCT02588287. Accessed July 2017.

9

Diagnostic accuracy of tests to detect Hepatitis C antibody

Weiming Tang[1,2,3,4†], Wen Chen[5,6†], Ali Amini[7], Debi Boeras[7], Jane Falconer[7], Helen Kelly[7], Rosanna Peeling[7], Olivia Varsaneux[7], Joseph D. Tucker[1,3,4,7*] and Philippa Easterbrook[8]

Abstract

Background: Although direct-acting antivirals can achieve sustained virological response rates greater than 90% in Hepatitis C Virus (HCV) infected persons, at present the majority of HCV-infected individuals remain undiagnosed and therefore untreated. While there are a wide range of HCV serological tests available, there is a lack of formal assessment of their diagnostic performance. We undertook a systematic review and meta-analysis to evaluate he diagnostic accuracy of available rapid diagnostic tests (RDT) and laboratory based EIA assays in detecting antibodies to HCV.

Methods: We used the PRISMA checklist and Cochrane guidance to develop our search protocol. The search strategy was registered in PROSPERO (CRD42015023567). The search focused on hepatitis C, diagnostic tests, and diagnostic accuracy within eight databases (MEDLINE, EMBASE, the Cochrane Central Register of Controlled Trials, Science Citation Index Expanded, Conference Proceedings Citation Index-Science, SCOPUS, Literatura Latino-Americana e do Caribe em Ciências da Saúde and WHO Global Index Medicus. Studies were included if they evaluated an assay to determine the sensitivity and specificity of HCV antibody (HCV Ab) in humans. Two reviewers independently extracted data and performed a quality assessment of the studies using the QUADAS tool. We pooled test estimates using the DerSimonian-Laird method, by using the software R and RevMan. 5.3.

Results: A total of 52 studies were identified that included 52,673 unique test measurements. Based on five studies, the pooled sensitivity and specificity of HCV Ab rapid diagnostic tests (RDTs) were 98% (95% CI 98-100%) and 100% (95% CI 100-100%) compared to an enzyme immunoassay (EIA) reference standard. High HCV Ab RDTs sensitivity and specificity were observed across screening populations (general population, high risk populations, and hospital patients) using different reference standards (EIA, nucleic acid testing, immunoblot). There were insufficient studies to undertake subanalyses based on HIV co-infection. Oral HCV Ab RDTs also had excellent sensitivity and specificity compared to blood reference tests, respectively at 94% (95% CI 93-96%) and 100% (95% CI 100-100%). Among studies that assessed individual oral RDTs, the eight studies revealed that OraQuick ADVANCE® had a slightly higher sensitivity (98%, 95% CI 97-98%) compared to the other oral brands (pooled sensitivity: 88%, 95% CI 84-92%).

Conclusions: RDTs, including oral tests, have excellent sensitivity and specificity compared to laboratory-based methods for HCV antibody detection across a wide range of settings. Oral HCV Ab RDTs had good sensitivity and specificity compared to blood reference standards.

Keywords: Diagnostic accuracy, Diagnostic tests, Hepatitis C, HCV antibody, Rapid diagnostic tests

* Correspondence: jdtucker@med.unc.edu
†Equal contributors
[1]University of North Carolina Project-China, No. 2 Lujing Road, Guangzhou 510095, China
[3]SESH Global, Guangzhou, China
Full list of author information is available at the end of the article

Background

Hepatitis C is a liver disease caused by the hepatitis C virus (HCV) that causes acute and chronic infection [1, 2]. An estimated 71 million people had chronic hepatitis C infection worldwide in 2015 [3]. Viral hepatitis caused 1.34 million deaths in 2015, a number comparable to deaths caused by tuberculosis and higher than those caused by HIV [3]. The introduction of direct-acting antivirals (DAAs) has led to a sustained virological response (SVR) in greater than 90% of treated individuals [4, 5]. DAAs are now recommended by the World Health Organization (WHO) [1] and many other HCV treatment guidelines [1]. DAAs will not only improve SVR rates but also may simplify HCV management algorithms and allow smaller health facilities to manage HCV-infected individuals [6]. Despite the availability of effective treatment, most HCV-infected individuals remain undiagnosed and untreated [7]. Left untreated, approximately 15–30% of individuals with chronic HCV infection progress to cirrhosis, leading to end-stage liver disease and hepatocellular carcinoma [1, 2].

In February 2016 the WHO updated the guidelines for the screening, care, and treatment of persons with chronic hepatitis C infection [1]. These guidelines included recommendations on whom to screen for HCV and how to confirm HCV infection, but not which tests are optimal for initial screening. Advances in HCV detection technology create new opportunities for enhancing screening, referral, and treatment. Previous systematic reviews on HCV infection have focused on treatment response [8, 9], clinical complications [10], and epidemiology [11, 12]. Two previous systematic reviews on hepatitis C testing have focused on evaluating point-of-care tests compared to EIAs and other reference tests [13, 14]. We have undertaken a further systematic review and meta-analysis to generate pooled sensitivity and specificity of rapid diagnostic tests used to detect HCV antibody (HCV Ab), and to inform the development of recommendations on serological testing in the 2017 WHO testing guidelines [15].

Methods

Research question

The main purpose of the review was to assess the diagnostic accuracy of available assays for detecting HCV Ab in persons identified for hepatitis C testing. The research question was structured in a PICO format (ie. population, intervention, comparisons and outcome).

P: Persons identified for HCV testing; I: Rapid diagnostic tests and enzyme immunoassays for HCV Ab detection; C: 1), EIA (with a subanalysis based on the last 10 years); 2), NAT (nucleic acid testing); 3), Immunoblot or similar assay; 4), A combination of 1,2,3 above; O: Diagnostic accuracy [Sensitivity (SE), Specificity (SP), Positive predictive value (PPV), Negative predictive value (NPV), True Negative, True Positive (TP), False negative (FN), and False positive (FP)].

Search strategy and identification of studies

Search strategies were developed by a medical librarian with expertise in designing systematic review searches. Our search algorithm consisted of the following components: hepatitis C, diagnostic tests, and diagnostic accuracy. We searched MEDLINE (OVID interface, 1946 onwards), EMBASE (OVID interface, 1947 onwards), the Cochrane Central Register of Controlled Trials (Wiley interface, current issue), Science Citation Index Expanded (Web of Science interface, 1970 onwards), Conference Proceedings Citation Index-Science (Web of Science interface, 1990 onwards), SCOPUS (1960 onwards), Literatura Latino-Americana e do Caribe em Ciências da Saúde (LILACS) (BIREME interface) and WHO Global Index Medicus. The search was supplemented by searching for ongoing studies in WHO's International Clinical Trials Registry. The literature search was limited to English language and human subjects that available until April 30th, 2015. In addition to searching databases, we contacted individual researchers and authors of major trials to address whether any relevant manuscripts are in preparation or in press. The references of published articles found in the above databases were searched for additional pertinent materials.

Study selection proceeded in three stages: 1) titles/abstracts were screened by a single reviewer according to standard inclusion and exclusion criteria; 2) full manuscripts were obtained and evaluated by two independent reviewers to include or not; 3) two independent reviewers extracted all data. Differences were resolved by a third independent reviewer.

Selection criteria

The inclusion criteria included the following: primary purpose was HCV Ab test evaluation, reported sensitivity and specificity of HCV Ab test kits, and studies published before May 2015. We included observational and randomised control trial (RCT) studies that provided original data from patient specimens. Studies that only reported sensitivity or specificity, conference abstracts, comments or review papers, panel studies, or those that only used reference assays for positive samples were excluded. In this manuscript, a hepatitis panel refers to a laboratory series test in which use the blood with confirmed hepatitis C serostatus to assess the accuracy of a testing kit.

Data extraction

Information on the following variables were extracted from each individual study: first author, total sample size, country (and city) of sampling, sample type (oral fluid, finger prick, venous blood), point-of-care (POC, defined as being able to give a result within 60 min and having the results to guide clinical management in the same encounter), eligibility criteria, reference standard, manufacturer, raw cell numbers (true positives, false negatives, false positives, true negatives), antibody-antigen combo (yes or no), sources of funding, reported conflict of interest, and study population (general population, high risk population and hospitalized population). The high risk population groups include men who have sex with men, sex workers and their clients, transgender people, people who inject drugs and prisoners and other incarcerated people [16]. The hospitalized population was defined as those admitted to a hospital for medical care or observation. We also verified whether assays evaluated in the studies were currently on the market (as of June 1st, 2017), and if this was the case, we also reported the available version of the testing kit (Table 1).

Assessment of methodological quality

Study quality was evaluated using the QUADAS-2 tool [17] and the STARD checklist [18]. QUADAS includes domains to evaluate bias in the following categories: risk of bias (patient selection, index test, reference standard, flow, and timing); applicability concerns (patient selection, index test, reference standard). The STARD checklist consists of a checklist of 25 items and flow diagram that authors can use to ensure that all relevant information is present.

Data analysis and synthesis

Data synthesis

Data were extracted to construct 2 × 2 tables. By comparing with reference standard results, the index test results were categorized as a true positive, a false positive, a false negative, or a true negative. Indeterminate test results were not included in pooled analyses.

Statistical analysis

To estimate test accuracy, we calculated sensitivity and specificity for each study and pooled statistics, along with 95% confidence intervals [19]. We pooled test estimates using the DerSimonian-Laird method, a bivariate random effect model. We did further subanalyses based on reference standard (EIA alone; NAT or immunoblot; EIA, NAT, or immunoblot), brand, sample type, and combination test. We performed all statistical analysis (including heterogeneity, through Q test) using the software R and RevMan 5.3.

Results

Study selection

A total of 11,163 citations were identified, and 6163 duplicates were removed. Each of the 5000 unique citations was examined. A total of 52 research studies were included in the final analysis (Fig. 1) [8, 16, 19–68]. Of the 52 studies, 32 studies evaluated the accuracy of 30 different rapid diagnostic tests (RDTs) [19–50], of which 5 evaluated RDTs compared to EIA alone [25, 26, 31, 34, 49], 13 compared RDT results to NAT or immunoblot [19–22, 27, 29, 32, 37, 42, 43, 45, 47, 50], and 14 focused on evaluating RDT by comparing with the results of EIA or immunoblot or NAT [23–26, 30, 34, 35, 38, 39, 41, 44, 48, 49, 51]. Eleven studies evaluated the diagnostic accuracy of oral fluid RDTs [22, 24, 27, 29, 33, 34, 43–45, 47, 52].

There were insufficient data to undertake a subanalysis based on HIV co-infection or other co-infections.

Study characteristics

Of the 52 included studies, nine were published before 2000 [37, 38, 42, 53–58], 12 studies reported evaluation using oral fluid samples, and 34 studies evaluated POC tests. Of the 52 studies, 41 different brands of testing kits were evaluated (Table 1).

Assessment of the quality of the studies

All studies used a cross-sectional or case–control design. The risk of bias in patient selection, index test, or reference standard was assessed using QUADAS-2 (Table 2). Among the included studies, 25 had at least one category that was considered high risk [19, 22, 25–28, 30, 31, 34, 36–39, 41, 45–50, 53, 55, 56, 58–62]. The risk of bias in patient selection usually came from a poor description of patient selection and clinical scenario. Bias in the index test was primarily due to a lack of reported blinding while reading test results. Bias in the reference standard was due to the use of multiple reference standards (EIA, NAT, and/or immunoblot). Bias in the flow and timing was primarily due to a lack of reported details.

Diagnostic accuracy

Overall clinical performance of assays

The 52 included studies contributed 127 data points from 52,273 unique test measurements. Some studies contributed additional data points by comparing the accuracy of two or more tests, reporting data from multiple study sites, or reporting the accuracy of a test in more than one type of specimen. The sample sizes of the included studies ranged from 37 to 17,894. Sensitivities of included studies ranged from 22 to 100%, and specificities ranged from 77 to 100%. The overall pooled sensitivity and specificity for all tests were 97% (95% CI: 97%–98%) and 99% (95% CI: 98%-99%) respectively. Figure 2 shows estimates of sensitivity and specificity from each study.

Manufacturers and accuracy of RDTs among included studies

Overall, 32 studies evaluated the accuracy of 30 different RDTs (Table 3). The most commonly evaluated test kit was the OraQuick ADVANCE® from OraSure Technologies.

Table 1 Characteristics of studies focused on evaluating diagnostic accuracy of HCV antibody tests

First author	Year	Settings	Sample type	Manufacturer	Study type	Sample size	POC (Y/N)	Reference standard	Still on the market? PRODUCT NAME
Al-Tahish et al.	2013	Egypt	Venous blood	HCV one step test device (ACON Laboratories, USA), Fourth- generation HCV TRI_DOT (J. Mitra Co, India) and ImmunoComb II HCV (Inverness Medical Innovations, USA)	CS	100	Y	PCR	Yes Foresight® HCV EIA test kit; Yes, HCV TRI_DOT
Bonacini et al.	2001	USA	Venous blood	Ortho Clinical Diagnostics (Raritan, NJ, USA)	CS	222	N	Chiron IMMUNOBLOT HCV 3.0 SIA	Not available
Buti et al.	2000	Sprain	Serum	Not available	CS	188	Y	IMMUNOBLOT	Not avaliable
Caudai et al.	1998	USA	Serum or plasma samples	ELISA 2nd generation Abbott Laboratories, Abbott park, IL, USA)	CS	682	N	PCR	Not avaliable
Cha et al.	2013	Korea	Oral fluids and serum	OraQuick (OraSure Technologies, PA USA)	CC	437	Y	PCR	Yes, The OraQuick® HCV
Croom et al.	2006	Austria	Venous blood	Monolisa anti-HCV PLUSVersion 2 EIA (Bio-Rad, France)	CS	182	N	EIA	Yes, MONOLISA™ Anti-HCV PLUS Assay Version 2
da Rosa et al.	2013	Brazil	Serum	Rapid Test Bioeasy® (Standard Diagnostics, Yongin, Korea) and Imuno-Rapido HCV® (Wama Diagnostica, Brazil).	CS	307	Y	Architect HCV, PCR	Not available for Rapid Test Bioeasy; Yes, Imuno-Rapido HCV
Daniel et al.	2005	India	Serum	TRI DOT (J. MITRA &Co. Ltd., New Delhi, India)	CS	2590	Y	EIA, IMMUNOBLOT, PCR	YES, HCV TRI_DOT
Denoyel et al.	2004	France and Germany	Serum or plasma samples	AxSYM HCV 3.0 (other information is not available)	CS	5700	N	IMMUNOBLOT	Yes, AXSYM HCV 3.0
Dokubo et al.	2014	USA	Blood	HCV Version 3.0 ELISA (Ortho®)	CS	132	N	PCR	Yes, ORTHO® HCV 3.0 Elisa
Drobnik et al.	2011	USA	Oral fluid	OraQuick (OraSure Technologies, PA USA)	CS	484	Y	EIA, IMMUNOBLOT	Yes, The OraQuick® HCV
Eroglu et al.	2000	Turkey	Plasma specimens	ELISA v3.0(Ortho®)	CS	160	N	PCR	Yes, ORTHO® HCV 3.0 Elisa
Feucht et al.	1995	Germany	Plasma specimens	Abbott HCV second-generation enzyme immunoassay (other information is not available)	CS	262	N	IMMUNOBLOT	Not avaliable
Gao et al.	2014	USA	Serum	OraQuick (OraSure Technologies, PA USA)	CS	289	Y	EIA	Yes, The OraQuick® HCV
Hess et al.	2014	USA	whole blood	DPP HIV-HCV-Syphilis Assay (Chembio Diagnostic Systems, Inc., Medford, NY)	CS	948	Y	EIA	Not avaliable
Hui et al.	2002	Hong kong, China	Whole blood	OraQuick (OraSure Technologies, PA USA)	CS	197	Y	EIA	Yes, The OraQuick® HCV
Ibrahim et al.	2015	Saudi Arabia	Oral fluid	OraQuick (OraSure Technologies, PA USA)	CC	160	Y	PCR	Yes, The OraQuick® HCV
Ivantes et al.	2010	Brazil	Whole blood	HCV Rapid Test Bioeasy (Bioeasy Diagnostica Ltda, Minas Gerais, Brazil)	CS	71	Y	CLIA	Not available

Table 1 Characteristics of studies focused on evaluating diagnostic accuracy of HCV antibody tests *(Continued)*

First author	Year	Settings	Sample type	Manufacturer	Study type	Sample size	POC (Y/N)	Reference standard	Still on the market? PRODUCT NAME
Jewett et al.	2012	USA	Oral fluids	Chembio DPP HCV test (Chembio Diagnostic Systems,USA) and Rapid HIV/HCV antibody test (Medmira Laboratories, Canada)	CS	407	Y	IMMUNOBLOT/NAT	Not available for Chembio DPP HCV test; Yes, Multiplo HBc/HIV/HCV
Kant et al.	2012	Germany	Whole blood	Toyo anti-HCV test (Turklab, Izmir, Turkey)	CS	185	Y	Architect HCV	Yes, anti-HCV TEST
Kaur et al.	2000	India	Serum	HCV Bidot (J. Mitra Co., India)	CS	2754	Y	EIA 3rd generation	YES, DIAGNOS HCV BI-DOT
Kim et al.	2013	Republic of Korea	Serum	GENEDIA® HCV Rapid LF (Green Cross medical science corp., Korea)	CC	200	Y	IMMUNOBLOT	Yes, GENEDIA HCV Rapid LF test kit
Kosack et al.	2014	Germany	Serum	The ImmunoFlow HCV test (Core Diagnostics,United Kingdom)	CS	81	Y	IMMUNOBLOT	Yes, ImmunoFlow HCV
Lakshmi et al.	2007	India	Blood	Beijing United Biomedical, Ortho Clinical Diagnostics, General Biologicals; other information is not avaliable	CS	69	N	PCR	Not avaliable
Larrat et al.	2012	France	FSB (fingerstick blood) and oral fluid	cEIA: the Monolisa® HCV-Ag-Ab-ULTRA (Bio-Rad, Marnes-la-Coquette, France)	CC	201	Y	PCR	Yes, MONOLISA™ HCV Ag-Ab ULTRA
Lee et al.	2010	USA	Oral fluid	OraQuick (OraSure Technologies, PA USA)	CS	572	Y	EIA, IMMUNOBLOT	Yes, The OraQuick® HCV
Lee et al.	2011	USA	Serum, plasma, venous blood, figerstick blood and oral fluid	Or Quick (OraSure Technologies, PA USA)	CS	2183	Y	EIA, IMMUNOBLOT, PCR	Yes, The OraQuick® HCV
Lee et al.	2011	USA	Oral fluid	OraQuick (OraSure Technologies, PA USA)	CS	2180, 2178	Y	EIA	Yes, The OraQuick® HCV
Maity et al.	2012	India	Serum	J Mitra & Co. Pvt. Ltd., SPAN Diagnostics Ltd. and Standard Diagnostics, INC, other information is not available	CC	100	Y	EIA	Not avaliable
Montebugnoil et al.	1999	Italy	whole blood	Anti-HCV Ab rapid test (1st IRP 75/537 by Thema Ricerca, WHO Geneva)	CC	100	Y	EIA, IMMUNOBLOT	Not avaliable
Mvere et al.	1996	Zimbabwe	Serum	HCV-SPOT (Genelabs Diagnostics, Singapore)	CS	206	Y	EIA 2nd generation, INNO-LIA HCV ab III	Not avaliable
Nalpas et al.	1992	France	Serum	Ortho Diagnostics, other information is not available	CS	62	N	PCR	Not avaliable
Njouom et al.	2006	Cameroon	Plasma	ImmunoComb® II HCV assay (Orgenics Ltd.,);	CS	329	Y	EIA 3rd generation, PCR	Not avaliable

Table 1 Characteristics of studies focused on evaluating diagnostic accuracy of HCV antibody tests *(Continued)*

First author	Year	Settings	Sample type	Manufacturer	Study type	Sample size	POC (Y/N)	Reference standard	Still on the market? PRODUCT NAME
				ImmunoComb® II HCV assay (Orgenics Ltd., Not reported manufacturer located country)					
Nyirenda et al.	2008	Malawi	Serum	Monoelisa HCV Ag/Ab ultra-microplate EIA (Bio-Rad, France)	CS	202	Y	EIA	Yes, MONOLISA™ HCV Ag-Ab ULTRA
O'Connell et al.	2013	USA	Plasma, whole blood (normal) and whole blood (cold storge)	OraQuick (OraSure Technologies, PA USA); CORE (CORE Diagnostics, United Kingdom); Axiom (Axiom Diagnostics, Burstadt,Germany); FirstVue (AT First Diagnostic, Woodbury,NY, USA) and Instant View Cassette (Alfa Scientific Designs, Poway)	CC	674, 168	Y	EIA, IMMUNOBLOT, and when available viral load)	Yes, The OraQuick® HCV; Yes, Core HCV; Not avaliable for Axiom; Yes, FirstVue™ Hepatitis "C" Rapid Test; Yes, Instant-view™ Hepatitis C Virus (HCV) Serum Test
O'Flynn et al.	1997	Ireland, Germany, UK	Plasma and serum	AxSYM (Abbott Laboratories, other information is not available)	CC	5554, 1421, 643	N	ABBOTT MATRIX HCV, Chiron IMMUNOBLOT HCV 2.0 or 3.0	Yes, AXSYM HCV 3.0
Park et al.	2012	Korea	Serum	Vitros anti-HCV assay kits (Ortho-Clinical Diagnostics, Bucking-hamshire, UK) and Elecsys (Roche Diag-nostics GmbHMann-heim, Germany)	CS	1008	N	IMMUNOBLOT HCV 3.0 and Cobas Ampliprep/ Taqman HCV RNA	Not avaliable
Poovorawari et al.	1994	Thailand	Serum	HCV-SPOT assay (Genelabs Diagnostics Pty Ltd., Singapore)	CS	192	Y	EIA 2nd generation or IMMUNOBLOT	Not avaliable
Prayson et al.	1993	USA	Serum	C100-3 HCV EIA (Abbott Laboratories, other information is not available)	CS	123	N	IMMUNOBLOT 2.0	Not avaliable
Rihn et al.	2000	France	serum	MATRIX hcv2 (Abbott Laboratories, other information is not available)	CS	146	N	PCR	Not avaliable
Scalioni Lde et al.	2014	Brazil	Serum,whole blood and oral fluid	WAMA Imuno-Rápido HCV Kit (WAMA Diag-nóstica, Brazil); Bioeasy HCV Rapid Test, (Bioeasy Diagnóstica Ltd., Brazil) and Ora-Quick (OraSure Tech-nologies, PA USA)	CS	194 or 172	Y	PCR	Yes, Imuno-Rapido HCV; Not avaliable for Rapid Test Bioeasy; Yes, The OraQuick® HCV
Smith et al.	2011	USA	Whole blood, oral fluid	Multiplo Rapid HIV/ HCV Antibody Test (MedMira, Canada); Chembio DPP HCV test (Chembio Diagnostic Systems, USA) and OraQuick (OraSure Technologies, USA)	CS	476, 385, 432, 549, 266	Y	MEIA/EIA/CLIA, IMMUNOBLOT	Yes, Multiplo HBc/HIV/ HCV; Not avaliable for Chembio DPP HCV test; Yes, The OraQuick® HCV
Smith et al.	2011	USA	Oral fluid and blood	Multiplo Rapid HIV/ HCV Antibody Test	CS	1081	Y	Chiron IMMUNOBLOT HCV 3.0 SIA; Bayer	Yes, Multiplo HBc/HIV/ HCV; Not avaliable for

Table 1 Characteristics of studies focused on evaluating diagnostic accuracy of HCV antibody tests *(Continued)*

First author	Year	Settings	Sample type	Manufacturer	Study type	Sample size	POC (Y/N)	Reference standard	Still on the market? PRODUCT NAME
				(MedMira, Canada); Chembio DPP HCV test (Chembio Diagnostic Systems, USA)				Advia Centaur HCV Chemiluminescent immunoassay	Chembio DPP HCV test
Sommese et al.	2014	Italy	Blood	CMIA assays (Abbott Diagnostics, Wiesbaden, Germany)	CS	17,894	N	INNO-LIA (Innogenetics, Ghent, Belgium), NAT	Not avaliable
Tagny et al.	2014	Cameron	Plasma	HCV Ag/Ab combination assay (Monolisa HCV Ag-Ab Ultra, BioRad, Marnes La Coquette, France)	CS	1998	Y	EIA	Yes, MONOLISA™ HCV Ag-Ab ULTRA
Vrielink et al.	1996	Netherlands	Blood	Abbott HCV EIA 3.0 (Abbott laboratories, Murex anti-HCV VK47 (Murex Diagnostic) and Ortho HCV 3.0 elisa (Ortho Diagnostic Systems; other information is not available	CS	403, 212, 253 03 1055	N	PCR	Not available for Abbott HCV EIA 3.0; Yes, Murex anti-HCV (version 4); Yes, OR-THO® HCV 3.0 Elisa
Vrielink et al.	1995	Netherlands	Blood	Monolisa anti-HCV new antigens (Sanofi Diagnostics Pasteur), Abbott HCV EIA 3.0 (Abbott Laboratories); other information is not available	CS	403, 212, 253	N	PCR	Not avaliable
Yang et al.	2011	China	Serum	AxSYM HCV 3.0 (Abbott Laboratories), Murex Ag/Ab test (Abbott Laboratories); other information is not available	CC	101 or 100	N	HCV RNA test (COBAS AMPLICOR Hepatitis C Virus Test, version 2.0	Yes, AXSYM HCV 3.0; Not avaliable for Murex Ag/Ab test
Yang et al.	2013	China	Serum	Elecsys anti-HCV II (Roche Diagnostics GmbH), Architect anti-HCV (Abbott) and Vitros anti-HCV (Ortho-Clinical Diagnostics), other information is not available	CS	859 or 167	N	IMMUNOBLOT 3.0 test or the Realtime HCV RNA assay	Yes, Elecsys® Anti-HCV II; Yes, ARCHITECT i1000SR I; Not available for Ortho-Clinical Diagnostics
Yarri et al.	2006	Israel	Serum and oral fluid	ImmunoComb II HCV (Inverness Medical Innovations, USA)	CS	37	Y	PCR	Not avaliable
Yoo et al.	2015	South Korea; China; China/Taiwan; Thailand; Australia; Malaysia; Indonesia	Serum	Elecsys® Anti-HCV II assay; (Roche Diagnostics GmbH, other information is not avaliable)	CS	7726	Y	1 or more of the following comparator assays at 9 centers: ARCHITECTTM Anti-HCV; Serodia®-HCV Particle Agglutination; Vitros® ECi Anti-HCV; Elecsys® Anti-HCV; ADVIA Centaur® HCV; InTec® HCV EIA; or Livzon® Anti-HCV.	Yes, Elecsys® Anti-HCV II
Yuen et al.	2001	China	Serum	SM-HCV Rapid Test (SERO-Med Laborspezialita¨ten GmbH, Eichsta ¨tt, Germany)	CC	290	Y	EIA, PCR	Not avaliable

Notes: *CC* case–control study, *CS* cross-sectional study

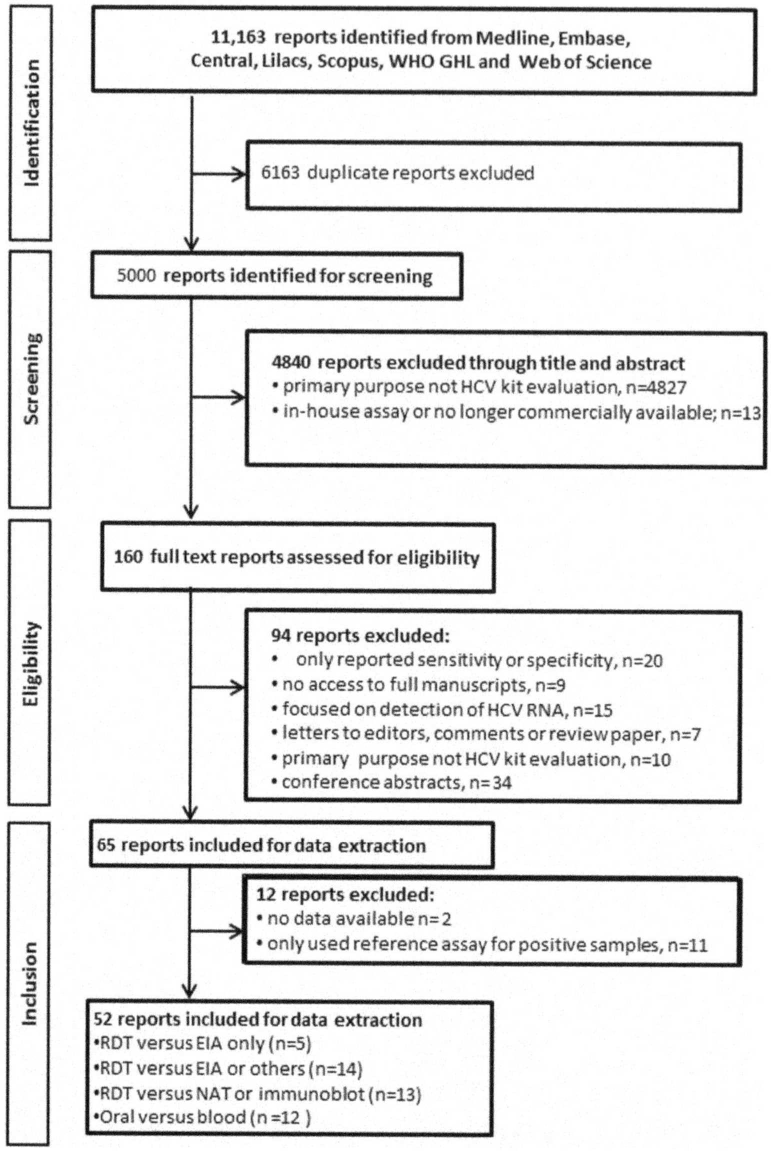

Fig. 1 PRISMA flow diagram outlining study selection examining the diagnostic accuracy of HCV antibody tests

Pooled test accuracy for RDT versus EIA alone

Overall, five studies evaluated RDTs compared to the EIA alone, with a total sample of 15,943. Of the five studies, sample sizes ranged from 197 to 2754, sensitivities ranged from 83 to 100%, and specificities ranged from 99 to 100%. The pooled sensitivity and specificity were 98% (95% CI 98%-100%) and 100% (95% CI 100%-100%), respectively, while heterogeneity was observed in the included studies ($P < 0.001$) (Table 3, Additional file 1).

For the three studies that were conducted within the last 10 years [25, 49, 51], the total sample size was 12,992, with pooled sensitivity and specificity of 99% (95%CI 99%-100%) and 100% (95%CI 100%-100%), respectively.

RDT accuracy compared to NAT or immunoblot

Overall, 13 studies evaluated RDTs compared to NAT or immunoblot [19–22, 27, 29, 32, 37, 42, 43, 45, 47, 50], with a total sample of 7083. Among these studies, sample sizes ranged from 36 to 549, sensitivities ranged from 76 to 100%, and specificities ranged from 77% to 100%. The pooled sensitivity and specificity were 93% (95% CI 91%-95%) and 98% (95% CI 98%- 99%), respectively, while heterogeneity was observed in the included studies ($P < 0.001$) (Table 3, Additional file 2).

RDT test accuracy compared to EIA, NAT or Immunoblot

Overall, 14 studies evaluated RDTs by referencing to EIA with NAT and/or immunoblot [25, 26, 31, 33–35, 38, 39, 41, 45, 48, 49], with a total sample of 42,212. Of

Table 2 Quality assessment by QUADAS-2 of the included studies

Reports		Bias assessment/Risk of bias				Acceptability concerns		
		Patient selection	Index test	Reference Standard	Flow and timing	Patient selection	Index test	Reference Standard
Al-Tahish et al.	2013	UC	LR	LR	LR	LR	LR	LR
Bonacini et al.	2001	HR	LR	LR	LR	LR	LR	LR
Buti et al.	2000	UC	UC	LR	LR	HR	LR	LR
Caudai et al.	1998	HR	LR	LR	LR	UC	LR	LR
Cha et al.	2013	HR	LR	LR	LR	UC	LR	LR
Croom et al.	2006	LR	LR	LR	UC	LR	LR	LR
da Rosa et al.	2013	HR	UC	LR	LR	HR	UC	LR
Daniel et al.	2005	LR	LR	LR	LR	LR	LR	LR
Denoyel et al.	2004	UC	LR	LR	LR	UC	LR	HR
Drobnik et al.	2011	LR	UC	LR	UC	LR	UC	LR
Eroglu et al.	2000	LR	LR	LR	LR	LR	LR	LR
Feucht et al.	1995	HR	LR	LR	LR	HR	LR	LR
Gao et al.	2014	LR	LR	LR	HR	LR	LR	LR
Hess et al.	2014	LR	HR	LR	LR	LR	HR	LR
Hui et al.	2002	HR	LR	HR	LR	HR	LR	HR
Ivantes et al.	2010	LR	UC	HR	LR	LR	LR	HR
Jewett et al.	2012	LR	LR	LR	LR	LR	LR	LR
Dokuboa et al.	2014	UC	LR	LR	LR	UC	LR	LR
Kant et al.	2012	HR	UC	HR	LR	HR	UC	HR
Kaur et al.	2000	LR	UC	HR	LR	LR	LR	LR
Kim et al.	2013	UC	LR	LR	LR	UC	LR	LR
Kosack et al.	2014	HR	LR	LR	LR	HR	LR	LR
Lakshmi et al.	2007	UC	LR	LR	UC	HR	LR	LR
Larrat et al.	2012	LR	LR	LR	LR	LR	LR	LR
Lee et al.	2010	LR	UC	LR	LR	LR	UC	LR
Lee et al.	2011	HR	UC	LR	LR	LR	LR	LR
Maity et al.	2012	HR	UC	HR	LR	HR	UC	HR
Montebugnoil et al.	1999	HR	LR	LR	LR	HR	LR	LR
Mvere et al.	1996	HR	LR	LR	LR	HR	LR	LR
Nalpas et al.	1992	HR	LR	LR	UC	HR	LR	LR
Njouom et al.	2006	HR	UC	LR	LR	HR	UC	LR
Nyirenda et al.	2008	LR	UC	LR	LR	LR	LR	LR
O'Connell et al.	2013	HR	LR	HR	LR	HR	LR	LR
O'Flynn et al.	1997	UC	LR	LR	UC	LR	LR	LR
Park et al.	2012	UC	LR	LR	UC	LR	LR	LR
Poovorawari et al.	1994	LR	UC	LR	LR	LR	LR	LR
Prayson et al.	1993	UC	LR	LR	UC	UC	LR	LR
Rihn et al.	2000	UC	LR	LR	UC	UC	LR	LR
Scalioni et al.	2014	UC	LR	LR	UC	UC	LR	LR
Smith et al.	2011	LR	LR	LR	LR	LR	LR	LR
Smith et al.	2011	HR	LR	LR	LR	HR	LR	LR
Sommese et al.	2014	LR	LR	LR	LR	LR	LR	LR
Lee et al.	2010_2	LR	LR	LR	LR	LR	LR	LR

Table 2 Quality assessment by QUADAS-2 of the included studies *(Continued)*

Reports		Bias assessment/Risk of bias				Acceptability concerns		
		Patient selection	Index test	Reference Standard	Flow and timing	Patient selection	Index test	Reference Standard
Ibrahim et al.	2015	HR	LR	LR	LR	HR	LR	LR
Tagny et al.	2014	LR	UC	HR	LR	LR	UC	HR
Vrielink et al.	1995	UC	LR	LR	LR	UC	LR	LR
Vrielink et al.	1995_2	UC	LR	LR	LR	HR	LR	LR
Yang et al.	2011	UC	LR	LR	LR	UC	LR	LR
Yang et al.	2013	LR	LR	LR	UC	LR	LR	LR
Yarri et al.	2006	HR	LR	LR	LR	HR	LR	LR
Yoo	2015	UC	LR	LR	HR	UC	LR	LR
Yuen et al.	2001	HR	LR	LR	LR	HR	LR	LR

N;otes: *LR* low risk, *HR* high risk, *UC* unclear risk

the 14 studies, sample sizes ranged from 168 to 2754, sensitivities ranged from 29 to 100%, and specificities ranged from 90 to 100%. The pooled sensitivity and specificity were 97% (95% CI 96% -98%) and 100% (95% CI 100%-100%), respectively, while heterogeneity was observed in the included studies ($P < 0.001$) (Table 3, Additional file 3).

Pooled test accuracy for oral versus blood samples

EIAs using oral fluid samples

Overall, 11 studies compared the accuracy of EIAs using oral fluid samples to a blood sample as a reference, with a total sample size of 12,370 [22, 24, 27, 29, 33, 34, 43–45, 47, 52]. Of the 12 studies, sample sizes ranged from 37 to 2176, sensitivities ranged from 72 to 100%, and specificities ranged from 91 to 100%. The pooled sensitivity and specificity were 94% (95% CI 93%-96%) and 100% (95% CI 99%-100%), respectively. Heterogeneity was observed in the included studies ($P < 0.001$) (Table 3, Additional file 4).

Blood samples

Overall, 47 studies used blood samples for evaluations, with a total sample of 90,008. Sample sizes ranged from 37 to 17,894, sensitivities ranged from 29 to 100%, and specificities ranged from 18 to 100%. The pooled sensitivity and specificity were 98% (95% CI 97%-98%) and 98% (95% CI 98%- 98%), respectively. Heterogeneity was observed in the included studies ($P < 0.001$) (Table 3, Fig. 3).

Pooled test accuracy for OraQuick versus other brands on oral kits

OraQuick

Overall, eight studies reported sensitivity and specificity of OraQuick (OraSure Technologies, PA, USA), with a total sample of 9024 [22, 24, 27, 33–35, 43, 45]. The sample size of these studies ranged from 172 to 2183, sensitivities ranged from 90% to 100%, and specificities ranged from 95% to 100%. The pooled sensitivity and specificity were 98% (95% CI 97%-99%) and 100% (95% CI 90%-100%), respectively. Heterogeneity was observed in the included studies ($P < 0.001$) (Table 3, Additional file 5).

Overall, six studies reported sensitivity and specificity for other three brands of oral kits [29, 43–45, 47, 52], with a total sample of 6652. The sample size of these studies ranged from 37 to 1081, sensitivities ranged from 72 to 100%, and specificities ranged from 91 to 100%. The pooled sensitivity and specificity were 88% (95% CI 84%-92%) and 99% (95% CI 99%- 100%), respectively, while heterogeneity was observed between the included studies ($P < 0.001$) (Table 3, Additional file 6).

Other findings

Our study further found that the overall sensitivity and specificity of studies conducted among general populations were 95% (95% CI 94%-96%) and 99% (95% CI 98%-99%), among high risk populations were 97% (95% CI 96%-98%) and 94% (95% CI 94%-95%), and among hospital patients were 97% (95% CI 96%-98%) and 100% (95% CI 100%-100%), respectively. The overall sensitivity and specificity of the antibody and antigen combo test were 86% (95% CI 79%-99%) and 99% (95% CI: 98%-100%).

GRADE approach (Grading of Recommendations, Assessment, Development and Evaluation to assessing overall quality of evidence

GRADE for RDT versus EIA

HCV Ab RDTs showed comparable sensitivity and specificity compared to that of EIAs. Among the five studies that evaluated RDTs versus EIA, 15,943 of samples were evaluated, and moderate risk of bias was observed (Table 4), but there was a consistent high level of specificity. Since the unit of the analysis varied among studies (Table 4), indirectness was

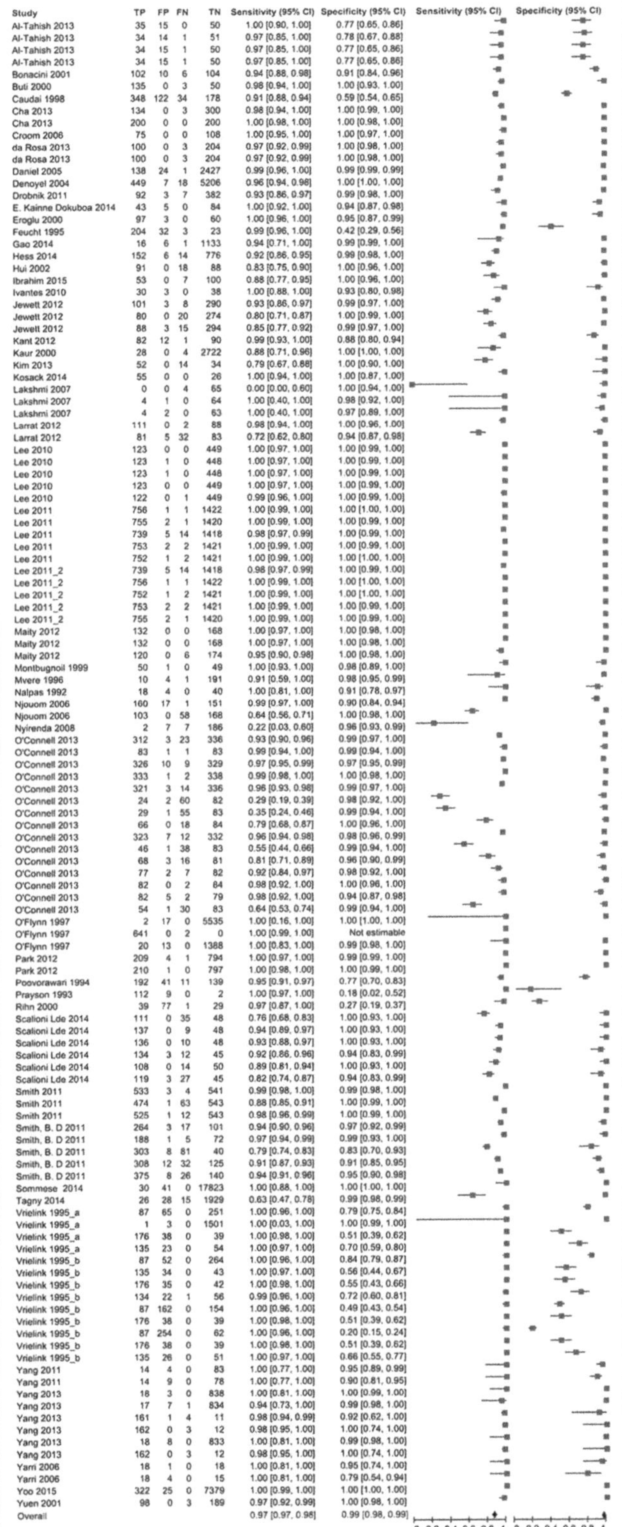

Fig. 2 Sensitivity and specificity of HCV Ab tests included in the review (n = 52)

observed. In addition, the overall strength of the pooled evaluation was moderate, with pooled sensitivity and specificity of 99% (95% CI 98%-100%) and 100% (95% CI 100%-100%), respectively. Under the pre-test probability of 5%, the post-test probability after a positive test result is 97%, and the post-test probability after a negative test result is 100%.

GRADE for oral RDT versus blood reference

The use of oral RDTs HCV Ab had comparable sensitivity and specificity compared to blood reference standards (Additional file 7). For the 12 studies evaluated oral RDT versus blood reference, 14,547 samples were evaluated. A moderate risk of bias was observed. Inconsistency was present for sensitivity, as the sensitivities of the included studies varied. But there was a consistent high level of specificity. Since the unit of the analysis varied with each other among the included studies (Table 4), indirectness was observed for included studies. In addition, the overall strength of the pooled evaluation was moderate, with pooled sensitivity and specificity of 94% (95% CI 93%-96%) and 100% (95% CI 100%-100%), respectively. Assuming a pre-test probability of 5%, the post-test probability after a positive test result was 94%, and the post-test probability after a negative test result was 100%.

Discussion

There is a global need to expand HCV diagnostic testing. In this meta-analysis, we found HCV Ab RDTs, including those using oral fluid, showed a high overall sensitivity and specificity compared to laboratory-based EIAs. This extends the literature by including several new studies that were not included in prior reviews, including a sub-analysis that focused on use of RDTs with oral fluid. In addition, the evidence collected from this review was used to inform recommendations in the 2017 WHO guidelines on testing for hepatitis B and C [15]. The evidence for generally high levels of diagnostic accuracy across most brands from this systematic review and meta-analysis supported a strong recommendation for the use of HCV RDTs in WHO testing guidelines [15].

Our data suggest that RDTs can be used for HCV Ab detection in a wide range of clinical settings. For example, for all the included studies, 17 were conducted among general populations, 20 were among high risk populations, and 17 were among hospitalized patients (two studies included two kinds of populations). High HCV Ab RDTs sensitivity and specificity were observed across multiple different populations (including general population, high risk populations, and hospital patients), which is consistent with previous systematic reviews [13, 14, 63]. The use of an EIA to detect HCV Ab followed

Table 3 Manufacturers and accuracy of RDTs among included studies

First author	Manufacturer	Sample size	TP	FP	TN	FN	SE	SP
Montbugnoil et al.	Anti-HCV Ab rapid test (1st IRP 75/537 by Thema Ricerca, WHO Geneva)	100	50	1	49	0	100%	98%
O'Connell, R. J. et al.	Axiom (Axiom Diagnostics, Burstadt,Germany)	674	326	10	329	9	97%	97%
O'Connell, R. J. et al.	Axiom (Axiom Diagnostics, Burstadt,Germany)	168	77	2	82	7	92%	98%
O'Connell, R. J. et al.	Axiom (Axiom Diagnostics, Burstadt,Germany)	168	82	5	79	2	98%	94%
Scalioni Lde, P et al.	Bioeasy HCV Rapid Test, (Bioeasy Diagnóstica Ltd., Brazil)	194	137	0	48	9	94%	100%
Scalioni Lde, P et al.	Bioeasy HCV Rapid Test (Bioeasy Diagnóstica Ltd., Brazil)	194	111	0	48	35	76%	100%
Scalioni Lde, P et al.	Bioeasy HCV Rapid Test (Bioeasy Diagnóstica Ltd., Brazil)	194	136	0	48	10	93%	100%
Jewett, A et al.	Chembio DPP HCV Test (Chembio Diagnostic Systems, USA)	407	101	3	290	8	93%	99%
Jewett, A et al.	Chembio DPP HCV test (Chembio Diagnostic Systems,USA)	400	88	3	294	15	85%	99%
Smith, B. D et al.	Chembio DPP HCV test (Chembio Diagnostic Systems, USA)	476	308	12	125	32	91%	91%
Smith, B. D et al.	Chembio DPP HCV test (Chembio Diagnostic Systems, USA)	385	264	3	101	17	94%	97%
Smith et al. et al.	Chembio DPP HCV test (Chembio Diagnostic Systems, USA)	1081	525	1	543	12	98%	100%
O'Connell, R. J. et al.	CORE (CORE Diagnostics, United Kingdom)	168	29	1	83	55	35%	99%
O'Connell, R. J et al.	CORE (CORE Diagnostics, United Kingdom)	168	24	2	82	60	29%	98%
O'Connell, R. J et al.	CORE (CORE Diagnostics, United Kingdom)	674	323	7	332	12	96%	98%
Maity et al.	Diagnostics Ltd. (other information is not available)	300	132	0	168	0	100%	100%
O'Connell, R. J. et al.	FirstVue (AT First Diagnostic, Woodbury,NY, USA)	168	66	0	84	18	79%	100%
O'Connell, R. J. et al.	FirstVue (AT First Diagnostic, Woodbury,NY, USA)	168	54	1	83	30	64%	99%
O'Connell, R. J. et al.	FirstVue (AT First Diagnostic, Woodbury,NY, USA)	674	312	3	336	23	93%	99%
Al-Tahish et al.	Fourth- generation HCV TRI_DOT (J. Mitra Co, India)	100	34	15	50	1	97%	77%
Daniel et al.	Fourth- generation HCV TRI_DOT (J. Mitra Co, India)	2590	138	24	2427	1	99%	99%
Kim, M. H. et al.	GENEDIA® HCV Rapid LF (Green Cross medical science corp., Korea)	100	52	0	34	14	79%	100%
Kaur et al.	HCV Bidot (J. Mitra Co., India)	2754	28	0	2722	4	88%	100%
Al-Tahish	HCV one step test device (ACON Laboratories, USA)	100	34	15	50	1	97%	77%
Ivantes et al.	HCV Rapid Test Bioeasy (Bioeasy Diagnostica Ltd., Brazil)	71	30	3	38	0	100%	93%
da Rosa et al.	HCV Rapid Test Bioeasy® (Standard Diagnostics, South Korea)	307	100	0	204	3	97%	100%
Poovoran et al.	HCV-SPOT assay (Genelabs Diagnostics Pty Ltd., Singapore)	192	41	11	139	1	98%	93%
Mvere et al.	HCV-SPOT assay (Genelabs Diagnostics Pty Ltd., Singapore)	206	10	4	191	1	91%	98%
Njouom et al.	Hexagon® HCV (Not reported manufacturer located country)	329	160	17	151	1	99%	90%
Al-Tahish et al.	ImmunoComb II HCV (Inverness Medical Innovations, USA)	100	34	14	51	1	97%	78%
Yarri et al.	ImmunoComb II HCV (Inverness Medical Innovations, USA)	37	18	4	15	0	100%	79%
Yarri et al.	ImmunoComb II HCV (Inverness Medical Innovations, USA)	37	18	1	18	0	100%	95%
Njouom et al.	ImmunoComb® II HCV assay (Orgenics Ltd., not reported manufacturer located country)	329	103	0	168	58	64%	100%
da Rosa et al.	Imuno-Rapido HCV® (Wama Diagnostica, Brazil).	307	100	0	204	3	97%	100%
	Instant View Cassette (Alfa Scientific Designs, Poway, CA, USA)	674	321	3	336	14	96%	99%

Table 3 Manufacturers and accuracy of RDTs among included studies *(Continued)*

First author	Manufacturer	Sample size	TP	FP	TN	FN	SE	SP
O'Connell, R. J. et al.								
O'Connell, R. J. et al.	Instant View Cassette (Alfa Scientific Designs, Poway, CA, USA)	168	68	3	81	16	81%	96%
O'Connell, R. J. et al.	Instant View Cassette (Alfa Scientific Designs, Poway, CA, USA)	168	46	1	83	38	55%	99%
Maity et al.	J Mitra Co. India other information is not available)	300	120	0	174	6	95%	100%
Jewett, A et al.	Rapid HIV/HCV antibody test (Medmira Laboratories, Canada)	374	80	0	274	20	80%	100%
Nyirenda et al.	Monoelisa HCV Ag/Ab ultra-microplate EIA (Bio-Rad, France)	202	2	7	186	7	22%	96%
Tagny et al.	Monolisa HCV Ag-Ab Ultra, (BioRad, France)	1998	26	28	1929	15	63%	99%
Smith et al.	Multiplo Rapid HIV/HCV Antibody Test (MedMira, Canada)	1081	474	1	543	63	88%	100%
Smith, B. D et al.	Multiplo Rapid HIV/HCV Antibody Test (MedMira, Canada)	432	303	8	40	81	79%	83%
Cha, Y. J. et al.	OraQuick (OraSure Technologies, PA USA)	437	134	0	300	3	98%	100%
Cha, Y. J. et al.	Architect (Abbott Laboratories, Abbott Park, IL, USA)	400	200	0	200	0	100%	100%
Lee, S. R et al.	OraQuick (OraSure Technologies, PA USA)	2183	756	1	1422	1	100%	100%
Lee, S. R et al.	OraQuick (OraSure Technologies, PA USA)	2183	755	2	1420	1	100%	100%
Lee, S. R et al.	OraQuick (OraSure Technologies, PA USA)	2183	753	2	1421	2	100%	100%
Lee, S. R et al.	OraQuick (OraSure Technologies, PA USA)	2183	752	1	1421	2	100%	100%
Lee, S. R et al.	OraQuick (OraSure Technologies, PA USA)	2183	739	5	1418	14	98%	100%
O'Connell, R. J et al.	OraQuick (OraSure Technologies, PA USA)	674	333	1	338	2	99%	100%
O'Connell, R. J et al.	OraQuick (OraSure Technologies, PA USA)	168	83	1	83	1	99%	99%
O'Connell, R. J et al.	OraQuick (OraSure Technologies, PA USA)	168	82	0	84	2	98%	100%
Smith, B. D et al.	OraQuick (OraSure Technologies, PA USA)	549	375	8	140	26	94%	.95%
Smith, B. D et al.	OraQuick (OraSure Technologies, PA USA)	266	188	1	72	5	97%	99%
Lee et al.	OraQuick (OraSure Technologies, PA USA)	572	122	0	449	1	99%	100%
Lee et al.	OraQuick (OraSure Technologies, PA USA)	572	123	0	449	0	100%	100%
Lee et al.	OraQuick (OraSure Technologies, PA USA)	572	123	0	449	0	100%	100%
Lee et al.	OraQuick (OraSure Technologies, PA USA)	572	123	1	448	0	100%	100%
Lee et al.	OraQuick (OraSure Technologies, PA USA)	572	123	1	448	0	100%	100%
Smith et al.	OraQuick (OraSure Technologies, PA USA)	1081	533	3	541	4	99%	99%
Drobnik et al.	OraQuick (OraSure Technologies, PA USA)	484	92	3	382	7	93%	99%
Stephen R. Lee et al.	OraQuick (OraSure Technologies, PA USA)	2180	756	1	1422	1	100%	100%
Stephen R. Lee et al.	OraQuick (OraSure Technologies, PA USA)	2178	755	2	1420	1	100%	100%
Stephen R. Lee et al.	OraQuick (OraSure Technologies, PA USA)	2178	753	2	1421	2	100%	100%
Stephen R. Lee et al.	OraQuick (OraSure Technologies, PA USA)	2176	752	1	1421	2	100%	100%
Stephen R. Lee et al.	OraQuick (OraSure Technologies, PA USA)	2176	739	5	1418	14	98%	100%
Gao et al.	OraQuick (OraSure Technologies, PA USA)	1156	16	6	1133	1	94%	99%
Ibrahim	OraQuick (OraSure Technologies, PA USA)	160	53	0	100	7	88%	100%
Scalioni Lde, P_2014	OraQuick (OraSure Technologies, PA USA)	172	108	0	50	14	89%	100%

Table 3 Manufacturers and accuracy of RDTs among included studies *(Continued)*

First author	Manufacturer	Sample size	TP	FP	TN	FN	SE	SP
Hess et al.	DPP HIV-HCV-Syphilis Assay (Chembio Diagnostic Systems, Inc., Medford, NY).	948	152	6	776	14	92%	99%
Buti et al.	Not available	188	135	0	50	3	98%	100%
Yuen et al.	SM-HCV Rapid Test (SERO-Med Laborspezialita¨ten GmbH, Eichsta ¨tt, Germany)	290	98	0	189	3	97%	100%
Maity et al.	SPAN Diagnostics, Indi, other information is not available	300	132	0	168	0	100%	100%
Kant et al.	Toyo anti-HCV test (Turklab, Izmir, Turkey)	185	82	12	90	1	99%	88%
Kosack, C. S. et al.	The ImmunoFlow HCV test (Core Diagnostics,United Kingdom)	82	55	0	26	0	100%	100%
Scalioni Lde et al.	WAMA Imuno-Rápido HCV Kit (WAMA Diagnóstica, Brazil)	194	119	3	45	27	82%	94%
Scalioni Lde, P et al.	WAMA Imuno-Rápido HCV Kit (WAMA Diagnóstica, Brazil)	194	134	3	45	12	92%	94%
Hui et al.	Not reported	197	91	0	88	18	83%	100%

by NAT to confirm active infection is standard practice for diagnosis of HCV infection and recommended by the US Centers for Disease Control and Prevention and the WHO [64, 65]. However, despite these recommendations, HCV Ab EIA assays have not been widely used because of the complexity of laboratory-based assays, long turnaround time, high cost and requirements for specialized apparatus and trained technicians [13]. To overcome these barriers, RDTs for HCV Ab screening were developed [66]. They obviate the need for multiple follow-up appointments, shorten wait times, and allow for the simplification and decentralization of testing (Additional file 8). However, it is essential for policymakers, government officials, and health care practitioners engaged in HCV screening, care, and treatment to be aware that the performance of individual RDTs for detection of HCV Ab vary widely. Individual diagnostic accuracy for specific brands should be examined to ensure acceptable performance.

Our data suggest that oral fluid RDTs have high sensitivity and specificity. This is consistent with other literature [67]. Tests that can be used with non-invasive samples allow testing to be decentralized further and can be used in outreach settings [68]. Our data suggest that oral tests have a slightly lower pooled sensitivity (94%, 95%CI: 93%-96%) compared to blood-based tests (98%, 95% CI: 97%-98%) but comparable specificity. Oral HCV Ab RDTs tests may be particularly useful in contexts where venepuncture may be difficult, such as subsets of people who inject drugs which have difficult veins to access.

With the increasing availability of DAAs, countries are seeking testing kits with high sensitivity and specificity, in order to allow them to scale up HCV Ab screening, especially among at-risk populations. The advantages and disadvantages of EIAs and RDTs are well established [15]. Performance, cost, and accessibility need to be considered. Determining which tests to deploy at which level of the health care system and for what settings require policy makers to consider the different attributes of laboratory-based EIA versus blood-based or oral RDTs. Potential trade-offs include slightly lower accuracy for greater uptake and acceptability of testing, provision of test results, and linkage to care. Each country needs to decide on which trade-offs or compromises are acceptable, based not only on disease prevalence and the health care infrastructure but also on technical, socioeconomic, cultural, behavioral considerations. For example, they need to be clear on whether it is acceptable to buy Test X which is 10% less accurate than Test Y but is considerably cheaper so that many more people can be tested. In addition, although oral RDTs are less accurate than blood-based RDTs, it may be that oral RDTs will be more acceptable for outreach testing and accessing at-risk populations and allow the control programs to identify more HCV cases. In a low prevalence setting, even a test with 98% specificity can yield more false positive than true positive results. All these trade-offs can be modeled to give an estimate of the cost-effectiveness and potential impact of different strategies for HCV Ab screening.

Our review also underlines some of the common methodological problems encountered in evaluating diagnostic accuracy. Cross-sectional or case–control designs were used by all 52 included studies, introducing a potential risk of bias. These studies used a broad range of reference standards, which makes the pooled performance data less meaningful. Within the evaluation of diagnostic accuracy, even cross-sectional studies in patients with diagnostic uncertainty and direct comparison of test results with an appropriate reference standard can be considered high quality [69]. The majority of the included studies used convenience sampling. In this review, we excluded panel studies because they are not based on clinical settings and our purpose was to generate data that would be relevant in clinical settings as part of detection of HCV Ab.

Study	TP	FP	FN	TN	Sensitivity (95% CI)	Specificity (95% CI)
Al-Tahish 2013	34	15	1	50	0.97 [0.85, 1.00]	0.77 [0.65, 0.86]
Al-Tahish 2013	34	15	1	50	0.97 [0.85, 1.00]	0.77 [0.65, 0.86]
Al-Tahish 2013	34	14	1	51	0.97 [0.85, 1.00]	0.78 [0.67, 0.88]
Al-Tahish 2013	35	15	0	50	1.00 [0.90, 1.00]	0.77 [0.65, 0.86]
Bonacini 2001	102	10	6	104	0.94 [0.88, 0.98]	0.91 [0.84, 0.96]
Buti 2000	135	0	3	50	0.98 [0.94, 1.00]	1.00 [0.93, 1.00]
Caudai 1998	348	122	34	178	0.91 [0.88, 0.94]	0.59 [0.54, 0.65]
Cha 2013	200	0	0	200	1.00 [0.98, 1.00]	1.00 [0.98, 1.00]
Croom 2006	75	0	0	108	1.00 [0.95, 1.00]	1.00 [0.97, 1.00]
da Rosa 2013	100	0	3	204	0.97 [0.92, 0.99]	1.00 [0.98, 1.00]
da Rosa 2013	100	0	3	204	0.97 [0.92, 0.99]	1.00 [0.98, 1.00]
Daniel 2005	138	24	1	2427	0.99 [0.96, 1.00]	0.99 [0.99, 0.99]
Denoyel 2004	449	7	18	5206	0.96 [0.94, 0.98]	1.00 [1.00, 1.00]
E. Kainne Dokuboa 2014	43	5	0	84	1.00 [0.92, 1.00]	0.94 [0.87, 0.98]
Eroglu 2000	97	3	0	60	1.00 [0.96, 1.00]	0.95 [0.87, 0.99]
Feucht 1995	204	32	3	23	0.99 [0.96, 1.00]	0.42 [0.29, 0.56]
Gao 2014	16	6	1	1133	0.94 [0.71, 1.00]	0.99 [0.99, 1.00]
Hess 2014	152	6	14	776	0.92 [0.86, 0.95]	0.99 [0.98, 1.00]
Hui 2002	91	0	18	88	0.83 [0.75, 0.90]	1.00 [0.96, 1.00]
Ivantes 2010	30	3	0	38	1.00 [0.88, 1.00]	0.93 [0.80, 0.98]
Jewett 2012	101	3	8	290	0.93 [0.86, 0.97]	0.99 [0.97, 1.00]
Jewett 2012	80	0	20	274	0.80 [0.71, 0.87]	1.00 [0.99, 1.00]
Kant 2012	82	12	1	90	0.99 [0.93, 1.00]	0.88 [0.80, 0.94]
Kaur 2000	28	0	4	2722	0.88 [0.71, 0.96]	1.00 [1.00, 1.00]
Kim 2013	52	0	14	34	0.79 [0.67, 0.88]	1.00 [0.90, 1.00]
Kosack 2014	55	0	0	26	1.00 [0.94, 1.00]	1.00 [0.87, 1.00]
Lakshmi 2007	4	2	0	63	1.00 [0.40, 1.00]	0.97 [0.89, 1.00]
Lakshmi 2007	0	0	4	65	0.00 [0.00, 0.60]	1.00 [0.94, 1.00]
Lakshmi 2007	4	1	0	64	1.00 [0.40, 1.00]	0.98 [0.92, 1.00]
Larrat 2012	111	0	2	88	0.98 [0.94, 1.00]	1.00 [0.96, 1.00]
Lee 2010	123	1	0	448	1.00 [0.97, 1.00]	1.00 [0.99, 1.00]
Lee 2010	123	0	0	449	1.00 [0.97, 1.00]	1.00 [0.99, 1.00]
Lee 2010	123	0	0	449	1.00 [0.97, 1.00]	1.00 [0.99, 1.00]
Lee 2010	123	1	0	448	1.00 [0.97, 1.00]	1.00 [0.99, 1.00]
Lee 2011	752	1	2	1421	1.00 [0.99, 1.00]	1.00 [1.00, 1.00]
Lee 2011	755	2	1	1420	1.00 [0.99, 1.00]	1.00 [0.99, 1.00]
Lee 2011	756	1	1	1422	1.00 [0.99, 1.00]	1.00 [1.00, 1.00]
Lee 2011	753	2	2	1421	1.00 [0.99, 1.00]	1.00 [0.99, 1.00]
Lee 2011_2	753	2	2	1421	1.00 [0.99, 1.00]	1.00 [0.99, 1.00]
Lee 2011_2	752	1	2	1421	1.00 [0.99, 1.00]	1.00 [1.00, 1.00]
Lee 2011_2	756	1	1	1422	1.00 [0.99, 1.00]	1.00 [1.00, 1.00]
Lee 2011_2	755	2	1	1420	1.00 [0.99, 1.00]	1.00 [0.99, 1.00]
Maity 2012	120	0	6	174	0.95 [0.90, 0.98]	1.00 [0.98, 1.00]
Maity 2012	132	0	0	168	1.00 [0.97, 1.00]	1.00 [0.98, 1.00]
Maity 2012	132	0	0	168	1.00 [0.97, 1.00]	1.00 [0.98, 1.00]
Montbugnoil 1999	50	1	0	49	1.00 [0.93, 1.00]	0.98 [0.89, 1.00]
Mvere 1996	10	4	1	191	0.91 [0.59, 1.00]	0.98 [0.95, 0.99]
Nalpas 1992	18	4	0	40	1.00 [0.81, 1.00]	0.91 [0.78, 0.97]
Njouom 2006	103	0	58	168	0.64 [0.56, 0.71]	1.00 [0.98, 1.00]
Njouom 2006	160	17	1	151	0.99 [0.97, 1.00]	0.90 [0.84, 0.94]
Nyirenda 2008	2	7	7	186	0.22 [0.03, 0.60]	0.96 [0.93, 0.99]
O'Connell 2013	326	10	9	329	0.97 [0.95, 0.99]	0.97 [0.95, 0.99]
O'Connell 2013	46	1	38	83	0.55 [0.44, 0.66]	0.99 [0.94, 1.00]
O'Connell 2013	82	5	2	79	0.98 [0.92, 1.00]	0.94 [0.87, 0.98]
O'Connell 2013	323	7	12	332	0.96 [0.94, 0.98]	0.98 [0.96, 0.99]
O'Connell 2013	321	3	14	336	0.96 [0.93, 0.98]	0.99 [0.97, 1.00]
O'Connell 2013	83	1	1	83	0.99 [0.94, 1.00]	0.99 [0.94, 1.00]
O'Connell 2013	333	1	2	338	0.99 [0.98, 1.00]	1.00 [0.98, 1.00]
O'Connell 2013	66	0	18	84	0.79 [0.68, 0.87]	1.00 [0.96, 1.00]
O'Connell 2013	82	0	2	84	0.98 [0.92, 1.00]	1.00 [0.96, 1.00]
O'Connell 2013	24	2	60	82	0.29 [0.19, 0.39]	0.98 [0.92, 1.00]
O'Connell 2013	68	3	16	81	0.81 [0.71, 0.89]	0.96 [0.90, 0.99]
O'Connell 2013	77	2	7	82	0.92 [0.84, 0.97]	0.98 [0.92, 1.00]
O'Connell 2013	312	3	23	336	0.93 [0.90, 0.96]	0.99 [0.97, 1.00]
O'Connell 2013	54	1	30	83	0.64 [0.53, 0.74]	0.99 [0.94, 1.00]
O'Connell 2013	29	1	55	83	0.35 [0.24, 0.46]	0.99 [0.94, 1.00]
O'Flynn 1997	641	0	2	0	1.00 [0.99, 1.00]	Not estimable
O'Flynn 1997	2	17	0	5535	1.00 [0.16, 1.00]	1.00 [1.00, 1.00]
O'Flynn 1997	20	13	0	1388	1.00 [0.83, 1.00]	0.99 [0.98, 1.00]
Park 2012	209	4	1	794	1.00 [0.97, 1.00]	0.99 [0.99, 1.00]
Park 2012	210	1	0	797	1.00 [0.98, 1.00]	1.00 [0.99, 1.00]
Poovorawari 1994	41	11	1	139	0.98 [0.87, 1.00]	0.93 [0.87, 0.96]
Prayson 1993	112	9	0	2	1.00 [0.97, 1.00]	0.18 [0.02, 0.52]
Rihn 2000	39	77	1	29	0.97 [0.87, 1.00]	0.27 [0.19, 0.37]
Scalioni Lde 2014	137	0	9	48	0.94 [0.89, 0.97]	1.00 [0.93, 1.00]
Scalioni Lde 2014	136	0	10	48	0.93 [0.88, 0.97]	1.00 [0.93, 1.00]
Scalioni Lde 2014	134	3	12	45	0.92 [0.86, 0.96]	0.94 [0.83, 0.99]
Smith, B. D 2011	264	3	17	101	0.94 [0.90, 0.96]	0.97 [0.92, 0.99]
Smith, B. D 2011	303	8	81	40	0.79 [0.74, 0.83]	0.83 [0.70, 0.93]
Smith, B. D 2011	188	1	5	72	0.97 [0.94, 0.99]	0.99 [0.93, 1.00]
Sommese 2014	30	41	0	17823	1.00 [0.88, 1.00]	1.00 [1.00, 1.00]
Tagny 2014	26	28	15	1929	0.63 [0.47, 0.78]	0.99 [0.98, 0.99]
Vrielink 1995_a	87	65	0	251	1.00 [0.96, 1.00]	0.79 [0.75, 0.84]
Vrielink 1995_a	135	23	0	54	1.00 [0.97, 1.00]	0.70 [0.59, 0.80]
Vrielink 1995_a	176	38	0	39	1.00 [0.98, 1.00]	0.51 [0.39, 0.62]
Vrielink 1995_a	1	3	0	1501	1.00 [0.03, 1.00]	1.00 [0.99, 1.00]
Vrielink 1995_b	135	26	0	51	1.00 [0.97, 1.00]	0.66 [0.55, 0.77]
Vrielink 1995_b	176	38	0	39	1.00 [0.98, 1.00]	0.51 [0.39, 0.62]
Vrielink 1995_b	176	38	0	39	1.00 [0.98, 1.00]	0.51 [0.39, 0.62]
Vrielink 1995_b	176	35	0	42	1.00 [0.98, 1.00]	0.55 [0.43, 0.66]
Vrielink 1995_b	87	52	0	264	1.00 [0.96, 1.00]	0.84 [0.79, 0.87]
Vrielink 1995_b	135	34	0	43	1.00 [0.97, 1.00]	0.56 [0.44, 0.67]
Vrielink 1995_b	87	254	0	62	1.00 [0.96, 1.00]	0.20 [0.15, 0.24]
Vrielink 1995_b	87	162	0	154	1.00 [0.96, 1.00]	0.49 [0.43, 0.54]
Vrielink 1995_b	134	22	1	56	0.99 [0.96, 1.00]	0.72 [0.60, 0.81]
Yang 2011	14	4	0	83	1.00 [0.77, 1.00]	0.95 [0.89, 0.99]
Yang 2011	14	9	0	78	1.00 [0.77, 1.00]	0.90 [0.81, 0.95]
Yang 2013	162	0	3	12	0.98 [0.95, 1.00]	1.00 [0.74, 1.00]
Yang 2013	161	1	4	11	0.98 [0.94, 0.99]	0.92 [0.62, 1.00]
Yang 2013	18	3	0	838	1.00 [0.81, 1.00]	1.00 [0.99, 1.00]
Yang 2013	17	7	1	834	0.94 [0.73, 1.00]	0.99 [0.98, 1.00]
Yang 2013	162	0	3	12	0.98 [0.95, 1.00]	1.00 [0.74, 1.00]
Yang 2013	18	8	0	833	1.00 [0.81, 1.00]	0.99 [0.98, 1.00]
Yarri 2006	18	4	0	15	1.00 [0.81, 1.00]	0.79 [0.54, 0.94]
Yoo 2015	322	25	0	7379	1.00 [0.99, 1.00]	1.00 [1.00, 1.00]
Yuen 2001	98	0	3	189	0.97 [0.92, 0.99]	1.00 [0.98, 1.00]
Overall					0.98 [0.91, 0.95]	0.99 [0.98, 0.99]

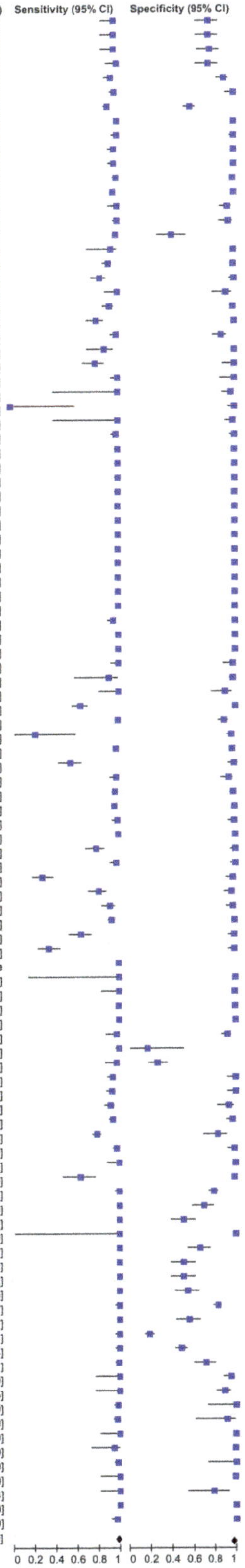

Fig. 3 Pooled HCV Ab test accuracy for blood samples (n = 47 studies)

Table 4 Pooled test accuracy for different testing strategies (n = 52 studies)*

Comparison	Pooled SE	95%CI		Tau-square *P*-value for hetero-geneity	Pooled SP	95%CI		Tau-square *P*-value for hetero-geneity
RDT versus EIA only (n = 5)	99%	98%	100%	<0.001	100%	100%	100%	<0.001
RDT versus NAT or Immunoblot (n = 13)	93%	91%	95%	<0.001	98%	97%	99%	<0.001
RDT versus EIA, NAT or Immunoblot (n = 14)	97%	96%	098%	<0.001	100%	100%	100%	<0.001
Oral RDT versus blood reference (n = 12)	94%	93%	96%	<0.001	100%	100%	100%	<0.001
Sample type								
Blood samples (n = 45)	98%	97%	98%	<0.001	98%	98%	99%	
Oral samples (n = 12)	94%	93%	96%	<0.001	100%	100%	100%	<0.001
Source population								
General screening (n = 17)	95%	94%	96%	<0.001	99%	98%	99%	<0.001
High risk population (n = 19)	97%	96%	98%	<0.001	94%	94%	95%	<0.001
Hospital patients (n = 16)	97%	96%	98%	<0.001	100%	100%	100%	<0.001
Antibody and Antigen Combo testing (n = 6)	86%	79%	94%	<0.001	99%	98%	100%	<0.001
Oral kits brand							100%	
OraQuick (n = 8)	98%	97%	99%	<0.001	100%	100%	100%	<0.001
Other brands (n = 6)	88%	84%	92%	<0.001	99%	99%	100%	<0.001

Notes: *Studies conducted in both LMIC and high-income countries were not included here
Studies conducted cross these regions were not included here
SE sensitivity, *SP* specificity

Most studies that reported HIV or HBV co-infection only reported the test performance of the kits among all samples, instead of disaggregated diagnostic accuracy. There were insufficient data from two studies to undertake a subanalysis based on HIV co-infection. It may be important for policymakers to know the diagnostic accuracy of HCV Ab tests among individuals with co-infections, particularly HIV co-infection [70], and this requires further research among co-infected individuals.

Our study is subject to several limitations. First, we included studies conducted among the general population, hospital patients, and high risk populations. Diagnostic performance can be influenced by disease prevalence and HCV prevalence is variable among these different populations [71, 72]. Second, we detected substantial heterogeneity that could influence our confidence in the review findings [73], but addressed this problem through a series of sub-group stratified analyses. Third, about 20 brands of RDT kits were used in the included studies, and their performance varies considerably. This limited our ability to summarize the accuracy of different brands, with the exception of comparing OraQuick to other brands. Another concern is publication bias, as studies with poor test performance may be less likely to be published, leading to distorted estimates of accuracy [74]. Fourth, since not all HCV RDTs can be performed from oral fluid/capillary whole blood (some require plasma/serum), and some of them require a cold chain for storage and transport, the direct comparison between EIA and RDTs in this meta-analysis would be less meaningful. Fifth, we should note that not all test kits are still on the market and that versions of the tests included in this meta-analysis may have since changed. Finally, statistical heterogeneity was present. But is common in meta-analyses of diagnostic studies. Additional research is important for understanding why the tests perform more poorly in certain populations or settings.

Conclusion

RDTs, including oral tests, have excellent sensitivity and specificity compared to laboratory-based methods for HCV antibody detection across a wide range of settings. National policymakers should consider the performance, cost and accessibility of RDTs into consideration, when selecting assays for use in their national testing algorithms.

Additional files

Additional file 1: Pooled test accuracy of HCV Ab RDTs compared to an EIA reference (5 studies).

Additional file 2: Pooled test accuracy of HCV Ab RDTs compared to a NAT or immunoblot reference (n = 13 studies).

Additional file 3: Pooled test accuracy of HCV Ab RDTs compared to EIA, NAT or immunoblot reference standards (n = 14 studies).

Additional file 4: Pooled test accuracy for oral HCV Ab RDTs compared to blood as a reference (n = 11 studies).

Additional file 5: Pooled test accuracy for HCV Ab OraQuick kits ($n = 8$ studies).

Additional file 6: Pooled test accuracy for other brands of oral HCV Ab test kits ($n = 6$ studies).

Additional file 7: Grade Table.

Additional file 8: Advantages and Disadvantages of Laboratory based EIAs vs RDTs.

Abbreviations

CI: Confidence interval; DAAs: Direct acting antivirals; EIA: Enzyme immunoassay; FN: False negative; FP: False positive; HCV Ab: HCV antibody; HCV: Hepatitis C Virus; NAT: Nucleic acid testing; NPV: Negative predictive value; POC: Point-of-care; PPV: Positive predictive value,; RCT: Randomised control trial; RDTs: Rapid diagnostic tests; SE: Sensitivity; SP: Specificity; TN: True negative; TP: True Positive; WHO: World Health Organization

Acknowledgements

The authors acknowledge the support of WHO, London School of Hygiene & Tropical Medicine, SESH Global and UNC Project China.

Funding

This work was supported by the National Institutes of Health National Institute of Allergy and Infectious Diseases 1R01AI114310-01 to JT, UNC-South China STD Research Training Centre Fogarty International Centre 1D43TW009532-01 to JT, and the World Health Organization. Publication of this article was funded by the World Health Organization.

About this supplement

This article has been published as part of BMC Infectious Diseases Volume 17 Supplement 1, 2017: Testing for chronic hepatitis B and C – a global perspective. The full contents of the supplement are available online at https://bmcinfectdis.biomedcentral.com/articles/supplements/volume-17-supplement-1.

Authors' contributions

All authors have read and approved the final manuscript. This review was prepared by WT, WC, RP and JDT. AA, DB, OV and JF helped on build searching algorism and performed the literature search. RP and JDT designed the study, and RP, JDT, AA, DB, OV and PE reviewed the manuscript.

Consent for publication

Not applicable.

Competing interests

The authors declare that they have no competing interests.

Author details

[1]University of North Carolina Project-China, No. 2 Lujing Road, Guangzhou 510095, China. [2]Guangdong Provincial Dermatology Hospital (Dermatology Hospital, Southern Medical University), Guangzhou, China. [3]SESH Global, Guangzhou, China. [4]School of Medicine, University of North Carolina at Chapel Hill, Chapel Hill, NC, USA. [5]School of Public Health, Sun Yat-sen University, Guangzhou, China. [6]Center for Migrant Health Policy, Sun Yat-sen University, Guangzhou, China. [7]London School of Hygiene and Tropical Medicine, Keppel St, London, UK. [8]Global Hepatitis Programme, HIV Department, World Health Organization, Geneva, Switzerland.

References

1. World Health Organization. New recommendations in the updated WHO guidelines for the screening, care and treatment of persons with chronic hepatitis C infection. Geneva: WHO; 2016. http://www.who.int/hepatitis/publications/hepatitis-c-guidelines-2016/en/.
2. Lavanchy D. The global burden of hepatitis C. Liver Int. 2009;29(s1):74–81.
3. World Health Organization. Global Hepatitis Report, 2017. Geneva; 2017. http://www.who.int/hepatitis/publications/global-hepatitis-report2017/en/. Accessed 6 Oct 2017.
4. Feeney ER, Chung RT. Antiviral treatment of hepatitis C. BMJ (Clinical research ed). 2014;348:g3308.
5. Pawlotsky JM. New hepatitis C therapies: the toolbox, strategies, and challenges. Gastroenterology. 2014;146(5):1176–92.
6. Soriano V, Labarga P, Fernández-Montero JV, Benito JM, Poveda E, Rallon N, Sánchez C, Vispo E, Barreiro P. The changing face of hepatitis C in the new era of direct-acting antivirals. Antivir Res. 2013;97(1):36–40.
7. Papatheodoridis G, Tsochatzis E, Hardke S, Wedemeyer H. Barriers to care and treatment for patients with chronic viral hepatitis in europe: a systematic review. Liver Int. 2014;34(10):1452–63.
8. Zheng H, Li M, Chi B, Wu XX, Wang J, Liu DW. IL28B rs12980275 variant as a predictor of sustained virologic response to pegylated-interferon and ribavirin in chronic hepatitis C patients: a systematic review and meta-analysis. Clin Res Hepatol Gastroenterol. 2015;35(5):576–83.
9. Manzano-Robleda Mdel C, Ornelas-Arroyo V, Barrientos-Gutierrez T, Mendez-Sanchez N, Uribe M, Chavez-Tapia NC. Boceprevir and telaprevir for chronic genotype 1 hepatitis C virus infection. A systematic review and meta-analysis. Ann Hepatol. 2015;14(1):46–57.
10. Ambrosino P, Lupoli R, Tarantino P, Di Minno A, Tarantino L, Di Minno MN. Viral hepatitis and anti-phospholipid antibodies positivity: a systematic review and meta-analysis. Dig Liver Dis. 2015;47(6):478–87.
11. Khodabandehloo M, Roshani D. Prevalence of hepatitis C virus genotypes in Iranian patients: a systematic review and meta-analysis. Hepat Mon. 2014; 14(12):e22915.
12. Khodabandehloo M, Roshani D, Sayehmiri K. Prevalence and trend of hepatitis C virus infection among blood donors in Iran: a systematic review and meta-analysis. J Res Med Sci. 2013;18(8):674–82.
13. Khuroo MS, Khuroo NS, Khuroo MS. Diagnostic accuracy of point-of-care tests for hepatitis C virus infection: a systematic review and meta-analysis. PLoS One. 2015;10(3):e0121450.
14. Shivkumar S, Peeling R, Jafari Y, Joseph L, Pant Pai N. Accuracy of rapid and point-of-care screening tests for hepatitis C: a systematic review and meta-analysis. Ann Intern Med. 2012;157(8):558–66.
15. World Health Organization. Guidelines on hepatitis B and C testing. Geneva; 2017. Available: http://www.who.int/hepatitis/publications/guidelines-hepatitis-c-b-testing/en/. Accessed 6 Oct 2017.
16. UNAIDS. Unaids terminology guidelines. Geneva: UNADIS; 2015.
17. Whiting PF, Rutjes AW, Westwood ME, Mallett S, Deeks JJ, Reitsma JB, Leeflang MM, Sterne JA, Bossuyt PM, Group Q. QUADAS-2: a revised tool for the quality assessment of diagnostic accuracy studies. Ann Intern Med. 2011;155(8):529–36.
18. Bossuyt PM, Reitsma JB, Bruns DE, Gatsonis CA, Glasziou PP, Irwig LM, Moher D, Rennie D, de Vet HC, Lijmer JG, et al. The STARD statement for reporting studies of diagnostic accuracy: explanation and elaboration. Ann Intern Med. 2003;138(1):W1-12.
19. da Rosa L, Dantas-Correa EB, Narciso-Schiavon JL, Schiavon LL. Diagnostic performance of two point-of-care tests for anti-HCV detection. Hepat Mon. 2013;13(9):e12274.
20. Al-Tahish G, El-Barrawy MA, Hashish MH, Heddaya Z. Effectiveness of three types of rapid tests for the detection of hepatitis C virus antibodies among blood donors in Alexandria, Egypt. J Virol Methods. 2013;189(2):370–4.
21. Buti M, Cotrina M, Chan H, Jardi R, Rodriguez F, Costa X, Esteban R, Guardia J. Rapid method for the detection of anti-HCV antibodies in patients with chronic hepatitis C. Rev Esp Enferm Dig. 2000;92(3):140–6.
22. Cha YJ, Park Q, Kang ES, Yoo BC, Park KU, Kim JW, Hwang YS, Kim MH. Performance evaluation of the OraQuick hepatitis C virus rapid antibody test. Ann Lab Med. 2013;33(3):184–9.
23. Daniel HD, Abraham P, Raghuraman S, Vivekanandan P, Subramaniam T, Sridharan G. Evaluation of a rapid assay as an alternative to conventional enzyme immunoassays for detection of hepatitis C virus-specific antibodies. J Clin Microbiol. 2005;43(4):1977–8.

24. Drobnik A, Judd C, Banach D, Egger J, Konty K, Rude E. Public health implications of rapid hepatitis C screening with an oral swab for community-based organizations serving high-risk populations. Am J Public Health. 2011;101(11):2151.
25. Hess KL, Fisher DG, Reynolds GL. Sensitivity and specificity of point-of-care rapid combination syphilis-HIV-HCV tests. PLoS One. 2014;9(11):e112190.
26. Hui AY, Chan FK, Chan PK, Tam JS, Sung JJ. Evaluation of anew rapid whole-blood serological test for hepatitis c virus. Acta Virol. 2002;46(1):47–8.
27. Ibrahim S, Al Attas SA, Mansour GA, Ouda S, Fallatah H. Accuracy of rapid oral HCV diagnostic test among a Saudi sample. Clin Oral Investig. 2015;19(2):475–80.
28. Ivantes CA, Silva D, Messias-Reason I. High prevalence of hepatitis C associated with familial history of hepatitis in a small town of south Brazil: efficiency of the rapid test for epidemiological survey. Braz J Infect Dis. 2010;14(5):483–8.
29. Jewett A, Smith BD, Garfein RS, Cuevas-Mota J, Teshale EH, Weinbaum CM. Field-based performance of three pre-market rapid hepatitis C virus antibody assays in STAHR (study to assess hepatitis C risk) among young adults who inject drugs in San Diego, CA. J Clin Virol. 2012;54(3):213–7.
30. Kant J, Moller B, Heyne R, Herber A, Bohm S, Maier M, Liebert UG, Mossner J, Berg T, Wiegand J. Evaluation of a rapid on-site anti-HCV test as a screening tool for hepatitis C virus infection. Eur J Gastroenterol Hepatol. 2013;25(4):416–20.
31. Kaur H, Dhanao J, Oberoi A. Evaluation of rapid kits for detection of HIV, HBsAg and HCV infections. Indian J Med Sci. 2000;54(10):432–4.
32. Kim MH, Kang SY, Lee WI. Evaluation of a new rapid test kit to detect hepatitis C virus infection. J Virol Methods. 2013;193(2):379–82.
33. Lee SR, Kardos K, Yearwood G, Kurtz L, Roehler M, Feiss G. Results of a multi-center evaluation of a new rapid test for detection of HCV infection using whole blood, serum, plasma and oral fluid. J Hepatol. 2010;52:S271.
34. Lee SR, Kardos KW, Schiff E, Berne CA, Mounzer K, Banks AT, Tatum HA, Friel TJ, Demicco MP, Lee WM, et al. Evaluation of a new, rapid test for detecting HCV infection, suitable for use with blood or oral fluid. J Virol Methods. 2011;172(1–2):27–31.
35. Lee SR, Yearwood GD, Guillon GB, Kurtz LA, Fischl M, Friel T, Berne CA, Kardos KW. Evaluation of a rapid, point-of-care test device for the diagnosis of hepatitis C infection. J Clin Virol. 2010;48(1):15–7.
36. Maity S, Nandi S, Biswas S, Sadhukhan SK, Saha MK. Performance and diagnostic usefulness of commercially available enzyme linked immunosorbent assay and rapid kits for detection of HIV, HBV and HCV in India. Virol J. 2012;9:290.
37. Montebugnoli L, Borea G, Miniero R, Sprovieri G. A rapid test for the visual detection of anti-hepatitis C virus antibodies in whole blood. Clin Chim Acta. 1999;288(1–2):91–6.
38. Mvere D, Constantine NT, Katsawde E, Tobaiwa O, Dambire S, Corcoran P. Rapid and simple hepatitis assays: encouraging results from a blood donor population in Zimbabwe. Bull World Health Organ. 1996;74(1):19–24.
39. Njouom R, Tejiokem MC, Zanga MC, Pouillot R, Ayouba A, Pasquier C, Nerrienet E. A cost-effective algorithm for the diagnosis of hepatitis C virus infection and prediction of HCV viremia in Cameroon. J Virol Methods. 2006; 133(2):223–6.
40. Nyirenda M, Beadsworth MB, Stephany P, Hart CA, Hart IJ, Munthali C, Beeching NJ, Zijlstra EE. Prevalence of infection with hepatitis B and C virus and coinfection with HIV in medical inpatients in Malawi. J Infect. 2008;57(1):72–7.
41. O'Connell RJ, Gates RG, Bautista CT, Imbach M, Eggleston JC, Beardsley SG, Manak MM, Gonzales R, Rentas FJ, Macdonald VW, et al. Laboratory evaluation of rapid test kits to detect hepatitis C antibody for use in predonation screening in emergency settings. Transfusion. 2013;53(3):505–17.
42. Poovorawan Y, Theamboonlers A, Chumdermpadetsuk S, Thong CP. Comparative results in detection of HCV antibodies by using a rapid HCV test, ELISA and immunoblot. Southeast Asian J Trop Med Public Health. 1994;25(4):647–9.
43. Scalioni Lde P, Cruz HM, de Paula VS, Miguel JC, Marques VA, Villela-Nogueira CA, Milagres FA, Cruz MS, Bastos FI, Andrade TM, et al. Performance of rapid hepatitis C virus antibody assays among high- and low-risk populations. J Clin Virol. 2014;60(3):200–5.
44. Smith BD, Drobeniuc J, Jewett A, Branson BM, Garfein RS, Teshale E, Kamili S, Weinbaum CM. Evaluation of three rapid screening assays for detection of antibodies to hepatitis C virus. J Infect Dis. 2011;204(6):825–31.
45. Smith BD, Teshale E, Jewett A, Weinbaum CM, Neaigus A, Hagan H, Jenness SM, Melville SK, Burt R, Thiede H, et al. Performance of premarket rapid hepatitis C virus antibody assays in 4 national human immunodeficiency virus behavioral surveillance system sites. Clin Infect Dis. 2011;53(8):780–6.
46. Tagny CT, Mbanya D, Murphy EL, Lefrere JJ, Laperche S. Screening for hepatitis C virus infection in a high prevalence country by an antigen/antibody combination assay versus a rapid test. J Virol Methods. 2014;199:119–23.
47. Yaari A, Tovbin D, Zlotnick M, Mostoslavsky M, Shemer-Avni Y, Hanuka N, Burbea Z, Katzir Z, Storch S, Margalith M. Detection of HCV salivary antibodies by a simple and rapid test. J Virol Methods. 2006;133(1):1–5.
48. Yuen MF, Hui CK, Yuen JC, Young JL, Lai CL. The accuracy of SM-HCV rapid test for the detection of antibody to hepatitis C virus. Am J Gastroenterol. 2001;96(3):838–41.
49. Gao F, Talbot EA, Loring CH, Power JJ, Dionne-Odom J, Alroy-Preis S, Jackson P, Bean CL. Performance of the OraQuick HCV rapid antibody test for screening exposed patients in a hepatitis C outbreak investigation. J Clin Microbiol. 2014;52(7):2650–2.
50. Kosack CS, Nick S, Shanks L. Diagnostic accuracy evaluation of the ImmunoFlow HCV rapid immunochromatographic test for the detection of hepatitis C antibodies. J Virol Methods. 2014;204:6–10.
51. Lee SR, Kardos K, Yearwood G, Kurtz L, Roehler M, Feiss G. Results of a multi-center evaluation of a new rapid test for detection of HCV infection using whole blood, serum, plasma and oral fluid. J Hepatol. 2011;52:S271.
52. Larrat S, Bourdon C, Baccard M, Garnaud C, Mathieu S, Quesada JL, Signori-Schmuck A, Germi R, Blanc M, Leclercq P, et al. Performance of an antigen-antibody combined assay for hepatitis C virus testing without venipuncture. J Clin Virol. 2012;55(3):220–5.
53. Nalpas B, Thiers V, Pol S, Driss F, Thepot V, Berthelot P, Brechot C. Hepatitis-C Viremia and anti-Hcv antibodies in alcoholics. J Hepatol. 1992;14(2–3):381–4.
54. Prayson RA, Proffitt MR, Sharp DE, Carey WD. Application of a 2nd-generation recombinant Immunoblot assay to assess hepatitis-C infection. Lab Med. 1993;24(11):732–8.
55. Feucht HH, Zollner B, Polywka S, Laufs R. Study on reliability of commercially available hepatitis C virus antibody tests. J Clin Microbiol. 1995;33(3):620–4.
56. Vrielink H, Zaaijer HL, Reesink HW, van der Poel CL, Cuypers HT, Lelie PN. Sensitivity and specificity of three third-generation anti-hepatitis C virus ELISAs. Vox Sang. 1995;69(1):14–7.
57. O'Flynn N, Jilg W, McQuillan T, Bauer I, Heyermann M, Schulte-Kellinghaus B, Moller D. New HCV assay on the Abbott AxSYM random access analyzer. Clin Lab. 1997;43(5):403–9.
58. Caudai C, Padula MG, Bastianoni I, Valensin PE, Shyamala V, Han J, Boggiano CA, Almi P. Antibody testing and RT-PCR results in hepatitis C virus (HCV) infection: HCV-RNA detection in PBMC of plasma viremia-negative HCV-Seropositive persons. Infection. 1998;26(3):151–4.
59. Bonacini M, Lin HJ, Hollinger FB. Effect of coexisting HIV-1 infection on the diagnosis and evaluation of hepatitis C virus. J Acquir Immune Defic Syndr. 2001;26(4):340–4.
60. Yang JF, Lin YY, Hsieh MH, Tsai CH, Liu SF, Yu ML, Dai CY, Huang JF, Lin WY, Lin ZY, et al. Performance characteristics of a combined hepatitis C virus core antigen and anti-hepatitis C virus antibody test in different patient groups. Kaohsiung J Med Sci. 2011;27(7):258–63.
61. Yang R, Guan W, Wang Q, Liu Y, Wei L. Performance evaluation and comparison of the newly developed Elecsys anti-HCV II assay with other widely used assays. Clin Chim Acta. 2013;426:95–101.
62. Yoo SJ, Wang LL, Ning HC, Tao CM, Hirankarn N, Kuakarn S, Yang R, Han TH, Chan RC, Hussain BM, et al. Evaluation of the Elecsys anti-HCV II assay for routine hepatitis C virus screening of different Asian Pacific populations and detection of early infection. J Clin Virol. 2015;64:20–7.
63. Aspinall EJ, Doyle JS, Corson S, Hellard ME, Hunt D, Goldberg D, Nguyen T, Falck-Ytter Y, Morgan RL, Smith B, Stoove M, Wiktor SZ, Hutchinson S. Targeted hepatitis C antibody testing interventions: a systematic review and meta-analysis. Eur J Epidemiol. 2015;30(2):115–29.
64. Alter MJ, Kuhnert WL, Finelli L Centers for Disease Control and Prevention. Guidelines for laboratory testing and result reporting of antibody to hepatitis C virus. Centers for Disease Control and Prevention. MMWR Recomm Rep. 2003;52:1-13, 15.
65. World Health Organization. Guidelines for the screening, care, and treatment of persons with hepatitis C infection. Geneva; 2014. Available: http://www.who.int/hiv/pub/hepatitis/hepatitis-c-guidelines/en/. Accessed 6 Oct 2017.
66. St John A, Price CP. Economic evidence and point-of-care testing. Clin Biochem Rev. 2013;34(2):61.
67. D'Angelo RG, Klepser M, Woodfield R, Patel H. Hepatitis C virus screening a review of the OraQuick hepatitis C virus rapid antibody test. J Pharm Technol. 2015;31(1):13–9.

68. Parisi MR, Soldini L, Vidoni G, Mabellini C, Belloni T, Brignolo L, Negri S, Schlusnus K, Dorigatti F, Lazzarin A. Point-of-care testing for HCV infection: recent advances and implications for alternative screening. New Microbiol. 2014;37(4):449–547.
69. Schünemann HJ, Oxman AD, Brozek J, Glasziou P, Jaeschke R, Vist GE, Williams JW Jr, Kunz R, Craig J, Montori VM. Grading quality of evidence and strength of recommendations for diagnostic tests and strategies. BMJ (Clinical research ed). 2008;336(7653):1106–10.
70. Operskalski EA, Kovacs A. HIV/HCV Co-infection: Pathogenesis, Clinical Complications, Treatment, and New Therapeutic Technologies. Curr HIV/AIDS Rep. 2011;8:12.
71. Shepard CW, Finelli L, Alter MJ. Global epidemiology of hepatitis C virus infection. Lancet Infect Dis. 2005;5(9):558–67.
72. Leeflang MM, Moons KG, Reitsma JB, Zwinderman AH. Bias in sensitivity and specificity caused by data-driven selection of optimal cutoff values: mechanisms, magnitude, and solutions. Clin Chem. 2008;54(4):729–37.
73. Irwig L, Macaskill P, Glasziou P, Fahey M. Meta-analytic methods for diagnostic test accuracy. J Clin Epidemiol. 1995;48(1):119–30.
74. Rothstein HR, Sutton AJ, Borenstein M. Publication bias in meta-analysis: Prevention, assessment and adjustments. John Wiley & Sons; 2006.

10

Current challenges and possible solutions to improve access to care and treatment for hepatitis C infection in Vietnam

Alessandra Berto[1,2*], Jeremy Day[1,2], Nguyen Van Vinh Chau[3], Guy E. Thwaites[1,2], Ngoc Nghiem My[1], Stephen Baker[1,2,4] and Thomas C. Darton[1,5]

Abstract

Background: Hepatitis C infection is a major public health concern in low- and middle-income countries where an estimated 71.1 million individuals are living with chronic infection. The World Health Organization (WHO) has recently released new guidance for hepatitis C virus (HCV) treatment programs, which include improving the access to new direct-acting antiviral agents. In Vietnam, a highly populated middle-income country, the seroprevalence of HCV infection is approximately 4% and multiple genotypes co-circulate in the general population. Here we review what is currently known regarding the epidemiology of HCV in Vietnam and outline options for reducing the significant burden of morbidity and mortality in our setting.

Methods: We performed a systematic review of the currently available literature to evaluate what has been achieved to date with efforts to control HCV infection in Vietnam.

Results: This search retrieved few publications specific to Vietnam indicating a significant gap in baseline epidemiological and public health data. Key knowledge gaps identified included an understanding of the prevalence in specific high-risk groups, characterization of circulating HCV genotypes in the population and likely response to treatment, and the extent to which HCV treatment is available, accessed and utilized.

Conclusions: We conclude that there is an urgent need to perform up to date assessments of HCV disease burden in Vietnam, especially in high-risk groups, in whom incidence is high and cross infection with multiple genotypes is likely to be frequent. Coordinating renewed surveillance measures with forthcoming HCV treatment studies should initiate the traction required to achieve the WHO goal of eliminating HCV as a public health threat by 2030, at least in this region.

Keywords: Hepatitis C virus, Treatment access, Low and middle-income countries, Epidemiology, Vietnam

Background

Approximately 71.1 million people worldwide have chronic hepatitis C virus infection, resulting in over 500,000 deaths each year and creating a substantial burden on healthcare services [1–4]. The prevalence of hepatitis C infection is estimated to be 1%, although the highest burden (85%) of chronic infection is in low and middle income countries (LMICs) [1–4].

Hepatitis C virus (HCV), a single-stranded positive RNA virus, can cause individual infection with multiple subtypes, and therefore knowledge of viral genotype is particularly important for predicting virological and clinical treatment response. Genotype distribution varies geographically and is known to be particularly diverse in Southeast Asia [1].

Recently, the treatment options available for chronic hepatitis C infection have undergone a revolution with

* Correspondence: aberto@oucru.org
[1]Oxford University Clinical Research Unit, Vietnam Wellcome Trust Major Overseas Programme, 764 Vo Van Kiet, District 5, Ho Chi Minh City, Vietnam
[2]Centre for Tropical Medicine and Global Health, Nuffield Department of Clinical Medicine, University of Oxford, Oxford, UK
Full list of author information is available at the end of the article

development of the direct-acting antivirals (DAAs) [5]. Treatment regimes containing drugs from this new class have demonstrated significantly higher rates of sustained virological response (SVR) compared to standard interferon- (IFN) and ribavirin-focused regimes [6, 7]. Additional benefits of this class include shorter treatment durations, oral administration and fewer side-effects. It has been estimated that, with unrestricted access to these costly DAA-containing regimes, more than 90% of HCV infected patients could attain SVR and thus achieve a definitive cure [8].

In May 2016, the World Health Organisation (WHO) launched a new global strategy to eliminate viral hepatitis as public health threat by 2030 [9]. A key priority in these recommendations is to ensure open access to the DAAs [10]. However, individuals living in LMICs, are unlikely to be able to afford regimes containing these new costly treatments [10]. Ongoing efforts to ensure equity of access include the development of generic drug formulations [10, 11].

The Socialist Republic of Vietnam has a population exceeding 93 million people. Since the mid-1980s there have been dramatic improvements in the key development indicators of this Southeast Asian country, including increases in life expectancy, gross-domestic product and expanding state and private healthcare provision [12]. This includes a new national strategy to improve access to viral hepatitis diagnostic and treatment services [12]. To achieve the WHO stated goal of HCV elimination as a public health problem, understanding how the control of HCV in countries such as Vietnam could be improved, is vital. This article aims to review the currently available published literature regarding the epidemiology, virological features and the current treatment options available for hepatitis C infection in Vietnam. We use these data to propose measures which could help in reducing the burden of HCV infections in Vietnam.

Methods

Search strategy and selection criteria

We searched PubMed-, MEDLINE- and Embase®-indexed articles for English-Vietnamese languages articles in June 2016, according to the PRISMA guidelines (Fig. 1) [13].

Databases were searched using a combination of the following MeSH terms and keywords, including (Hepatitis C virus OR HCV) AND Vietnam AND (Prevalence OR Epidemiology OR Surve* OR Seroprevalence) (OR hepatitis C). No date restriction was used although included articles/data were restricted to original research articles relating to hepatitis C infection and HCV in Vietnam only, and on those published in either English or Vietnamese. We further searched the clinical trials registry *http:/ClinicalTrial.gov* for treatment trials

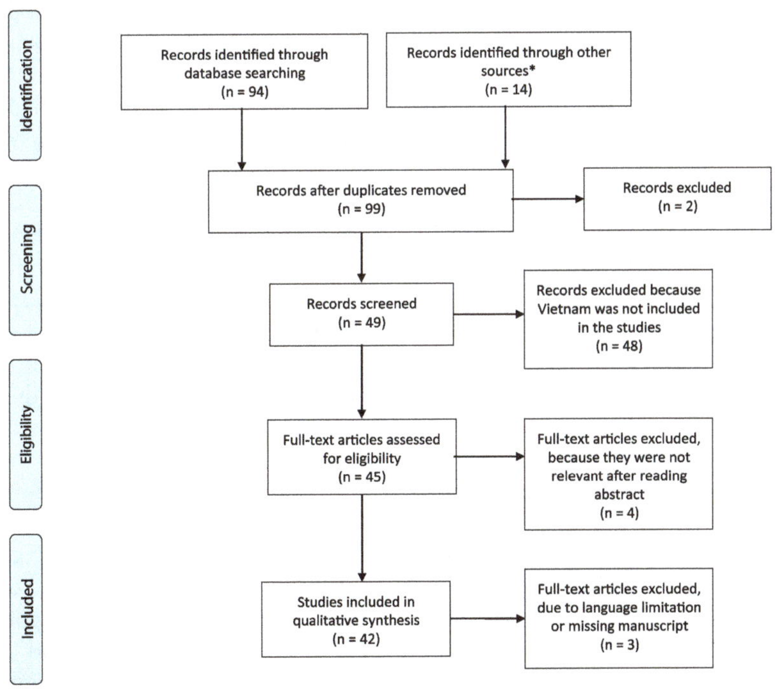

Fig. 1 Flow chart of studies included in data synthesis. * Other sources from which records were obtained include *Clinicaltrials.gov* (*n* = 9, see Table 2) and Standard Operating Procedures for the identification, diagnosis and management of Hepatitis C infection published in Vietnamese and identified through web searches (*n* = 5)

currently underway or completed in Vietnam using the search term "Hepatitis C" AND "Vietnam".

After performing the literature searches, one author (AB) extracted and screened the titles and abstracts before selecting and reviewing the full-text articles. The following data were extracted from each article: first author's name, publication year, country of origin, date of study, type of patient group, and additional details of epidemiology, seroprevalence, HCV RNA positivity figures, treatment availability etc.

Results

Search results

A total of 99 abstracts for manuscripts published between September 1990 and June 2016 were identified. Of these, 42 contained information relevant for our review and full texts were retrieved [11, 14–60] (Table 1 and Fig. 1). The majority of publications (73.8%, 31/42) assessed the prevalence of HCV infection specifically in high-risk groups, including HIV infected patients, injecting drug users (IDU), community sex workers (CSW), men that have sex with men (MSM) and renal haemodialysis patients [11, 17, 21–23, 25, 26, 28, 29, 31, 32, 34, 36, 37, 39, 41–47, 51–53, 55–60] (Table 1). Online search for Vietnamese articles retrieved one research publication and four Standard Operating Procedures (SOPs); only the Vietnamese research paper retrieved from a Vietnamese journal was included in this analysis [38].

Twenty one percent (9/42) of the publications reported data from Ho Chi Minh City (HCMC) or from the southern Vietnam region (Table 1), while 52.3% (22/42) reported studies conducted in the north of the country, principally in Hanoi and surrounding provinces [18, 22, 27, 32, 36, 47, 49, 52, 53] (Table 1). Eight of forty two retrieved publications characterized the diversity of HCV genotypes in Vietnam [14, 16, 21, 33, 34, 48, 50, 51] (Table 1). Two manuscripts were reviews assessing risk factors associated with HCV acquisition in Vietnam [11, 24]. One article, retrieved from a Vietnamese website assessed the prevalence of HCV in the Vietnamese ethnic minority [38].

Nine clinical trials were found registered with *ClinicalTrials.com* (see Table 2). Five out of nine were completed but no results have been published to-date, two are completed with results available, one is active but no recruiting, while one is actively recruiting (Fig. 1). Only the two clinical trials that had published results were included in the review, the remaining seven studies have been excluded.

The epidemiology of hepatitis C in Vietnam

In Vietnam, the background prevalence of HCV infection in the general population, at least historically, appears to vary depending on the region studied. In 1994 it was estimated that the seroprevalence in individuals without liver disease was 9% (43/491; 95% CI, 6.4%–11.5%) and 4% (18/511; 95% CI, 2.3%–5.6%) in HCMC and Hanoi, respectively [53] (Fig. 2). By 1998 it was estimated that in HCMC, the HCV seroprevalence in patients with underlying liver disease was 23% (69/289; 95% CI, 18.1%–27.8%) and in this population, HCV RNA was detectable in blood of 61% (42/69; 95% CI, 49.4%–72.5%) of the individuals [47]. This same study reported an HCV seroprevalence in healthy individuals in Da Lat (in the Southern Highlands) of 1% (9/890; 95% CI, 0.9%–1.0%); HCV RNA was detected in 44% (4/9) of these individuals [47]. Four years later in 2002, HCV RNA detection in HCMC was estimated to be 2% (2/100; 95% CI, 1.3%–5.3%) in apparently healthy individuals and 33% (45/234; 95% CI, 27.0%–39.0%) in patients with liver disease [15]. In Binh Thuan province (212 km northeast of HCMC) HCV seroprevalence in the general population between 2005 and 2007 was estimated to be 3.3% (17/509; 95% CI, 1.7%–4.8%); the male population exhibited a higher burden of seropositive samples (3.3%) than women (1.8%), and HCV RNA was detected in 52.9% (9/17) of the identified anti-HCV positive individuals (Fig. 2) [30]. Furthermore, one article was retrieved from a Vietnamese journal. The original manuscript was in Vietnamese and only the abstract was translated in English. The manuscript assessed the seroprevalence of HCV in the Vietnamese ethnic minority in the north of Vietnam and the detected seroprevalence in 1305 individuals was 1.22% (95% CI, 0.6%–1.7%) in 2011 [38].

The majority of the remaining publications evaluated HCV prevalence in specific high-risk groups (Table 1). These data estimated that 89% (1255/1434; 95% CI, 87.3%–90.6%) of IDU in Nguyen province (Northern Vietnam) were HCV RNA positive between 2005 and 2007 and 35% (502/1434; 95% CI, 32.5%-37.4) were HIV/HCV co-infected [29]. Similar figures were reported in Hai Phong province (northern Vietnam) in 2014 (Fig. 2), where the prevalence of HCV in HIV-infected individual was 89.4% (93/104; 95% CI, 82.1%–96.6%). This study also reported that the majority of HCV cases presented with clinical features of advanced liver fibrosis and cirrhosis [26].

Between 2005 and 2012, several studies were conducted around Vietnam (including HCMC, Hanoi, Hai Phong Province, Da Nang, Khanh Hoa Province and Can Tho), which aimed to determine HCV seroprevalence in patients undergoing renal haemodialysis or receiving multiple blood transfusions [23, 37]. These six hospital-based studies found an apparent iatrogenic HCV seroprevalence of 26% (n = 153/575; 95% CI, 22.4%–29.5%) and was similar at all sites assessed.

Table 1 Characteristics population-based studies reporting prevalence of HCV in Vietnam

Year	First Author	Prevalence	Group Type	Sample Size	Reference
1998	Kakumu	1%	General Population	1179	[47]
2007	Nguyen	1%	General Population	837	[45]
2015	Quesada	4.7%	General Population	27/571	[27]
2015	Do	3.3% 1.3%*	General population	509	[30]
2003	Tran	2%	General population	334	[15]
1996	Corwin	2%	General population	188	[49]
2012	Sereno	0.38–4.3%	General population	NA[b]	[21]
2016	Martinello	42.5%	HIV	89.452[a]	[24]
2015	Nadol	53.3%	HIV/IDU	3010	[32]
2015	Zang	88%	HIV	1434	[29]
1999	Follézou	>80%	HIV	280	[18]
2012	Durier	22.9%	HIV	110	[20]
2016	Nguyen	89%	HIV	104	[26]
2016	Hser	74%	HIV/IDU	NA[b, c]	[11]
2012	Sereno	95.8%	HIV/IDU	NA[b]	[21]
2012	Gish	87%	IDU	NA[b]	[36]
1998	Kakumu	47%	Liver Disease	1179	[47]
2003	Tran	10%	Liver disease	334	[15]
1996	Corwin	10%	Liver Disease	188	[49]
2004	Buchy	9%	Liver disease	45	[46]
2012	Gish	23%	Liver disease	NA[b]	[36]
1993	Cordier	2%	Hepatocarcinoma	152	[54]
2010	Bjoerkvoll	12.7%	Blood donors	1305	[38]
2012	Viet	76.4%	Blood Donors	1200[a]	[40]
1994	Song	20.6%	Blood Donors	491	[52]
2012	Dunford	26.6%	Dialysis	8652[a]	[37]
2016	Duong	8%	Dialysis	142	[22]
2015	Duong	6%	Dialysis	113	[31]
2012	Gish	54%	Hemodialysis	NA[b]	[36]
2016	Nadol	28.4%	MSM	1588	[25]
2012	Dunford	8.7%	CSW	8652[a]	[37]

*Presence of HCV RNA
[a]Multi countries study
[b]*NA* Not applicable
[c]Estimate

In 2010, a study estimated the prevalence of HCV infection in MSM in the south of Vietnam (Can Tho and HCMC) and in the north of Vietnam (Hai Phong Province and Hanoi) [25]. The overall seroprevalence of infection in 1588 male participants was 28.4% (95% CI, 26.1%–30.6%) [25]; 29% of the individuals were co-infected with HIV and more northerly regions observed a higher HCV and HCV/HIV co-infection prevalence [25]. A single publication from 1997 assessed the frequency of HCV infection in patients with chronic hepatitis in HCMC, and concluded that HCV was the underlying etiology in 19–27% of chronic hepatitis cases [19]. However, no indication of the sample size used to derive this estimate was provided.

The molecular epidemiology of HCV in Vietnam

A study conducted in four major conurbations in Vietnam – Hanoi, Hai Phong Province, Da Nang, Khanh Hoa Province and Can Tho, identified HCV genotypes 1, 6, 3 and 2 in 59.9% (n = 169), 37.9% (n = 107), 1.8% (n = 5) and 0.4% (n = 1) of samples collected from mixed healthy and high-risk populations, respectively

Table 2 List of the clinical trials conducted in Vietnam to date [a]

Year	Title	City	Sponsor	Status
2010–2016	Hepatic Safety of Raltegravir Versus Efavirenz as HIV Therapy for Patients With HIV and HCV Coinfection	Ho Chi Minh City, Hai Phong	University of Hawaii	Active, not recruiting
2014–2016	The Study of Safety, Pharmacokinetics, Pharmacodynamics of Peglamda (Peginterferon Lamda 1) on Healthy Volunteers and the Preliminary Evaluation of Peglamda and Hepasig (Ribavirin) Treatment's Effects on Chronic Hepatitis C Patients	Unknown	Nanogen Pharmaceutical Biotechnology Co., Ltd	Completed
2015–2016	Feasibility of Interventions on People Who Inject Drugs in Vietnam			
	Implementation of a Sexual Health Intervention for Young Men Who Have Sex With Men (MSM) in Two Vietnamese Cities	Ho Chi Minh City, Hanoi	Inserm-ANRS	Completed
2013–2016	HCV Treatment in HIV Co-Infected Patients in Asia	Hanoi	amfAR,	Completed
2016	Long Term Follow-up Study to Assess Durability of Sustained Virologic Response in Alisporivir-treated Hepatitis C Patients	Unknown	Debiopharm International SA	Completed, has results
2011–2016	Efficacy and Safety of Alisporivir Triple Therapy in Chronic Hepatitis C Genotype 1 Treatment-naïve Participants	Unknown	Debiopharm International SA	Completed, has results
2016–2017	Efficacy and Safety of Sofosbuvir/Velpatasvir Fixed Dose Combination for 12 Weeks in Participants With Chronic HCV	Unknown	Gilead Sciences	Recruiting
2015	3-year Follow-up Study to Assess the Viral Activity in Hepatitis C Patients Who Failed Feeder DEB025/Alisporivir Study		Novartis Pharmaceuticals	Completed
2014–2016	Implementation of a Sexual Health Intervention for Young Men Who Have Sex With Men (MSM) in Two Vietnamese Cities	Hanoi	National Development and Research Institutes, Inc.	Completed

[a]For further details please see the following website: ClinicalTrials.gov

[37]. While genotype 1 was the most prevalent HCV genotype in all four areas, the genotype distribution ranged from 47% in Khanh Hoa Province to 81% in Da Nang [37]. These four genotypes (1–3, 6, and) were identified in dialysis and multi-transfused individuals with nine recognized subtypes (1a, 1b, 2a, 3a, 3b, 6a, 6e, 6 h, 6 l) [39]. A further study similarly identified HCV genotype 1 as the predominant virus circulating in MSM in Hanoi, Hai Phong Province, HCMC and Can Tho [25]. Additionally, plasma samples from 97 HCV infected individuals were molecularly characterized between 2003 and 2010 in HCMC. The RNA sequences obtained from these samples suggested that genotypes 1b and 2a were imported from East Asia, 1a from the United States, 2i, 2j and 2 m imported from France [33, 58]. They also identified an additional 4 subtypes of genotype 6 (6a, 6ax, 6xb and 6xc) with no obvious international link [34].

Clinical trials

Of the nine trials registered on *ClinicalTrials.gov*, only two had published results available at time of review [61, 62]. Both studies were sponsored by Debiopharm International SA and neither the source country information nor the locations where trial participant recruitment was performed within the country have been specified. Both studies were multicenter international trials to assess the treatment responses (SVR to single agent or combination treatment) to the synthetic cyclosporine-like agent, Alisporivir, a novel host-targeting antiviral (HTA) agent [61, 62].

Discussion

Our literature search identified a paucity of published data regarding the nature or burden of HCV infection in Vietnam. Studies in the publications identified were generally conducted in high-risk populations and focused in the more populous northern provinces (around Hanoi) and southern provinces (around HCMC) of the country. In addition, most studies have measured HCV antibody seroprevalence rather than HCV RNA prevalence, which would more reliably indicate the numbers of individuals with active infection. As elsewhere, the available literature suggested that blood transfusions, intravenous drug use, and unsafe therapeutic injections were a likely common source of HCV infection in the Vietnamese populations studied. Furthermore, the data suggests while the HCV seroprevalence in the general population is approximately 4% (18/511; 95% CI, 2.3%–5.6%) in Hanoi and 9% (43/491; 95% CI, 6.4%–11.5%) in Ho Chi Minh City, which is high in comparison to America or Europe [63, 64], this is likely to be even higher in IDU (55.6%, n = 556/1000; 95% CI, 52.8%–58.3%), MSM (38.8%; n = 1558; 95% CI, 36.3%–41.2%), and hemodialysis patients (26.6%, n = 153/575; 95% CI, 22.4%–29.5%) [23, 31, 53, 57] . There are still substantial gaps in our understanding of the molecular epidemiology of HCV infection in Vietnam, however the limited findings from the few studies that have been conducted suggest that multiple (≥4) HCV genotypes and subtypes are circulating in the population [25, 37].

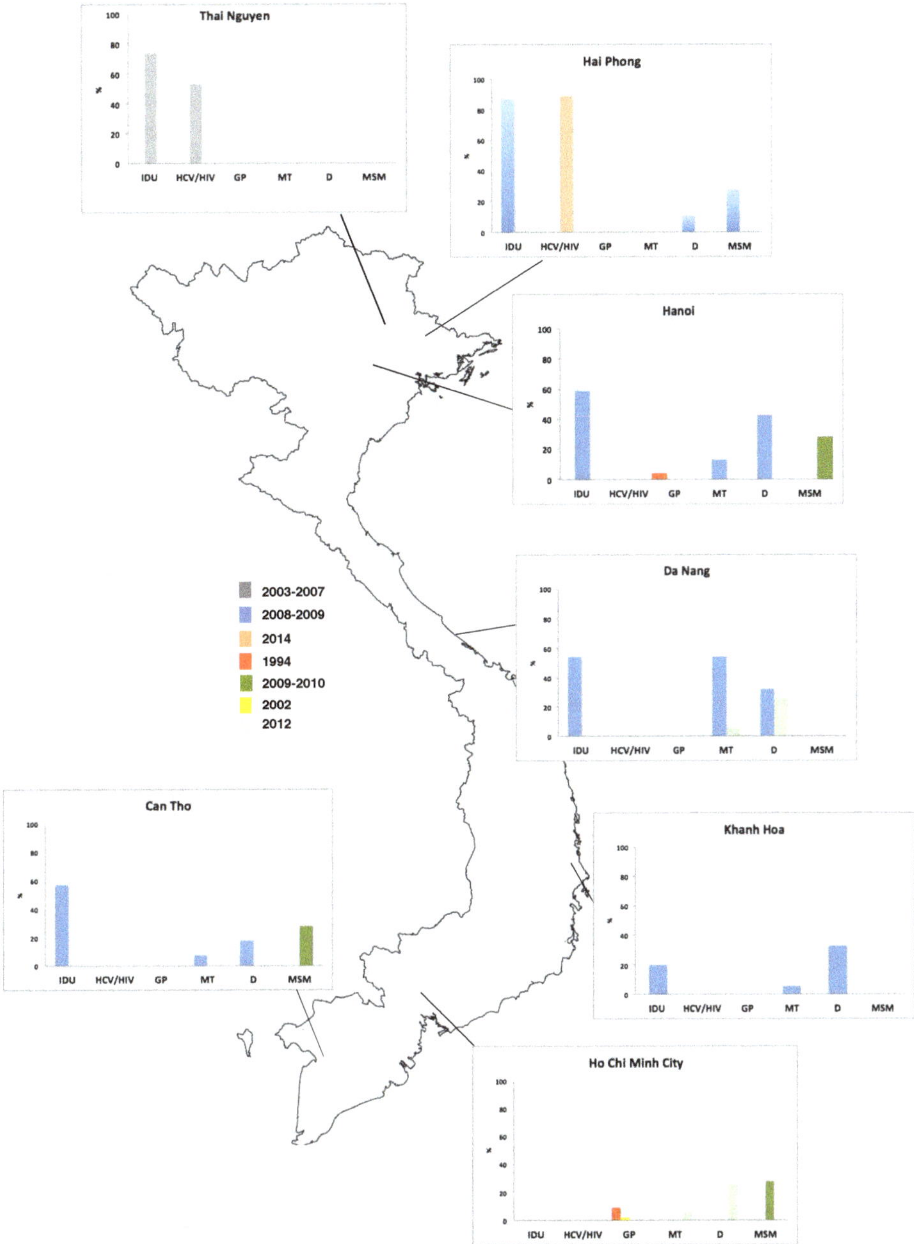

Fig. 2 Vietnam Map and summary of the main studies conducted so farA summary of the main studies performed in Vietnam to-date measuring the prevalence of HCV viral detection (PCR positivity) in selected populations by year of study publication and geographic location. * Data for 'General adult healthy populations' is for measured anti-HCV antibody seroprevalence. The map represents the location where the main studies have been conducted and summarized the HCV prevalence or seroprevalence observed during the studies in different groups, such as IDU, MSM, liver disease, hemodialysis and multi-blood transfusion and general population

Ascertaining the burden of hepatitis C in Vietnam

Ascertaining the true likely burden of infection in Vietnam would facilitate advocacy for the implementation of disease specific strategies and guidelines, and provide useful baseline data for further epidemiological measurements. Our search identified that HCV seroprevalence in the population may be high (1–4%) compared to other countries in the region [3, 27, 53]. For example, several large-scale seroprevalence studies have reported HCV estimates of asymptomatic Chinese ranging from 0.39 to 3.2% depending of the region [65]. Other Asian countries such as Japan, India or Indonesia reported an HCV seroprevalence of between 2.3, 0.9 and 2.1% respectively [4].

Observations supporting the speculation that the true seroprevalence might be underestimated include data from neighboring countries such as China, where the reported rate of HCV infections increased more than 10-fold (from 21,000 reported cases/year to 210,000 reported cases/year) between 2003 and 2011 [66]. Reasons for this increase may include an increase in life expectancy and/or the increased detection/occurrence of new infections due to better surveillance and improved diagnostics. The ageing of the population creates two potentially major pressures on health care finances: increased utilization of health services and decreased revenues (as a declining share of the population is economically active).

Further insights into the current HCV situation in Vietnam may be provided by two non-resident populations; data on HCV infection in USA veterans after the Vietnam/American war suggest that returning veterans had a higher risk (10–17%) of being HCV infected than the general North American population (1.3%) [63, 64, 67]. This conflict was associated with the highest rate of HCV acquisition in comparison to any that the US has been engaged in. More recently, it was observed that Vietnamese migrants to other countries have a higher prevalence (5.8%) of HCV infection when compared to the autochthonous population (1.3%) [60, 68].

The transmission of HCV infection in clinical settings is still particularly concerning in Vietnamese healthcare facilities; the high HCV prevalence (26%) in haemodialysis patients [23, 31, 57] has not been observed in other Asian-Pacific countries (0.7–18.1%) [69]. This literature review also found a high seroprevalence (27%) in other high-risk populations including IDU, MSM, and CSW, similar data has been reported from studies conducted between the Myanmar and Chinese border region [70].

We therefore speculate that the seroprevalence in the general population might be higher than that currently estimated as the limited data currently available (only 42 publications published in over two decades) is from studies performed in only a few locations across Vietnam and which mostly had relatively small sample sizes upon which to base these calculations. Of note, the two most recent and larger studies performed to estimate seroprevalence in the general population have found an HCV prevalence of 3.3 and 4.7%, respectively [27, 30].

Identifying the genetic characteristics of HCV to improve public health

In addition to assessing the burden of HCV disease, further data is required regarding HCV genotype, viral mutations and viral loads in HCV infected patients in order to assess how to implement the recent HCV treatment guidance, and to estimate the cost-benefit of an integrated HCV control program.

While currently available data are limited, they imply a broad genetic diversity within circulating HCV strains in all parts of the country [33, 34, 37, 39, 58]. More detailed phylogenetic approaches have proposed that the HCV population has been influenced by the international turmoil of the past, with importation of genotypes that are more typically associated with North America, Europe and other parts of Asia [34]. This genetic variation can also be observed in high-risk groups, meaning that the formation of a local treatment policy may be more complex than in other locations. For example, the distribution of HCV genotype in haemodialysis patients is variable according to the geographical region, this may be due to a lack of infection control and or point source outbreaks [37]. This genotype distribution is in contrast to other countries in Asia, such as China, where hemodialysis patients are predominantly affected by genotype 2 HCV [71, 72]. An improved understanding of the genotype distribution and frequency of viral treatment mutations among Vietnamese patients will facilitate the development of appropriate local guidelines.

Current treatment options, molecular challenges and social taboos

Early diagnosis and access to treatment are essential components for an effective HCV control program in Vietnam. As in most LMICs, current treatment for HCV infection in Vietnam is limited to interferon-based (IFN-gamma and pegylated-IFN) therapy [10]. More recently, some patients have been treated with newer DAA agents at the Hospital for Tropical Diseases (HTD) in HCMC, where more than 18,000 patients with viral hepatitis are assessed each year. Further clinical treatment studies have received funding and are planned to commence in the near future [73].

The more widespread introduction of the DAAs is hindered by a lack of data regarding HCV genotype distribution and viral treatment mutations [74]. This lack of data is especially problematic for the early detection of treatment resistance mutations, which occurred previously with hepatitis B treatment and HCV treatment in Japan and North America [75–77]. Furthermore, the efficacy of DAAs against some of the less common genotypes, such as genotype 6 which was frequently identified in previously studies, is not well established [78].

Other barriers to increasing the utilization of HCV treatment in resource-limited settings such as Vietnam include high costs, a perceived complexity in treatment regimes and bureaucratic support for importation, licensing and distribution of medicines for which specific clinical trial data in the local populations is lacking. Vietnam is a rapidly developing country, whose GDP per-capita has increased from $1095 to $1684 from 2004 until 2014 [79]. However, the per capita income remains low (~ $1024) [80] with limited annual spending on healthcare (according to WHO, approximately $264 in 2006) [80]. A large proportion of people in Vietnam do not invest in health insurance and even those who do may not have full coverage to expensive treatment courses: pegylated-interferon courses are reimbursed at 30% ($10,000–18,000 for a 48 week treatmentcourse), and this partial reimbursement is based on doctor opinion only, with no allowance given for those in high-risk populations such as haemodialysis patients [81, 82].

While the treatment of HCV infection requires prescription from a medical practitioner, a further concern is the non-completion of treatment courses due to high costs and changes in family/patient financial circumstances. Some patients may also travel to other countries in the region where medications, which may be substandard, might be more affordable. Incomplete or inadequate treatment courses are likely to lead to increased rates of viral resistance, which has been previously widely observed in hepatitis B treatment programs in Vietnam [83, 84]. Further, PEG + INF + RBV remains (as 2016) the first line of therapy for chronic patients in many part of Asia, Vietnam included [85].

Study limitations

The majority of the studies included here had small sample sizes and concentrated on groups of individuals at known high-risk of acquiring HCV infection thus risking an overestimation bias. Given the heterogeneity of the study populations sampled, in addition to the broad time period and diverse geographic locations described, more accurate meta-analysis is not currently feasible. Thus, a considerable knowledge gap remains regarding the likely true burden of chronic HCV infection in the general, healthy adult Vietnamese population.

Conclusions

Relatively little is known regarding the burden of HCV infection in the general population in Vietnam. Available data suggest that the seroprevalence could be higher than previously assumed, especially in known high-risk groups such as patients undergoing haemodialysis. Limited data predict a broad distribution of HCV genotypes and, to-date, very few HCV treatment trials have been performed in Vietnam. While HCV control programs in Vietnam are in their infancy, there is an urgent need for more detailed disease burden and viral genotyping data, which, in addition to planned treatment studies, could be used to inform the development of local HCV treatment strategies and thus eventual attainment of the 2030 elimination target.

Abbreviations

HCV: Hepatitis C virus; DAA: Direct acting anti-viral; HTD: Hospital for Tropical Diseases; HCMC: Ho Chi Minh City; IFN: Interferon-based; LMIC: Low to middle income countries; WHO: World Health organization; IDU: Injecting drug users; MSM: Men that have sex with men; CSW: Commercial sex workers; SVR: Sustained virological response

Funding

No funding was used for this manuscript.

Authors' contributions

AB performed the literature search and wrote the draft manuscript. TD made substantial contributions to conception and design; JD, SB and GET contributed with study revision and gave final approval. NG helped to retrieve data from HTD hospital. All authors contributed to this paper with revision editing, and final approval.

Competing interests

The authors declare that they have no competing interests.

Consent for publication

"Not applicable".

Author details

[1]Oxford University Clinical Research Unit, Vietnam Wellcome Trust Major Overseas Programme, 764 Vo Van Kiet, District 5, Ho Chi Minh City, Vietnam. [2]Centre for Tropical Medicine and Global Health, Nuffield Department of Clinical Medicine, University of Oxford, Oxford, UK. [3]Hospital for Tropical Diseases, Ho Chi Minh City, Vietnam. [4]The London School of Hygiene and Tropical Medicine, London, UK. [5]Department of Infection, Immunity and Cardiovascular Disease, University of Sheffield, Sheffield, UK.

References

1. Gower E, Estes C, Blach S, Razavi-Shearer K, Razavi H. Global epidemiology and genotype distribution of the hepatitis C virus infection. J Hepatol. 2014; 61(1 Suppl):S45–57.
2. Simmonds P. Genetic diversity and evolution of hepatitis C virus–15 years on. J Gen Virol. 2004;85(Pt 11):3173–88.
3. Blach S, Zeuzem S, Manns M, Altraif I, Duberg A-S, Muljono DH, et al. Global prevalence and genotype distribution of hepatitis C virus infection in 2015: a modelling study. Lancet Gastroenterol Hepatol. 2016;2(3):161–76.
4. Shepard CW, Finelli L, Alter MJ. Global epidemiology of hepatitis C virus infection. Lancet Infect Dis. 2005;5(9):558–67.
5. Poordad F, Dieterich D. Treating hepatitis C: current standard of care and emerging direct-acting antiviral agents. J Viral Hepat. 2012;19(7):449–64.
6. Jacobson IM, McHutchison JG, Dusheiko G, Di Bisceglie AM, Reddy KR, Bzowej NH, et al. Telaprevir for previously untreated chronic hepatitis C virus infection. N Engl J Med. 2011;364(25):2405–16.
7. Poordad F, McCone JJ, Bacon BR, Bruno S, Manns MP, Sulkowski MS, et al. Boceprevir for untreated chronic HCV genotype 1 infection. N Engl J Med. 2011;364(13):1195–206.
8. Hezode C, Bronowicki JP. Ideal oral combinations to eradicate HCV: the role of ribavirin. J Hepatol. 2016;64(1):215–25.
9. WHO. Combating hepatitis B and C to reach elimination by 2030. World Health Organisation; 2016.
10. World Health Organization. Guidelines for the screening, care and treatment of persons with hepatitis C infection; 2016. p. 1–135.
11. Hser Y-I, Liang D, Lan Y-C, Vicknasingam BK, Chakrabarti A. Drug abuse, HIV, and HCV in Asian countries. J NeuroImmune Pharmacol. 2016;11:383.
12. Ministry of Health. Plan of preventing viral Hepatits Deseases in Vietnam 2015–2019. 2015.
13. Moher D, Liberati A, Tetzlaff J, Altman DG. Preferred reporting items for systematic reviews and meta-analyses: the PRISMA statement. PLoS Med. 2009;6(7):e1000097.

14. Nakano T, Lu L, Liu P, Pybus OG. Viral gene sequences reveal the variable history of hepatitis C virus infection among countries. J Infect Dis. 2004; 190(6):1098–108.
15. Tran HT-T, Ushijima H, Quang VX, Phuong N, Li TC, Hayashi S, et al. Prevalence of hepatitis virus types B through E and genotypic distribution of HBV and HCV in ho chi Minh City. Vietnam Hepatol Res. 2003;26(4):275–80.
16. Tran HT-T, Ushijima H, Ngoc TT, Ha LD, Hayashi S, Sata T, et al. Recombination of genotypes B and C in hepatitis B virus isolated from a Vietnamese patient with fulminant hepatitis. Jpn J Infect Dis. 2003;56(1):35–7.
17. Nerurkar VR, Woodward CL, Nguyen HT, DeWolfe MF, Tashima LT, Zalles-Ganley A, et al. Lack of association between acquisition of TT virus and risk behavior for HIV and HCV infection in Vietnam. Int J Infect Dis. 1999;3(4):181–5.
18. Follezou JY, Lan NY, Lien TX, Lafon ME, Tram LT, Hung PV, et al. Clinical and biological characteristics of human immunodeficiency virus-infected and uninfected intravascular drug users in ho chi Minh City, Vietnam. AmJTrop Med Hyg. 1999;61(3):420–4.
19. Ha MV. Some peculiarities of hepatobiliary diseases in Vietnam. J Gastroenterol Hepatol. 1997;12(5):S15–8.
20. Durier N, Nguyen C, White LJ. Treatment of hepatitis C as prevention: a modeling case study in Vietnam. PLoS One. 2012;7(4):e34548.
21. Sereno L, Mesquita F, Kato M, Jacka D, Van Nguyen TT, Nguyen TN. Epidemiology, responses, and way forward: the silent epidemic of viral hepatitis and HIV coinfection in Vietnam. J Int Assoc Physicians AIDS Care (Chic). 2012;11(5):311–20.
22. Duong CM, Olszyna DP, Nguyen PD, ML ML. Challenges of hemodialysis in Vietnam: experience from the first standardized district dialysis unit in ho chi Minh City. BMC Nephrol. 2015;16:122.
23. Duong CM, McLaws M-L. An investigation of an outbreak of hepatitis C virus infections in a low-resourced hemodialysis unit in Vietnam. Am J Infect Control. 2016;44(5):560–6.
24. Martinello M, Amin J, Matthews GV, Dore GJ. Prevalence and disease burden of HCV Coinfection in HIV cohorts in the Asia Pacific region: a systematic review and meta-analysis. AIDS Rev. 2016;18(2):68–80.
25. Nadol P, O'Connor S, Duong H, Mixson-Hayden T, Tram TH, Xia G-L, et al. High hepatitis C virus (HCV) prevalence among men who have sex with men (MSM) in Vietnam and associated risk factors: 2010 Vietnam Integrated Behavioural and Biologic Cross-Sectional Survey. Sex Transm Infect. 2016.
26. Nguyen Truong T, Laureillard D, Lacombe K, Duong Thi H, Pham Thi Hanh P, Truong Thi Xuan L, et al. High proportion of HIV-HCV Coinfected patients with advanced liver fibrosis requiring hepatitis C treatment in Haiphong, northern Vietnam (ANRS 12262). PLoS One. 2016;11(5):e0153744.
27. Quesada P, Whitby D, Benavente Y, Miley W, Labo N, Chichareon S, et al. Hepatitis C virus seroprevalence in the general female population from 8 countries. J Clin Virol. 2015;68:89–93.
28. Wasitthankasem R, Vongpunsawad S, Siripon N, Suya C, Chulothok P, Chaiear K, et al. Genotypic distribution of hepatitis C virus in Thailand and Southeast Asia. PLoS One. 2015;10(5):e0126764.
29. Zhang L, Celentano DD, Le Minh N, Latkin CA, Mehta SH, Frangakis C, et al. Prevalence and correlates of HCV monoinfection and HIV and HCV coinfection among persons who inject drugs in Vietnam. Eur J Gastroenterol Hepatol. 2015;27(5):550–6.
30. Do SH, Yamada H, Fujimoto M, Ohisa M, Matsuo J, Akita T, et al. High prevalences of hepatitis B and C virus infections among adults living in Binh Thuan province, Vietnam. Hepatol Res. 2015;45(3):259–68.
31. Duong CM, Olszyna DP, ML ML. Hepatitis B and C virus infections among patients with end stage renal disease in a low-resourced hemodialysis center in Vietnam: a cross-sectional study. BMC Public Health. 2015;15:192.
32. Nadol P, O'connor S, Duong H, Le L-VN, Thang PH, Tram TH, et al. Findings from integrated behavioral and biologic survey among males who inject drugs (MWID) - Vietnam, 2009-2010: evidence of the need for an integrated response to HIV, hepatitis B virus, and hepatitis C virus. PLoS One. 2015; 10(2):e0118304.
33. Li C, Yuan M, Lu L, Lu T, Xia W, Pham VH, et al. The genetic diversity and evolutionary history of hepatitis C virus in Vietnam. Virology. 2014;468–470:197–206.
34. Li C, Pham VH, Abe K, Lu L. Nine additional complete genome sequences of HCV genotype 6 from Vietnam including new subtypes 6xb and 6xc. Virology. 2014;468–470:172–7.
35. Viet L, Lan NTN, Ty PX, Bjorkvoll B, Hoel H, Gutteberg T, et al. Prevalence of hepatitis B & hepatitis C virus infections in potential blood donors in rural Vietnam. Indian J Med Res. 2012;136(1):74–81.
36. Gish RG, Bui TD, Nguyen CTK, Nguyen DT, Tran HV, Tran DMT, et al. Liver disease in Viet Nam: screening, surveillance, management and education: a 5-year plan and call to action. J Gastroenterol Hepatol. 2012;27(2):238–47.
37. Dunford L, Carr MJ, Dean J, Waters A, Nguyen LT, Ta Thi TH, et al. Hepatitis C virus in vietnam: high prevalence of infection in dialysis and multi-transfused patients involving diverse and novel virus variants. PLoS One. 2012;7(8):1–10.
38. Nguyễn ThịLan Anh, Dương ThịThu Thủy, Nguyễn Thùy Linh Bùi ThịLan Anh, Nguyễn Tuấn Nghĩa NTH. Tình trạng nhiễm vi rút viêm gan B và Cởcộng đồng dân tộc thiểu sốxã MỏVàng, huyện Văn Yên, tỉnh Yên Bái. Vietnamese J Prev Med. 2013;49(147):1.
39. Pham VH, Nguyen HDP, Ho PT, Banh DV, Pham HLT, Pham PH, et al. Very high prevalence of hepatitis C virus genotype 6 variants in southern Vietnam: large-scale survey based on sequence determination. Jpn J Infect Dis. 2011;64(6):537–9.
40. Bjoerkvoll B, Viet L, Ol HS, Lan NTN, Sothy S, Hoel H, et al. Screening test accuracy among potential blood donors of HBsAg, anti-HBc and anti-HCV to detect hepatitis B and C virus infection in rural Cambodia and Vietnam. Southeast Asian J Trop Med Public Health. 2010;41(5):1127–35.
41. Tanimoto T, Nguyen HC, Ishizaki A, Chung PTT, Hoang TTH, Nguyen VT, et al. Multiple routes of hepatitis C virus transmission among injection drug users in Hai Phong, northern Vietnam. J Med Virol. 2010;82(8):1355–63.
42. Clatts MC, Colon-Lopez V, Giang LM, Goldsamt LA. Prevalence and incidence of HCV infection among Vietnam heroin users with recent onset of injection. J Urban Health. 2010;87(2):278–91.
43. Pham DA, Leuangwutiwong P, Jittmittraphap A, Luplertlop N, Bach HK, Akkarathamrongsin S, et al. High prevalence of hepatitis C virus genotype 6 in Vietnam. Asian Pac J Allergy Immunol. 2009;27(2–3):153–60.
44. Quan VM, Go VF, Nam L Van, Bergenstrom A, Thuoc NP, Zenilman J, et al. Risks for HIV, HBV, and HCV infections among male injection drug users in northern Vietnam: a case-control study. AIDS Care; 2009;21(1):7–16.
45. Nguyen VTT, McLaws M-L, Dore GJ. Prevalence and risk factors for hepatitis C infection in rural north Vietnam. Hepatol Int. 2007;1(3):387–93.
46. Buchy P, Monchy D, An TTN, Srey CT, Tri DV, Son S, et al. Prevalence of hepatitis a, B, C and E virus markers among patients with elevated levels of Alanine aminotransferase and Aspartate aminotransferase in Phnom Penh (Cambodia) and Nha Trang (Central Vietnam). Bull Soc Pathol Exot. 2004; 97(3):165–71. Article in Russian
47. Kakumu S, Sato K, Morishita T, Trinh KA, Nguyen HB, Banh VD, et al. Prevalence of hepatitis B, hepatitis C, and GB virus C/hepatitis G virus infections in liver disease patients and inhabitants in ho chi Minh, Vietnam. J Med Virol. 1998;54(4):243–8.
48. Simmonds P, Mellor J, Sakuldamrongpanich T, Nuchaprayoon C, Tanprasert S, Holmes EC, et al. Evolutionary analysis of variants of hepatitis C virus found in South-East Asia: comparison with classifications based upon sequence similarity. J Gen Virol. 1996 Dec;77(Pt 12):3013–24.
49. Corwin AL, Dai TC, Duc DD, Suu PI, Van NT, Ha LD, et al. Acute viral hepatitis in Hanoi, Viet Nam. Trans R Soc Trop Med Hyg. 1996;90(6):647–8.
50. Mellor J, Walsh EA, Prescott LE, Jarvis LM, Davidson F, Yap PL, et al. Survey of type 6 group variants of hepatitis C virus in Southeast Asia by using a core-based genotyping assay. J Clin Microbiol. 1996;34(2):417–23.
51. Tokita H, Okamoto H, Tsuda F, Song P, Nakata S, Chosa T, et al. Hepatitis C virus variants from Vietnam are classifiable into the seventh, eighth, and ninth major genetic groups. Proc Natl Acad Sci U S A. 1994;91(23):11022–6.
52. Song P, Duc DD, Hien B, Nakata S, Chosa T, Watanabe J, et al. Markers of hepatitis C and B virus infections among blood donors in ho chi Minh City and Hanoi, Vietnam. Clin Diagn Lab Immunol. 1994;1(4):413–8.
53. Nakata S, Song P, Duc DD, Nguyen XQ, Murata K, Tsuda F, et al. Hepatitis C and B virus infections in populations at low or high risk in ho chi Minh and Hanoi, Vietnam. J Gastroenterol Hepatol. 1994;9(4):416–9.
54. Cordier S, Le TB, Verger P, Bard D, Le CD, Larouze B, et al. Viral infections and chemical exposures as risk factors for hepatocellular carcinoma in Vietnam. Int J Cancer. 1993;55(2):196–201.
55. Toan NL, Song LH, Kremsner PG, Duy DN, Binh VQ, Koeberlein B, et al. Impact of the hepatitis B virus genotype and genotype mixtures on the course of liver disease in Vietnam. Hepatology. 2006;43(6):1375–84.
56. Phung TBT, Alestig E, Nguyen TL, Hannoun C, Lindh M. Genotype X/C recombinant (putative genotype I) of hepatitis B virus is rare in Hanoi, Vietnam-genotypes B4 and C1 predominate. J Med Virol. 2010;82(8):1327–33.

57. Dunford L, Carr MJ, Dean J, Waters A, Nguyen LT, Ta Thi TH, et al. Hepatitis C virus in Vietnam: high prevalence of infection in dialysis and multi-transfused patients involving diverse and novel virus variants. PLoS One. 2012;7(8):e41266.
58. Fu Y, Qin W, Cao H, Xu R, Tan Y, Lu T, et al. HCV 6a prevalence in Guangdong province had the origin from Vietnam and recent dissemination to other regions of China: phylogeographic analyses. PLoS One. 2012;7(1):e28006.
59. Sy BT, Nguyen HM, Toan NL, Song LH, Tong HV, Wolboldt C, et al. Identification of a natural intergenotypic recombinant hepatitis delta virus genotype 1 and 2 in Vietnamese HBsAg-positive patients. J Viral Hepat. 2015;22(1):55–63.
60. Caruana S, Bowden S, Kelly H. Transmission of HCV in the Vietnamese community. Aust N Z J Public Health. 2001;25:276.
61. ClinicalTrails.gov. No Title. Efficacy and Safety of Alisporivir Triple Therapy in Chronic Hepatitis C Genotype 1 Treatment-naïve Participants. 2016.
62. ClinicalTrials.gov. No Title. Long Term Follow-up Study to Assess Durability of Sustained Virologic Response in Alisporivir-treated Hepatitis C Patients. 2016.
63. Zuniga IA, Chen JJ, Lane DS, Allmer J, Jimenez-Lucho VE. Analysis of a hepatitis C screening programme for US veterans. Epidemiol Infect. 2006; 134(2):249–57.
64. Roselle GA, Danko LH, Kralovic SM, Simbartl LA, Kizer KW. National Hepatitis C Surveillance day in the veterans health Administration of the Department of veterans affairs. Mil Med. 2002;167(9):756–9.
65. Qin Q, Smith MK, Wang L, Su Y, Wang L, Guo W, et al. Hepatitis C virus infection in China: an emerging public health issue. J Viral Hepat. 2015;22(3): 238–44.
66. Duan Z, Jia J-D, Hou J, Lou L, Tobias H, Xu XY, et al. Current challenges and the management of chronic hepatitis C in mainland China. J Clin Gastroenterol. 2014;48(8):679–86.
67. Brau N, Bini EJ, Shahidi A, Aytaman A, Xiao P, Stancic S, et al. Prevalence of hepatitis C and coinfection with HIV among United States veterans in the new York City metropolitan area. Am J Gastroenterol. 2002;97(8):2071–8.
68. Richter C, Ter Beest G, Gisolf EH, VAN Bentum P, Waegemaekers C, Swanink C, et al. Screening for chronic hepatitis B and C in migrants from Afghanistan, Iran, Iraq, the former soviet republics, and Vietnam in the Arnhem region, The Netherlands. Epidemiol Infect. 2014;142(10):2140–6.
69. Johnson DW, Dent H, Yao Q, Tranaeus A, Huang C-C, Han D-S, et al. Frequencies of hepatitis B and C infections among haemodialysis and peritoneal dialysis patients in Asia-Pacific countries: analysis of registry data. Nephrol Dial Transplant. 2009;24(5):1598–603.
70. Li L, Assanangkornchai S, Duo L, McNeil E, Li J. Risk behaviors, prevalence of HIV and hepatitis C virus infection and population size of current injection drug users in a China-Myanmar border city: results from a respondent-driven sampling survey in 2012. PLoS One. 2014;9(9):e106899.
71. Khan S, Attaullah S, Ali I, Ayaz S, Naseemullah, Khan SN, et al. Rising burden of hepatitis C virus in hemodialysis patients. Virol J. 2011;8:438.
72. Pybus OG, Barnes E, Taggart R, Lemey P, Markov PV, Rasachak B, et al. Genetic history of hepatitis C virus in East Asia. J Virol. 2009;83(2):1071–82.
73. DNDI. An alternative reseach and development strategy to deliver aforadble treatments for hepatitis C patients. The Drugs for Neglected Diseases initiative' s 2016.
74. Pawlotsky J, REVIEWS IN. BASIC AND CLINICAL GASTROENTEROLOGY AND HEPATOLOGY in Interferon-Free Regimens. Gastroenterology. 2016;151(1): 70–86.
75. Gu L, Han Y, Li Y, Zhu T, Song X, Huang Y, et al. Emergence of Lamivudine-Resistant HBV during antiretroviral therapy including Lamivudine for patients Coinfected with HIV and HBV in China. PLoS One. 2015;10(8): e0134539.
76. Cento V, Chevaliez S, Perno CF. Resistance to direct-acting antiviral agents: clinical utility and significance. Curr Opin HIV AIDS. 2015;10(5):381–9.
77. Chayama K, Hayes CN. HCV drug resistance challenges in Japan: the role of pre-existing variants and emerging Resistant strains in direct acting antiviral therapy. Viruses. 2015;7(10):5328–42.
78. Antaki N, Craxi A, Kamal S, Moucari R, Van der Merwe S, Haffar S, et al. The neglected hepatitis C virus genotypes 4, 5 and 6: an international consensus report. Liver Int. 2010;30(3):342–55.
79. WBG. The Word bank Country Srurvey FY14. Word Bank Group; 2014.
80. Res JMB, SP S, Shyamala R, JR R, RRM V, Dwivedi M, et al. Global policy report on the prevention and control of viral hepatitis IN WHO MEMBER STATES. Indian J Gastroenterol. 2012;2(2):146–9.
81. Mohamed R, Desmond P, Suh D-J, Amarapurkar D, Gane E, Guangbi Y, et al. Practical difficulties in the management of hepatitis B in the Asia-Pacific region. J Gastroenterol Hepatol. 2004;19(9):958–69.
82. Hipgrave DB, Van NT, Vu MH, Hoang TL, Do TD, Tran NT, et al. Hepatitis B infection in rural Vietnam and the implications for a national program of infant immunization. AmJTrop Med Hyg. 2003;69(3):288–94.
83. Ding CM, Sung JJY, Chan HLY, Luan J. Viral mutant discovery in hepatitis B virus quasi-species in patients undergoing long-term lamivudine treatment. Hong Kong Med J. 2015;21(Suppl 4):31–4.
84. Yin F, Wu Z, Fang W, Wu C, Rayner S, Han M, et al. Resistant mutations and quasispecies complexity of hepatitis B virus during telbivudine treatment. J Gen Virol. 2015;96(11):3302–12.
85. Younossi ZM, Tanaka A, Eguchi Y, Lim YS, Yu ML, Kawada N, et al. The impact of hepatitis C virus outside the liver: Evidence from Asia. Liver Int. 2016;37(2):159-172.

11

Hepatitis virus (HCV) diagnosis and access to treatment in a UK cohort

Emily Adland[1], Gerald Jesuthasan[2], Louise Downs[2], Victoria Wharton[3], Gemma Wilde[3], Anna L. McNaughton[4], Jane Collier[3], Eleanor Barnes[3,4,5], Paul Klenerman[2,3,4,5], Monique Andersson[2], Katie Jeffery[2] and Philippa C. Matthews[2,4*]

Abstract

Background: As direct acting antiviral (DAA) therapy is progressively rolled out for patients with hepatitis C virus (HCV) infection, careful scrutiny of HCV epidemiology, diagnostic testing, and access to care is crucial to underpin improvements in delivery of treatment, with the ultimate goal of elimination.

Methods: We retrospectively studied microbiology records from a large UK teaching hospital in order to compare the performance of HCV screening and diagnostic tests (antibody, antigen and HCV RNA detection). Having described a local cohort of adults with active HCV infection, we investigated the proportion who attended hospital appointments, were prescribed direct acting antiviral (DAA) therapy, and cleared HCV RNA following treatment.

Results: Over a total time period of 33 months between 2013 and 2016, we tested 38,509 individuals for HCV infection and confirmed a new diagnosis of active HCV infection (HCV-Ag + and/or HCV RNA+) in 353 (positive rate 0.9%). Our in-house HCV-Ab screening test had a positive predictive value of 87% compared to repeat HCV-Ab testing in a reference laboratory, highlighting the potential for false positives to arise using this test. HCV-Ag had 100% positive predictive value compared to detection of HCV RNA. There was a strong correlation between quantitative HCV-Ag and HCV RNA viral load ($p < 0.0001$). Among the cases of infection, genotype-1 and genotype-3 predominated, the median age was 37 years, 84% were male, and 36% were in prison. Hepatology review was provided in 39%, and 22% received treatment. Among those who received DAA therapy with 12 weeks of follow-up, 93% achieved a sustained virologic response (SVR_{12}).

Conclusions: HCV-Ag performs well as a diagnostic test compared to PCR for HCV RNA. Active HCV infection is over-represented among men and in the prison population. DAA therapy is successful in those who receive it, but a minority of patients with a diagnosis of HCV infection access clinical care. Enhanced efforts are required to provide linkage to clinical care within high risk populations.

Keywords: HCV, Antigen, Antibody, Screening, Genotype, Epidemiology, Prison, Diagnosis, Ethnicity, DAA, Treatment, Cure, Sustainable development goals

Background

The World Health Organization (WHO) estimates that 71 million people are chronically infected with the Hepatitis C Virus (HCV), and 0.4 million people die each year as a consequence [1, 2]. International targets have been set for the elimination of viral hepatitis as a public health threat by the year 2030 [2, 3], underscoring an urgent need for improved case-finding. The need for enhancing HCV diagnosis has also become more pertinent as a result of the increasing availability and success of Direct Acting Antiviral (DAA) treatment [4–7]. Globally, only 15–20% of individuals with chronic HCV infection are currently thought to be aware of their diagnosis, with even fewer receiving treatment [5, 8, 9].

Streamlined, accurate and accessible HCV diagnosis is important not only as a pathway to treatment for individual patients, but also to allow confident estimates of the true prevalence of chronic HCV infection in different settings. Epidemiologic data are crucial to underpin

* Correspondence: philippa.matthews@ndm.ox.ac.uk
[2]Department of Infectious Diseases and Microbiology, John Radcliffe Hospital, Headley Way, Headington, Oxford OX3 9DU, UK
[4]Nuffield Department of Medicine, Peter Medawar Building for Pathogen Research, South Parks Road, Oxford OX1 3SY, UK
Full list of author information is available at the end of the article

appropriate allocation of resources and development of infra-structure for treatment [10]. Screening and diagnosis of HCV infection is based on three different approaches, which may be used alone or in combination. These are (i) detection of an IgG antibody by ELISA (HCV-Ab); (ii) detection of HCV core antigen (HCV-Ag); (iii) Nucleic acid testing (NAT) to detect HCV RNA by PCR (Table 1). Of these, only (ii) and (iii) can confirm active infection.

Reliance upon HCV-Ab screening has potentially distorted epidemiological data upon which resource-planning depends [11], as this approach includes detection of individuals who have cleared infection either spontaneously or through treatment (estimating exposure as well as active infection), and also includes false positives. As a result, there has been a progressive move towards using HCV-Ag and/or HCV PCR to determine accurately the population prevalence of active infection [1, 12, 13]. Although sensitivity and specificity of HCV-Ag testing appears to perform well when compared head-to-head with PCR [10, 13, 14], there are still potential doubts over whether this test is sufficiently sensitive to be widely implemented as a primary screening tool, and recent WHO guidelines continue to recommend use of the HCV-Ab test for first line screening [12]. A careful balance must be struck between managing cost and optimising specificity without sacrificing sensitivity [15–18].

We here set out to assess our progress in diagnosing and treating HCV infection in a tertiary referral UK hospital. We reviewed the performance of our local HCV testing protocol in two different time periods, first when screening was undertaken using an HCV-Ab test only, and subsequently following the introduction of a combined approach using HCV-Ab screening and HCV-Ag diagnostic confirmation. In each period, we went on to evaluate further using PCR for HCV RNA. Collating these data allowed us to evaluate the performance of different screening and diagnostic tests, to describe the characteristics of our local cohort, and to determine the proportion of those with active HCV infection who attend a hepatology clinic and receive treatment.

Methods

Setting and cohort

Our microbiology laboratory in the South East of the UK is located in a large tertiary referral teaching hospital (http://www.ouh.nhs.uk/) that provides one million patient contacts a year, and handles samples referred from the community as well as four in-patient sites.

We retrospectively interrogated electronic microbiology records for all HCV assays performed within two defined time-intervals, during which different diagnostic algorithms were operating, in each case starting with a screening test and then proceeding to confirm active infection. These are summarized in Fig. 1 and outlined as follows:

i. **Group 1** (18 months; January 2013–June 2014). Samples were screened for HCV-Ab using an ADVIA Centaur automated immunoassay (Bayer). HCV-Ab-positive samples (excluding repeat samples from patients with a pre-existing HCV diagnosis) were sent for confirmatory testing by the regional reference laboratory (Public Health England, Colindale), using two further ELISA tests (Ortho and BioRad). Antibody positive samples (based on sample:cut-off ratio > 1) were tested for HCV RNA.
ii. **Group 2** (15 months; January 2015–March 2016). HCV testing was undertaken using a combination of HCV-Ab and HCV-Ag, using Abbott Architect i2000SR, with Diasorin Liason XL for confirmation

Table 1 Comparison of diagnostic laboratory tests used to detect exposure and activity of HCV infection

Screening tool	HCV-Ab	HCV-Ag	PCR for HCV RNA
Benefits	♦ Widely available; ♦ Inexpensive; ♦ Much experience and data for use as first-line approach to screening for HCV exposure (underpins many old seroprevalence studies).	♦ Diagnostic of active infection (not past exposure); ♦ Improved specificity and reduced window period compared to HCV-Ab [14, 29, 42–45].	♦ Accepted gold-standard diagnostic test for active infection (not past exposure); ♦ Allows quantitative monitoring of viraemia; useful for monitoring therapy; ♦ Genome amplification allows other information to be ascertained (e.g. genotype; drug resistance); ♦ Can potentially be applied to dried blood spots (DBS).
Challenges	♦ Subject to inter-assay variability and a variable rate of false positive results [46, 47]; false positive has been associated with ethnicity [48, 49], age [48], raised IgM and erythrocyte sedimentation rate (ESR) [46], auto-antibodies [50], and prosthetic devices [51]; ♦ Test of exposure, not of active infection, so should be followed up with a more specific diagnostic test.	♦ Not universally available; ♦ More expensive than HCV-Ab; ♦ Not consistently regarded as sufficiently sensitive to replace PCR.	♦ Not universally available; ♦ Expensive: beyond the financial reach of many resource-limited settings.

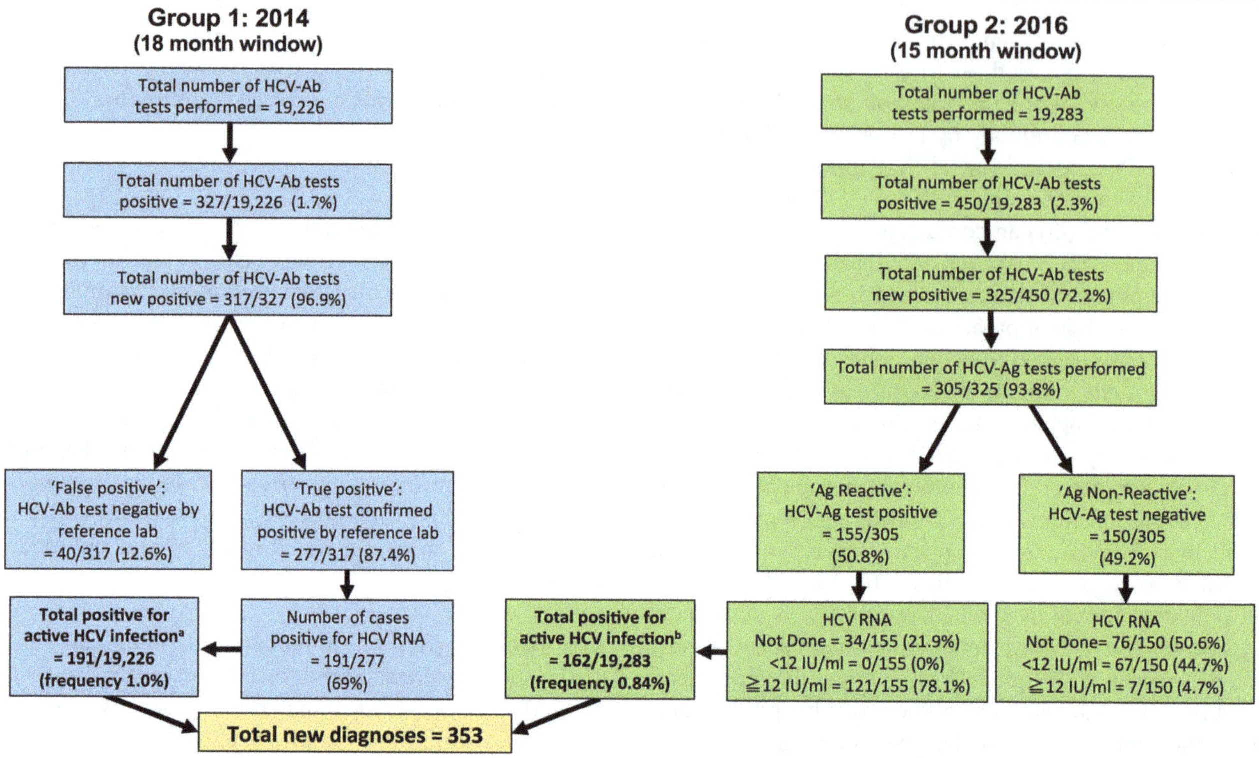

Fig. 1 Algorithms describing HCV screening and diagnosis in a UK teaching hospital laboratory in 2014 (Group 1) and 2016 (Group 2). [a]The total positive rate for Group 1 is defined as the number of samples that were HCV RNA positive (n = 191) divided by the total number of samples screened (n = 19,226). [b]The total positive rate for Group 2 is defined as samples that were deemed positive for active HCV infection based on interpretation of combined results (this includes HCV-Ag positive and not further screened (n = 34), plus any sample that was HCV-RNA positive irrespective of the HCV-Ag result (n = 128, comprising 121 HCV-Ag positive, and 7 HCV-Ag negative samples), divided by the total number of samples screened (n = 19,283). The lower limit of quantification for HCV RNA was 12 iU/ml. There was no case of detectable HCV RNA below the limit of quantification.

of HCV-Ab. The HCV-Ag assay provides a quantitative result up to an upper limit of 20,000 fmol/L. We classified values of ≥3 fmol/L as positive (as previously reported [19]). When we introduced the HCV-Ag assay, we tested the same sample for HCV RNA in parallel, for the puporses of validation. Following this validation period, we stopped routinely testing the same sample for HCV RNA, and changed the protocol to request a second sample for RNA testing (only in those that are HCV-Ag positive). This allows us to confirm the diagnosis using two separate samples, in keeping with good laboratory practice, and also provides material for genotyping.

For Groups 1 and 2, samples were tested for HCV RNA using the Abbott HCV M2000 assay.

Some individuals were tested for HCV infection on > 1 occasion; we removed duplicate tests from our overall positive cohort using unique identifiers (hospital number or NHS number). We recorded patient age, sex, and the location from which the sample was sent. Treatment data were captured and recorded from an electronic database within the Hepatology Department. Response to treatment was defined as sustained virologic response (undetectable HCV RNA using PCR) at ≥12 weeks following the end of therapy (SVR_{12}).

Ethnic origin is not routinely captured data in hospital electronic systems. Prior to anonymisation, we therefore used an analytical tool to estimate ethnicity, applying Onolytics software for all patients for whom a full name was part of the electronic record (https://onolytics.com [20–22]). This software was developed in 2006–7 funded by Economic and Social Research Council (ESRC) Knowledge Transfer Partnerships, and sets out to determine probable ethnic origin based on name.

Data analysis

Statistical analysis was performed using GraphPad Prism v.7.0b and Googlesheets (https://docs.google.com/spreadsheets). We compared binary values using Fisher's Exact Test, Mann-Whitney U test for continuous non-parametric data, chi-square for analysis of categorical data, and linear regression for correlation between continuous variables.

Ethics approval

Ethics approval was not required, as this study was undertaken as a departmental quality improvement exercise within microbiology using anonymised patient data, and completed the audit cycle for previously approved audit projects [23, 24]. Data for Onolytics analysis were handled separately, subject to a confidential disclosure agreement drawn up by University of Oxford Research Services (February 2016).

Results

HCV testing: Frequency and characteristics of infection

In total, we present data for 38,509 HCV tests done during the two intervals reviewed. On average we performed an average of 1068 tests / month during the earlier phase of the study (Group 1) and 1286 tests / month in the later time period (Group 2); Fig. 1.

We identified 353 active HCV infections across Group 1 and Group 2, using a combination of HCV-Ag and/or HCV RNA testing. We estimated the frequency of active HCV infection within this cohort at 0.9% based on a combined numerator ($n = 353$), and using the total number of samples tested as the denominator ($n = 38{,}509$); Fig. 1. Comparing the two time periods, there was no change in the frequency of positive HCV-Ab testing: HCV-Ab frequency 317 / 19,226 (1.6% in Group 1) vs. 325 / 19,283 (1.7% in Group 2); $p = 0.8$, chi-sqaure test. There was also no significant difference in the frequency of confirmed active HCV infection (based on HCV-Ag and/or HCV RNA PCR): 191 / 19,226 (1.0% in Group 1) vs. 162 /19,283 (0.8% in Group 2); $p = 0.13$, chi-square test.

Characteristics of the 353 individuals with active HCV infection are summarised in Table 2, and the complete metadata are available on-line (https://doi.org/10.6084/m9.figshare.5355097). The median age was 37 years (IQR 31–48). Men accounted for 55% of all individuals tested, but 84% of all new diagnoses (Table 2) [23]. Over one-third (36%) of new diagnoses were made in prison. Genotype was available in 186 cases (53% of new diagnoses), with genotype 1 ($n = 84$) and genotype 3 ($n = 80$) accounting for the majority (45% and 43%, respectively); Fig. 2.

Table 2 Characteristics of individuals screened for HCV infection in a UK teaching hospital in two time windows between 2014 and 2016

	Group 1 (2014)	Group 2 (2016)	Group 1 + Group 2 (2014–2016)
Total number HCV-Ab positive	317	325	642
Total number confirmed positive for active HCV infection (HCV-Ag/ HCV RNA positive)	191	162	353
Number male (% of active infections)[a,b]	165 (86.3%)	132 (81.5%)	297 (84.1%)
Age in years (median and IQR)[a]	39 (31–49)	36 (30–46)	37 (31–48)
Location[a, c]			
- Primary Care	64 (33.5%)	46 (28.4%)	110 (31.2%)
- Hospital out-patient	17 (8.9%)	17 (5.2%)	34 (9.6%)
- Prison	61 (31.9%)	66 (40.7%)	127 (35.9%)
- Hospital in-patient[d]	22 (11.5%)	9 (5.5%)	31 (8.8%)
- Emergency Dept.	5 (2.6%)	6 (3.7%)	11 (3.1%)
- Sexual health clinic	16 (8.4%)	13 (8.0%)	29 (8.2%)
- Occupational health	2 (1.0%)	1 (0.6%)	3 (0.8%)
- Other locations[e]	4 (2.1%)	4 (2.5%)	8 (2.3%)
Ethnic origin[a]			
- Black	5 (2.6%)	1 (0.6%)	6 (1.7%)
- Asian	17 (8.9%)	7 (4.3%)	24 (6.8%)
- European	149 (78.0%)	100 (61.7%)	249 (70.5%)
- Unknown	20 (10.5%)	54 (33.3%)	74 (21.0%)

[a]Breakdown of characteristics is shown for the individuals who have confirmed active HCV infection, based on HCV-Ag and/or HCV RNA PCR
[b]Numbers of positive tests are shown with percentage of positive tests in brackets
[c]We did not have access to data for PWID, but prison location may be an important surrogate marker for this group
[d]Hospital in-patient locations include general surgery, orthopaedics, transplant, renal, haematology, intensive care, unspecified ward locations in the hospital, and in-patients in community hospitals
[e]Other locations include paediatrics, psychiatry, fertility and pathology

Outcomes and performance of HCV-ab and HCV-ag assays

In the earlier testing period (Group 1), 277/317 HCV-Ab positive samples were positive on confirmatory testing for HCV-Ab at the reference laboratory (Fig. 1), giving our in-house test a positive predictive value (PPV) of 87.4% compared to a regionally accepted standard. We used these results to investigate whether any host factors were associated with false positive antibody tests, and found that individuals identified as African have a higher chance of a false-positive HCV Ab test (Fig. 3). We confirmed this result by multivariate logistic regression analysis, in which African ethnicity was significantly associated with a false positive Ab test result ($p = 0.0004$), but age > 60 years and sex were not. Prison location was associated with a true positive Ab-test result ($p = 0.01$). We did not have access to data on representation of PWID in this cohort, but recognise that prison location is a likely surrogate marker for this risk factor for infection.

In the later testing period (Group 2), the PPV of the combined use of HCV-Ab plus HCV-Ag was 100% when compared to a gold-standard diagnostic test using PCR (Table 3).

Individuals with a positive HCV-Ag test had a median HCV viral load of 5.9×10^5 IU/ml (Fig. 4a), and there

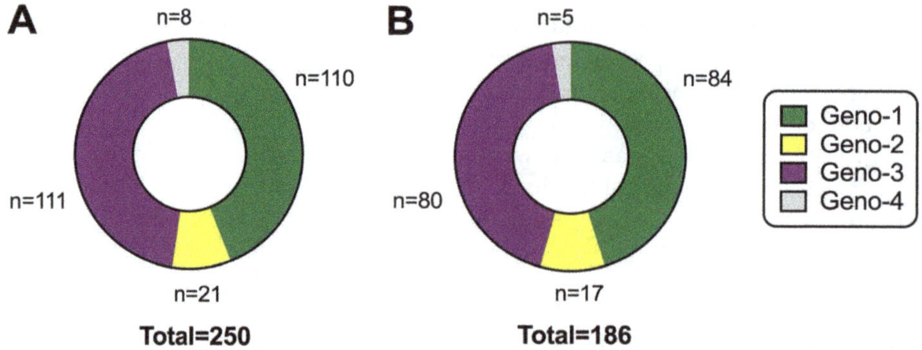

Fig. 2 Distribution of HCV genotypes in a UK cohort. **a** Data for an extended cohort of 250 individuals for whom HCV genotyping was undertaken in our laboratory between 2014 and 2016 (includes the 186 individuals represented in panel **b**, plus an additional 64 individuals who had genotyping undertaken within this time period but were not captured within Group 1 or Group 2). **b** Data for 186 individuals for whom genotype was determined from among the cohort of 353 new HCV diagnoses within Group 1 and Group 2 of this study. There was no enrichment of a specific genotype in the prison population (prison population accounted for 30/84 geno-1 infections, and 34/80 geno-3 infections; $p = 0.4$ Fisher's Exact Test)

was a significant positive correlation between quantitative antigenaemia and viral load ($r^2 = 0.3$, $p < 0.0001$; Fig. 4b). However, in a small proportion of cases, the HCV-Ag test was falsely negative (Table 4).

Based on the strong correlation between HCV-Ag and viral load (Fig. 4b), and on a previous analysis that documents HCV-Ag down to a level equivalent to viral load 3000 IU/ml [13], we sought to determine whether the false negative HCV-Ag tests ($n = 7$) were associated with low viraemia. Indeed, in 5/7 cases, HCV RNA was $< 10^4$ IU/ml, one of which had HCV RNA as low as 25 IU/ml. Among 128 samples for which we had both an HCV-Ag and HCV RNA assay result, the false-negative tests were significantly enriched in the group with HCV RNA $< 10^4$ IU/ml ($p < 0.0001$, Fig. 4c).

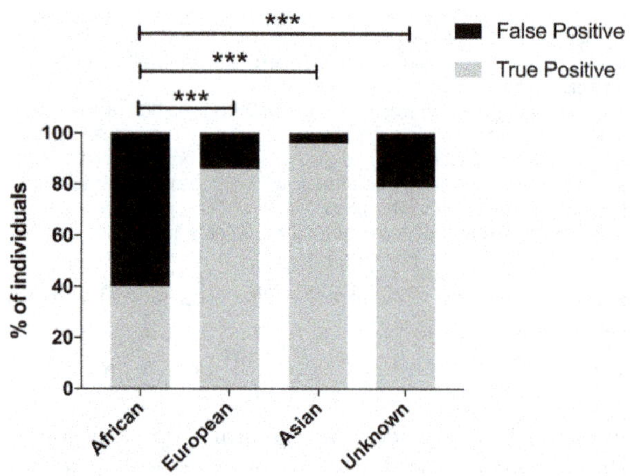

Fig. 3 False positive HCV IgG antibody results according to ethnic origin in a UK cohort. Ethnicity was estimated using Onolytics software [26, 27]. Data shown are for a cohort recruited starting in 2014 (designated Group 1), screened using an in-house HCV-Ab (ADVIA Centaur automated immunoassay; Bayer) and confirmed using two further ELISA tests (Ortho and BioRad). 'False positives' are defined as those screening positive on ADVIA but subsequently negative, 'true positives' are defined as samples positive on all three tests. *P*-values obtained by Fishers Exact Test; *** $p < 0.0005$

Clinical management and outcomes

Of 353 patients with a new HCV diagnosis, 142 (40%) attended a hepatology clinic appointment, 79 were treated (22% of the cohort) and 66 met the SVR_{12} criterion (19% of the whole cohort; 84% of all those treated). Among those treated with a DAA-based regimen ($n = 59$), a treatment endpoint was documented in 54, of which 50 were classified as SVR_{12} (93%). For individual treatment regimens, see full clinical metadata available on-line.

This study was not designed to examine or report on the outcomes of treatment. However, we examined existing treatment data to look for evidence of different outcomes between genotypes 1 and 3. Among treated genotype 1 infections with outcome data ($n = 34$), we recorded 32 cases of SVR_{12}, and two cases of relapse. For treated genotype 3 ($n = 30$), there were 25 cases of SVR_{12} and five relapses, but this difference did not reach statistical significance (relapse rate 2/34 (6%) for geno-1 vs. 5/30 (17%) for geno-3; $p = 0.2$, Fisher's Exact Test).

Discussion

Summary comments

Careful scrutiny of HCV screening, diagnosis and treatment is important so that enhanced efforts can be made to identify individuals with active infection in order to provide access to DAA therapy, and to move towards international elimination goals [3, 9, 13].

In our setting in the UK, 0.9% of all samples submitted for HCV testing had evidence of active HCV infection.

Table 3 Outcome of diagnostic testing for HCV infection using core antigen detection (HCV-Ag) compared to gold standard PCR for HCV RNA

Outcome	Result (n)*
True positive	121
False negative	7
False positive	0
True negative	67
Test characteristic	Result (%)
Sensitivity	94.5
Specificity	100
Positive predictive value	100
Negative predictive value	90.5

*Results pertain to all HCV-antibody individuals in 'Group 2', based on samples that were tested with assays for both HCV-Ag and HCV RNA, defined as follows: true positives (HCV-Ag + and HCV RNA+); false negatives (HCV Ag- and HCV RNA+); false positives (HCV Ag + and HCV RNA-); true negatives (HCV Ag- and HCV RNA-). These groups are also shown in Fig. 4a. Threshold for positive HCV-Ag was 3 fmol/L

Following the implementation of HCV-Ag testing as part of the diagnostic algorithm, the PPV of a positive test increased to 100%, slightly exceeding that reported by other recently published studies [14]. The close correlation between HCV-Ag and HCV RNA viral load suggests that, in the absence of having access to a quantitative PCR result, HCV-Ag may be a useful surrogate marker of viraemia, particularly at higher viral loads (e.g. if HCV RNA > 10^4 IU/ml). Genotypes 1 and 3 predominated (in keeping with other published studies in this setting [25, 26]).

Our data confirm the success of DAA treatment, with SVR_{12} documented in 93%. However, this cohort also highlights the substantial loss of patients at each step of the clinical 'cascade' (Fig. 5; Table 5). This is due to a combination of factors that include poor linkage between services (community, prisons, sexual health and secondary care), itinerant populations, specific challenges in providing follow-up for those in prison and PWID, and deaths.

Relevance to laboratory and clinical practice

Although HCV-Ag testing can potentially replace a nucleic acid test for HCV diagnosis or monitoring in some settings [14, 27, 28], guidelines from the UK [29], North America [30] and the WHO [12] still advocate use of PCR as a definitive test following HCV-Ab (± HCV-Ag) screening. RNA PCR also remains the gold-standard approach to monitoring progress during and after treatment and is currently still recommended for genotyping, to underpin optimum choice of DAA regimen [31]. However, as we move towards pan-genotype treatments for HCV, a single diagnostic test, with the potential to be applied at the point-of-care, is an appealing strategy [13].

The small proportion of all diagnosed patients who access clinical care and receive successful treatment is in keeping with that reported in other centres [5, 32], reflecting many challenges for HCV elimination. Our data highlight the particular vulnerability of the prison population, in keeping with a worldwide estimate of 15% HCV prevalence in prisoners [33]. Offering treatment within the prison system has now become a realistic

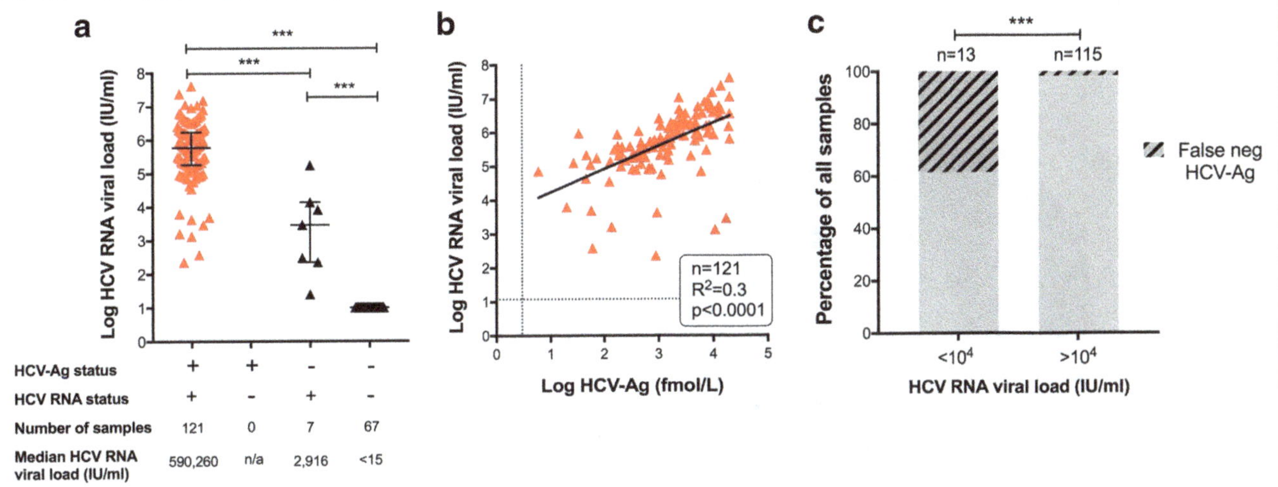

Fig. 4 Relationship between HCV Antigen test and quantitative PCR for HCV RNA viral load. **a** Range of HCV RNA viral loads for samples testing HCV-Ag positive (*n* = 121) and HCV-Ag negative (*n* = 74). Median and interquartile range shown. *P*-values by Mann-Whitney U test; ****p* < 0.0001. **b** Relationship between between HCV-Ag and HCV RNA viral load for all samples testing HCV-Ag positive (n = 121). Dashed lines represent threshold for detection for HCV RNA (12 IU/ml) and HCV-Ag (3 fmol/L). Solid line represents linear regression analysis; R^2 = 0.3, p < 0.0001. **c** Percentage of samples testing false-negative for HCV-Ag according to HCV RNA viral load. *P*-value by Fisher's Exact test ****p* < 0.0001. Data are shown for 128 samples for which both HCV RNA and HCV-Ag testing was undertaken. HCV-Ag was falsely negative (< 3 fmol/L) in 5/13 cases with HCV RNA < 10^4 IU/ml, and in 2/115 cases with HCV RNA > 10^4 IU/ml

Table 4 Summary of seven adults in whom HCV core antigen (HCV-Ag) assay was falsely negative, as compared to PCR for HCV RNA as a gold-standard reference test

Age group (years)	Sex	Patient location	Ethnicity	HIV status	HCV Ag (fmol/L)	HCV Ab (sample/ cut-off ratio)	Genotype	HCV viral load (IU/ml)
30–39	F	Sexual health	Unknown	negative	0.0	11.8	N/A	25
40–49	M	Primary care	European	negative	0.0	12.2	N/A	226
50–59	F	Hospital in-patient (General Medicine)	European	positive	0.0	3.1	N/A	302
20–29	M	Prison	European	negative	0.62	14.2	2b	2916
20–29	M	Prison	European	N/A	0.00	12.6	N/A	8232
30–39	F	Hospital out-patient	European	N/A	1.98	15.8	1b	13,860
30–39	M	Prison	European	negative	0.00	12.2	3a	174,834

N/A = not available. Total number of HCV-Ag tests carried out in this period $n = 305$. None of the patients with a false negative result underwent a repeat Ag test so laboratory error cannot be ruled out in this instance. Threshold for positive HCV-Ag defined as ≥3 fmol/L. Samples are ranked in ascending viral load order

possibility, on the basis of oral DAA therapy, shortened treatment regimens, and a low rate of side-effects [34, 35].

In the longer term, bigger datasets are required to improve our insights into the HCV-infected population [32], and health economics analyses should be used to support optimum deployment of resources in different settings [36, 37]. On the global stage, optimization of laboratory testing and reduction of costs are essential to improve access to accurate diagnosis, advocacy for better testing and treatment for populations in resource-limited settings, and especially for targeting interventions at high-risk populations including MSM, PWID and prisons.

Performance of HCV-ag test

Our calculated PPV of 100% for the HCV-Ag test exceeds a previous estimation of the PPV of the Ag test (94.7%) calculated from assimilation of data from other comparable reports [14]. However, PPV is dependent on the overall prevalence of infection, and will therefore vary between settings.

A recent meta-analysis concludes that the HCV-Ag test performs similarly to HCV RNA PCR when viral load is > 3000 iu/ml [13]. Thus this diagnostic tool provides a high sensitivity without unduly influencing specificity. The HCV-Ag assay is likely to perform less reliably at low viral loads, and a low threshold should be applied for using NAT to confirm a diagnosis in the setting of an equivocal HCV-Ag result (3–10 fmol/L). Another potential explanation for false negative HCV-Ag test is mutations in the core region of the HCV genome which could account for a failure of antigen detection [38], or potentially cause lack of PCR amplification if mutations occur in primer binding regions.

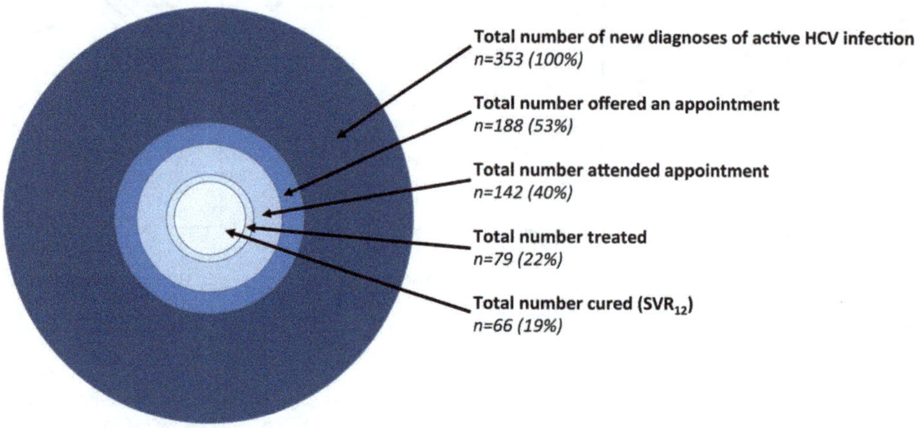

Fig. 5 Graphical representation of the disparity between the number of individuals diagnosed with active HCV infection and those who access clinical review, treatment, and achieve SVR_{12}. Summary of outcomes for the entire cohort is shown in Table 5. The percentages quoted in this figure represent the proportion of patients in each category from the total denominator of 353. Individuals diagnosed in prison were significantly less likely to attain an SVR_{12} endpoint (SVR_{12} was documented for 5/127 individuals in prison vs. 61/226 not in prison, $p < 0.0001$, Fisher's Exact test)

Table 5 Summary of clinical care outcomes in 353 individuals with a diagnosis of chronic HCV infection

Treatment Status	Patient Classification	Number	Percentage of treatment subgroup[a]	Percentage of total cohort
Not yet treated (n = 130)	Offered appointment but did not attend	46	35.4	13.0
	Seen in another clinic (sexual health, prison, paediatrics)	32	24.6	9.1
	Seen by hepatology but not on treatment waiting list	23	17.7	6.5
	Seen by hepatology and on treatment waiting list for DAA	3	2.3	0.9
	Died	11	8.5	3.1
	Transferred out of area	10	7.7	2.8
	Seen in clinic but lost to follow-up	2	1.5	0.6
	Spontaneous clearer	3	2.3	0.8
Treated with DAA (n = 59)	SVR_{12}	50	84.7	14.2
	Relapsed	4	6.8	1.1
	Outcome data pending	5	8.5	1.4
Treated with IFN/RBV (n = 20)	SVR_{12}	16	80.0	4.5
	Relapsed	3	15.0	0.8
	No outcome data	1	5.0	0.3
Unknown (n = 150)	Not known to local services	144	100	40.8
TOTAL		353	400	100

[a]Treatment subgroup is defined as the four categories listed in the first column of this table. The total of this column is 300%, as the total for each of three subgroups is 100%

DAA = direct acting antivirals, *IFN* = interferon, *RBV* = ribavirin; SVR_{12} = sustained viraemic response at ≥12 weeks following therapy

Caveats and limitations

Our analysis must be set in the overall context of the low prevalence of HCV in our setting, and the retrospective approach to data collection. We cannot comment on population level epidemiology, as a large pool of individuals who are HCV-infected never have a screening or diagnostic test [9]. Due to gaps in the laboratory data-set, in which not every sample was tested for HCV RNA, we adopted a pragmatic definition of active HCV infection based on the best laboratory evidence available (in some cases this was an assay for HCV-Ag without an accompanying NAT). Our analysis of sensitivity and specificity of HCV-Ag testing could only be assessed in the subset of samples that had undergone testing with assays for both HCV-Ag and HCV RNA quantification.

The rate of false negative HCV tests is our population is likely to be low, but quantifying this was not possible within this study, as we relied on identifying samples that initially tested positive. In order to ascertain the PPV of the HCV-Ab test in-house, we referred to a Reference Laboratory test as 'gold standard'. However, this repeat testing in a Reference Laboratory setting is itself subject to an error rate, and therefore may lead to a misrepresentation of our overall assay performance.

We found evidence that the HCV-Ab test performs poorly in individuals predicted to be of African origin. A similar high rate of false positive tests has previously been reported from Polynesia [39]. This illustrates how tests that have been validated in white European/Caucasian populations cannot necessarily be robustly applied in other settings. Although the tools used here have been validated [21, 22], use of name is an imperfect way to derive ethnic origin and is potentially confounded by a variety of factors, the most obvious of which is individuals who change their name through marriage.

In our setting, the sexual health clinic anonymises patient data, preventing robust linkage between services. We are therefore unable to trace outcomes for patients who were diagnosed via this route (8% of the total; Table 2). Likewise, consistent identification and tracing of individuals who use drugs and/or are in prison is challenging, and we cannot exclude the possibility of duplication of some of these individuals within our dataset.

In the context of this study we do not have prospective socio-demographic data that are required to investigate the reasons for the male excess we describe (e.g. MSM, PWID). Sex differences could also be accounted for by genuine biological discrepancies in susceptibility to, and outcomes of, infection between males and females [40, 41]. We have also not been able to characterise the prison population in detail; this group is difficult to treat and to follow-up, and so is at risk of worse outcomes, but we may have underestimated SVR_{12} due to missing data.

Conclusions

A sensitive, affordable point-of care test in the form of an HCV-Ag test is a desirable solution for HCV diagnosis in many settings, and we have shown this to be reliable in most cases, although with a reduced sensitivity in the context of HCV viral loads $< 10^4$ IU/ml. In concordance with other studies [5], our data highlight the ongoing need for multilateral efforts to provide access to diagnosis and routes into treatment, if success is to be achieved in the global targets for elimination of this infection as a threat to public health.

Abbreviations

DAA: Direct acting antiviral; ELISA: Enzyme linked immunosorbent assay; HCV RNA: Hepatitis C ribonucleic acid (viral load); HCV: Hepatitis C virus; HCV-Ab: IgG antibody to Hepatitis C virus; HCV-Ag: Hepatitis C virus core antigen; MSM: Men who have sex with men; NAT: Nucleic acid testing; PCR: Polymerase chain reaction (test for viral load); PPV: Positive predictive value; PWID: People who inject drugs; SDG: Sustainable Development Goals; SVR: Sustained virologic response; WHO: World Health Organisation

Acknowledgements

A subset of these data was presented as a poster at the UK Federation of Infection Societies (FIS) conference, November 2014 [23].

Funding

PCM received research salary from the NIHR during the course of this data collection and is now funded by the Wellcome Trust (grant number 110110). EB is supported by the MRC as a Senior Clinical Fellow. Oxford NIHR BRC has supported the development of the Oxford HCV cohort. No specific funding was allocated for this study. The funders had no role in the conception or design of the study, in the production of the manuscript or in the decision to publish.

Authors' contributions

Study conception and design: PK, KJ, PCM. Data collection: GJ, LD, VW, GW. Running and interpreting clinical laboratory tests: GJ, MA, KJ, PCM. Data analysis: EA, AM, PK, KJ, PCM. Involved in management of clinical cohort: JC, EB, PK, KJ, PCM. Wrote the manuscript: EA, PCM, with editorial input from AM, MA, KJ. All authors read and approved the final manuscript.

Authors' information

EB is the lead for the UK STOP-HCV program. PCM is a Wellcome Trust Clinical Research Fellow investigating chronic viral hepatitis infection.

Consent for publication

Not applicable.

Competing interests

MA has received research funding from Gilead. PCM is a member of BMC Infectious Diseases Editorial Board (assistant editor).

Author details

[1]Department of Paediatrics, Peter Medawar Building for Pathogen Research, South Parks Road, Oxford OX1 3SY, UK. [2]Department of Infectious Diseases and Microbiology, John Radcliffe Hospital, Headley Way, Headington, Oxford OX3 9DU, UK. [3]Department of Hepatology, John Radcliffe Hospital, Headley Way, Headington, Oxford OX3 9DU, UK. [4]Nuffield Department of Medicine, Peter Medawar Building for Pathogen Research, South Parks Road, Oxford OX1 3SY, UK. [5]Oxford NIHR Biomedical Research Centre, John Radcliffe Hospital, Headley Way, Headington, Oxford OX3 9DU, UK.

References

1. Chun HM, Fieberg AM, Hullsiek KH, Lifson AR, Crum-Cianflone NF, et al. Epidemiology of hepatitis B virus infection in a US cohort of HIV-infected individuals during the past 20 years. Clin Infect Dis. 2010;50:426–36.
2. Uneke CJ, Ogbu O, Inyama PU, Anyanwu GI, Njoku MO, et al. Prevalence of hepatitis-B surface antigen among blood donors and human immunodeficiency virus-infected patients in Jos, Nigeria. Mem Inst Oswaldo Cruz. 2005;100:13–6.
3. Griggs D, Stafford-Smith M, Gaffney O, Rockstrom J, Ohman MC, et al. Policy: sustainable development goals for people and planet. Nature. 2013; 495:305–7.
4. Pawlotsky JM, Feld JJ, Zeuzem S, Hoofnagle JH. From non-a, non-B hepatitis to hepatitis C virus cure. J Hepatol. 2015;62:S87–99.
5. Zuckerman A, Douglas A, Nwosu S, Choi L, Chastain C. Increasing success and evolving barriers in the hepatitis C cascade of care during the direct acting antiviral era. PLoS One. 2018;13:e0199174.
6. Lanini S, Scognamiglio P, Mecozzi A, Lombardozzi L, Vullo V, et al. Impact of new DAA therapy on real clinical practice: a multicenter region-wide cohort study. BMC Infect Dis. 2018;18:223.
7. Asselah T, Marcellin P, Schinazi RF. Treatment of hepatitis C virus infection with direct-acting antiviral agents: 100% cure? Liver Int. 2018;38 Suppl 1:7–13.
8. Smith BD, Jewett A, Drobeniuc J, Kamili S. Rapid diagnostic HCV antibody assays. Antivir Ther. 2012;17:1409–13.
9. WHO (2012) Hepatitis C Fact Sheet Number 164. http://www.who.int/mediacentre/factsheets/fs164/en/index.html.
10. Easterbrook PJ, Group WHOGD. WHO to test and how to test for chronic hepatitis C infection - 2016 WHO testing guidance for low- and middle-income countries. J Hepatol. 2016;65:S46–66.
11. Moorman AC, Drobenuic J, Kamili S. Prevalence of false-positive hepatitis C antibody results, National Health and nutrition examination study (NHANES) 2007-2012. Journal of clinical virology : the official publication of the Pan American Society for Clinical Virology. 2017;89:1–4.
12. World Health Organisation. (2017) Guidelines on Hepatitis B and Hepatitis C testing.
13. Freiman JM, Tran TM, Schumacher SG, White LF, Ongarello S, et al. Hepatitis C Core antigen testing for diagnosis of hepatitis C virus infection: a systematic review and meta-analysis. Ann Intern Med. 2016;165:345–55.
14. Khan H, Hill A, Main J, Brown A, Cooke G. Can hepatitis C virus antigen testing replace ribonucleic acid Polymearse chain reaction analysis for detecting hepatitis C virus? A systematic review. In: Open forum infect dis 4: ofw252; 2017.
15. Maasoumy B, Bremer B, Raupach R, Lehmann P, Manns MP, et al. How to interpret borderline HCV antibody test results: a comparative study investigating four different anti-HCV assays. Viral Immunol. 2014;27:7–13.
16. Maity S, Nandi S, Biswas S, Sadhukhan SK, Saha MK. Performance and diagnostic usefulness of commercially available enzyme linked immunosorbent assay and rapid kits for detection of HIV, HBV and HCV in India. Virol J. 2012;9:290.
17. Bloch EM, Shah A, Kaidarova Z, Laperche S, Lefrere JJ, et al. A pilot external quality assurance study of transfusion screening for HIV, HCV and HBsAG in 12 African countries. Vox Sang. 2014;107:333–42.
18. Contreras AM, Tornero-Romo CM, Toribio JG, Celis A, Orozco-Hernandez A, et al. Very low hepatitis C antibody levels predict false-positive results and avoid supplemental testing. Transfusion. 2008;48:2540–8.
19. Kesli R, Polat H, Terzi Y, Kurtoglu MG, Uyar Y. Comparison of a newly developed automated and quantitative hepatitis C virus (HCV) core antigen test with the HCV RNA assay for clinical usefulness in confirming anti-HCV results. J Clin Microbiol. 2011;49:4089–93.
20. Lakha F, Gorman DR, Mateos P. Name analysis to classify populations by ethnicity in public health: validation of Onomap in Scotland. Public Health. 2011;125:688–96.

21. Mateos P. Names, ethnicity and populations; tracing identity in space. Heidelberg: Springer; 2014.
22. Mateos P. A review of name-based ethnicity classification methods and their potential in population studies. Popul Space Place. 2007;13:243–63.
23. Matthews PC, Jesuthasan G, Jeffery K (2017) Hepatitis C in a teaching hospital trust: translating diagnosis into treatment [version 1]. Poster [not peer reviewed]. F1000Research 6:1147 (doi: https://doi.org/10.7490/f1000research.1114429.1).
24. Hodgekiss C, Shipman A, Jeffery K Outcome of hepatitis C testing in the pre-protease era 2008 – 2012 [version 1; not peer reviewed]. . F1000Research 2017, 6:1677 (poster).
25. Messina JP, Humphreys I, Flaxman A, Brown A, Cooke GS, et al. Global distribution and prevalence of hepatitis C virus genotypes. Hepatology. 2015;61:77–87.
26. England. Hepatitis C in the UK; 2015 report. Public Health England.
27. Duchesne L, Njouom R, Lissock F, Tamko-Mella GF, Rallier S, et al. HCV ag quantification as a one-step procedure in diagnosing chronic hepatitis C infection in Cameroon: the ANRS 12336 study. J Int AIDS Soc. 2017;20:1–8.
28. Cresswell FV, Fisher M, Hughes DJ, Shaw SG, Homer G, et al. Hepatitis C core antigen testing: a reliable, quick, and potentially cost-effective alternative to hepatitis C polymerase chain reaction in diagnosing acute hepatitis C virus infection. Clinical infectious diseases : an official publication of the Infectious Diseases Society of America. 2015;60:263–6.
29. Pan N, Jiang W, Sun H, Miao F, Qiu J, et al. KIR and HLA loci are associated with hepatocellular carcinoma development in patients with hepatitis B virus infection: a case-control study. PLoS One. 2011;6:e25682.
30. AASLD IDSA HCV Guidance Panel. Hepatitis C guidance: AASLD-IDSA recommendations for testing, managing, and treating adults infected with hepatitis C virus. Hepatology. 2015;62:932–54.
31. Weisberg IS, Jacobson IM. A pangenotypic, single tablet regimen of sofosbuvir/velpatasvir for the treatment of chronic hepatitis C infection. Expert Opin Pharmacother. 2017;18:535–43.
32. Jones CR, Glampson B, Shaw AT, Smith D, Barnes E, et al. (2017) The NIHR Heath Informatics Collaborative: sharing electronic NHS clinical information to capture the hepatitis C treatment revolution. [version 1; not peer reviewed]. F1000Research 2017, 6:1838 (poster) doi: https://doi.org/10.7490/f1000research.1114972.1.
33. Dolan K, Wirtz AL, Moazen B, Ndeffo-Mbah M, Galvani A, et al. Global burden of HIV, viral hepatitis, and tuberculosis in prisoners and detainees. Lancet. 2016;388:1089–102.
34. Martin NK, Vickerman P, Brew IF, Williamson J, Miners A, et al. Is increased hepatitis C virus case-finding combined with current or 8-week to 12-week direct-acting antiviral therapy cost-effective in UK prisons? A prevention benefit analysis. Hepatology. 2016;63:1796–808.
35. Kronfli N, Linthwaite B, Kouyoumdjian F, Klein MB, Lebouche B, et al. Interventions to increase testing, linkage to care and treatment of hepatitis C virus (HCV) infection among people in prisons: a systematic review. Int J Drug Policy. 2018;57:95–103.
36. Morgan JR, Servidone M, Easterbrook P, Linas BP. Economic evaluation of HCV testing approaches in low and middle income countries. BMC Infect Dis. 2017;17:697.
37. Julicher P, Galli C. Identifying cost-effective screening algorithms for active hepatitis C virus infections in a high prevalence setting. J Med Econ. 2018;21:1–10.
38. Nguyen LT, Dunford L, Freitas I, Holder P, Nguyen LA, et al. Hepatitis C virus Core mutations associated with false-negative serological results for genotype 3a Core antigen. J Clin Microbiol. 2015;53:2697–700.
39. Harrison GL, Pryor J, Malani J, Supuri M, Masta A, et al. Infection frequency of hepatitis C virus and IL28B haplotypes in Papua New Guinea, Fiji, and Kiribati. PLoS One. 2013;8:e66749.
40. Ubeda F, Jansen VA. The evolution of sex-specific virulence in infectious diseases. Nat Commun. 2016;7:13849.
41. Mori M, Adland E, Paioni P, Swordy A, Mori L, et al. Sex differences in antiretroviral therapy initiation in pediatric HIV infection. PLoS One. 2015;10: e0131591.
42. Reyes-Mendez MA, Juarez-Figueroa L, Iracheta-Hernandez P, Medina-Islas Y, Ruiz-Gonzalez V. Comparison of two diagnostic algorithms for the identification of patients with HCV viremia using a new HCV antigen test. Ann Hepatol. 2014;13:337–42.
43. Wang L, Lv H, Zhang G. Hepatitis C virus core antigen assay: an alternative method for hepatitis C diagnosis. Ann Clin Biochem. 2017;54:279–85.
44. Medici MC, Chezzi C, De Conto F, Ferraglia F, Pinardi F, et al. Evolving strategy for HCV testing in an Italian tertiary care hospital. Journal of clinical virology : the official publication of the Pan American Society for Clinical Virology. 2016;77:92–8.
45. Moini M, Ziyaeyan M, Aghaei S, Sagheb MM, Taghavi SA, et al. Hepatitis C virus (HCV) infection rate among seronegative hemodialysis patients screened by two methods; HCV Core antigen and polymerase chain reaction. Hepat Mon. 2013;13:e9147.
46. Sakiani S, Koh C, Heller T. Understanding the presence of false-positive antibodies in acute hepatitis. J Infect Dis. 2014;210:1886–9.
47. Narciso-Schiavon JL, Schiavon LL, Carvalho-Filho RJ, Cardoso JR, Freire FC, et al. Anti-HCV reactive blood donors: clinical and epidemiological factors associated with false-reactive results. Eur J Gastroenterol Hepatol. 2008;20: 1071–6.
48. Ownby HE, Korelitz JJ, Busch MP, Williams AE, Kleinman SH, et al. Loss of volunteer blood donors because of unconfirmed enzyme immunoassay screening results. Retrovirus epidemiology donor study. Transfusion. 1997; 37:199–205.
49. Seremba E, Ocama P, Opio CK, Kagimu M, Thomas DL, et al. Poor performance of hepatitis C antibody tests in hospital patients in Uganda. J Med Virol. 2010;82:1371–8.
50. Agha S, El-Mashad N, El-Malky M, El-Shony H, El-Sherif MZ, et al. Prevalence of low positive anti-HCV antibodies in blood donors: Schistosoma mansoni co-infection and possible role of autoantibodies. Microbiol Immunol. 2006; 50:447–52.
51. Srivastava AV, Hrobowski T, Krese L, Huang MA, Nemeh H, et al. High rates of false-positive hepatitis C antibody tests can occur after left ventricular assist device implantation. ASAIO J. 2013;59:660–1.

12

Adherence to response-guided pegylated interferon and ribavirin for people who inject drugs with hepatitis C virus genotype 2/3 infection

Evan B. Cunningham[1*], Behzad Hajarizadeh[1], Olav Dalgard[2], Janaki Amin[1], Margaret Hellard[14], Graham R Foster[3], Philip Bruggmann[4], Brian Conway[5], Markus Backmund[6], Geert Robaeys[7,8,9], Tracy Swan[10], Philippa S. Marks[1], Sophie Quiene[1], Tanya L Applegate[1], Martin Weltman[11], David Shaw[12], Adrian Dunlop[13], Julie Bruneau[15], Håvard Midgard[2], Stefan Bourgeois[16], Maria Christine Thurnheer[17], Gregory J Dore[1], Jason Grebely[1] and on behalf of the ACTIVATE Study Group

Abstract

Background: The aims of this analysis were to investigate treatment completion and adherence among people with ongoing injecting drug use or receiving opioid substitution therapy (OST) in a study of response-guided therapy for chronic HCV genotypes 2/3 infection.

Methods: ACTIVATE was a multicenter clinical trial recruited between 2012 and 2014. Participants with genotypes 2/3 were treated with directly observed peg-interferon alfa-2b (PEG-IFN) and self-administered ribavirin for 12 (undetectable HCV RNA at week 4) or 24 weeks (detectable HCV RNA at week 4). Outcomes included treatment completion, PEG-IFN adherence, ribavirin adherence, and sustained virological response (SVR, undetectable HCV RNA >12 weeks post-treatment).

Results: Among 93 people treated, 59% had recently injected drugs (past month), 77% were receiving OST and 56% injected drugs during therapy. Overall, 76% completed treatment. Mean on-treatment adherence to PEG-IFN and ribavirin were 98.2% and 94.6%. Overall, 6% of participants missed >1 dose of PEG-IFN and 31% took <95% of their prescribed ribavirin., Higher treatment completion was observed among those receiving 12 vs. 24 weeks of treatment (97% vs. 46%, $P < 0.001$) while the proportion of participants with 95% on-treatment ribavirin adherence was similar between groups (67% vs. 72%, $P = 0.664$). Receiving 12 weeks of therapy was independently associated with treatment completion. No factors were associated with 95% RBV adherence. Neither recent injecting drug use at baseline nor during therapy was associated with treatment completion or adherence to ribavirin. In adjusted analysis, treatment completion was associated with SVR (aOR 23.9, 95% CI 2.9–193.8).

Conclusions: This study demonstrated a high adherence to directly observed PEG-IFN and self-administered ribavirin among people with ongoing injecting drug use or receiving OST. These data also suggest that shortening therapy from 24 to 12 weeks can lead to improved treatment completion. Treatment completion was associated with improved response to therapy.

Keywords: Hepatitis C, Treatment, PWID, Injection drug use, Adherence

* Correspondence: ecunningham@Kirby.Unsw.Edu.Au
[1]The Kirby Institute, UNSW Sydney, Sydney, NSW, Australia
Full list of author information is available at the end of the article

Background

Among people who inject drugs (PWID), there is a substantial burden of hepatitis C virus (HCV) infection [1, 2]. Adherence [3–6] and treatment completion [3] are associated with sustained virologic response (SVR). Adherence to HCV therapy among PWID is of particular interest given the high cost of new direct-acting antiviral (DAA) therapies and the importance of maximizing the chance of successful therapy.

Adherence refers to the extent to which a person's behaviour, with respect to timing, dosage and frequency of taking medication, corresponds with agreed recommendations from a healthcare provider [7, 8]. Medication adherence research has been performed in a variety of medical conditions, including diabetes, hypertension, arthritis, pulmonary diseases, HIV and others [9] and on average, patients take 79% of prescribed doses of medications [7]. Adherence to HCV therapy is often defined measuring "80/80 adherence", or the receipt of ≥80% of scheduled doses for ≥80% of the scheduled treatment period [7]. However, this definition combines the two distinct concepts of treatment completion and missed doses during therapy. Understanding the two concepts individually is important for understanding adherence in this population of PWID.

Among health practitioners, HCV therapy is sometimes withheld from people with ongoing injecting drug use, based on concerns of poor adherence to therapy, and risk of reinfection [10]. However, there are few studies that have evaluated adherence to HCV therapy among people with ongoing injecting drug use. Understanding adherence to therapy among PWID is a key component to the scale-up of DAA therapy among this population.

ACTIVATE is a multicentre international trial evaluating the efficacy of response-guided directly observed pegylated-interferon and self-administered ribavirin therapy for chronic HCV genotypes 2/3 infection among people with ongoing injecting drug use or receiving opioid substitution therapy (OST). Participants with genotypes 2/3 were treated with directly observed peg-interferon alfa-2b and self-administered ribavirin for either 12 weeks (in those with undetectable HCV RNA at week 4, RVR) or 24 weeks (in those with detectable HCV RNA at week 4, no RVR). The primary analysis from this study demonstrated that cirrhosis (vs. no/mild fibrosis [adjusted odds ratio (aOR) 0.33, 95% CI 0.13, 0.86]) predicted reduced SVR, while response at week 4 was associated with increased SVR (aOR 8.11, 95% CI 2.73, 24.10) [11]. While the PEG-IFN based regimen used in this study has been replaced in many settings with new DAA therapies, data on adherence to HCV therapy among PWID is still needed. Given the increased tolerability and simplicity of new DAA regimens compared to PEG-IFN based therapies, results in this study likely represent a lower bound of adherence among PWID using new DAA therapies.

The primary aim of this analysis was to evaluate treatment completion, adherence to therapy and associated factors (including impact of treatment duration) in the ACTIVATE study. Further, this analysis also investigated the effect of treatment completion and on-treatment adherence on response to HCV therapy (as measured by SVR).

Methods

Study participants

From May 11 2012, to September 30 2014, participants were enrolled at 17 sites in Australia (n = 5), Belgium (n = 2), Canada (n = 3), Germany (n = 1), Norway (n = 2), Switzerland (n = 3) and the United Kingdom (n = 1). The last participant visit was July 15 2015. Study recruitment was conducted through a network of drug and alcohol clinics (n = 3), office-based practices (n = 2), hospital clinics (n = 9), and community clinics (n = 3).

Participants had to be more than 18 years of age, have chronic HCV genotype 2 or 3 infection, be HCV treatment-naïve, and have reported recent injecting drug use, defined as injecting drug use within 12 weeks of enrolment. Due to slower than anticipated recruitment, on June 26 2013, a study protocol amendment was implemented to also include people currently receiving OST with no recent injection drug use and people who had injected within 24 weeks prior to enrolment. Participants with HIV infection and decompensated liver disease were excluded. Full eligibility has been previously published [11].

Study design and intervention

ACTIVATE was an international, multicentre open-label study. Participants received directly observed pegylated interferon alfa-2b (PEG-IFN, 1.5 μg/kg/week) and self-administered ribavirin (RBV, 800–1400 mg daily, weight-based).

Participants with a rapid virological response [RVR, defined as non-quantifiable HCV RNA (<15 IU/ml detected and <15 IU/ml undetected) or undetectable HCV RNA on qualitative assay at week 4] received 12 weeks of therapy (shortened duration). Participants without an RVR [defined as quantifiable HCV RNA (≥15 IU/ml) or detectable HCV RNA on qualitative assay at week 4] received 24 weeks of therapy (standard duration).

Study assessments

Screening assessments included serum HCV RNA levels, HCV genotype, standard laboratory and clinical testing and self-reported behavioural questionnaires (details have been previously reported [11]).

HCV RNA levels and HCV genotype and subtype were measured as previously described [11]. HCV RNA testing was performed on samples collected at screening, baseline, and weeks 4, 12, 24, 36 and 48 (standard duration). All adverse events were recorded and graded according to a standard scale (details have been previously reported [11]).

Directly observed PEG-IFN adherence was recorded by the study nurse. RBV adherence was determined through the return of unused RBV pills. Self-reported RBV adherence was also measured monthly during study visits while on treatment by a patient-administered questionnaire and was used where returned pill counts were unavailable for that time point.

All participants completed a self-administered questionnaire at enrolment (pre-treatment assessment), at baseline (treatment commencement), every 4th week during treatment, and at 12 and 24 weeks of follow-up. The questionnaires collected information on demographics (age, gender, ethnicity, education level, housing status and history of imprisonment), drug and alcohol use, injecting risk behaviours (injection frequency, use of non-sterile needles, needle and syringe borrowing or lending, and injecting paraphernalia [spoons or mixing containers, drug solution/mix, water or filter] sharing), drug treatment, and symptoms of psychological distress (Depression Anxiety Stress Scale, DASS-21). Stable housing was defined as living in a rented or privately owned house or flat..

Social functioning was measured using the short-form Opioid Treatment Index Social Functioning Scale [12]. Social functioning are scored as a sum of the coded responses with higher scores indicating lower social functioning. Alcohol consumption was evaluated by the

Table 1 Baseline demographic and clinical characteristics stratified by 12 week and 24 week duration (n = 93)

Characteristic, n (%)	Overall (n = 93)	12 week (n = 61)	24 week (n = 26)
Age, median (25%, 75%)	41 (35–49)	41 (34–49)	40 (35–48)
Male sex, n (%)	77 (83)	49 (80)	23 (88)
Drug use in the last 6 months (injecting/non-injecting)	77 (83)	48 (79)	25 (96)
Injecting drug use in the last month	55 (59)	39 (64)	15 (58)
Heroin	33 (35)	23 (37)	10 (38)
Cocaine	10 (11)	7 (11)	3 (12)
Amphetamines	14 (15)	7 (11)	6 (23)
Other opiates	11 (12)	8 (13)	3 (12)
Benzodiazapines	2 (2)	2 (3)	0 (0)
Injecting drug use frequency in the last month			
Never	38 (41)	22 (36)	11 (42)
< daily	40 (43)	29 (48)	10 (38)
> daily	15 (16)	10 (16)	5 (19)
Opioid substitution treatment (ever)	82 (88)	56 (92)	21 (81)
OST and recent injecting (past month) at enrolment			
No OST, recent injecting	30 (32)	20 (33)	9 (33)
OST, no recent injecting	23 (25)	15 (25)	5 (19)
OST, recent injecting	40 (43)	26 (43)	12 (44)
OST and recent injecting (past month) at baseline			
No OST, recent injecting	21 (23)	14 (23)	6 (23)
OST, no recent injecting	34 (37)	21 (34)	8 (31)
OST, recent injecting	38 (41)	26 (43)	12 (46)
Stage of liver disease			
No or mild fibrosis (F0-F1)	63 (68)	44 (72)	16 (62)
Moderate or advanced fibrosis (F2-F3)	20 (22)	12 (20)	5 (19)
Cirrhosis (F4)	10 (11)	5 (8)	5 (19)
Study site distribution			
Europe	38 (41)	24 (39)	13 (50)
Australia	40 (43)	27 (44)	9 (35)
Canada	15 (16)	10 (16)	4 (15)

Alcohol Use Disorders Identification Test-Consumption (AUDIT-C), derived from the first three questions of the full AUDIT (scores ≥3 and ≥4 indicate hazardous consumption or active alcohol use disorders among women and men, respectively) [13]. Depression was measured using DASS 21 with a depression score of ≥10 indicating depression.

Study definitions

Treatment completion

Participants with no early discontinuation of PEG-IFN/RBV therapy prior to the per-protocol planned end of treatment (12 or 24 weeks for shortened or standard therapy respectively) were defined as having completed treatment. Participants were deemed to have discontinued treatment early if for any reason (e.g. physician advised treatment discontinuation, virological non-response, lost to follow up, patient decision, etc.) a participant did not reach the per protocol defined end of treatment.

On-treatment adherence

On-treatment adherence was calculated by determining the number of doses taken as proportion of the expected number of doses during the time on treatment. This measures the proportion of doses received from the time that treatment was initiated until treatment was discontinued or completed.

Dose modification

A physician directed increase or reduction in the dose at any time during treatment.

Study outcomes

The main study outcomes were to assess treatment completion, and on-treatment PEG-IFN and RBV adherence. Evaluation of adherence was based on all participants who received at least one injection of PEG-IFN. Treatment success was defined as undetectable qualitative HCV RNA rates at week 12 (SVR).

Statistical analysis

Treatment completion and 95% on-treatment adherence (at least 95% of scheduled doses were taken) were assessed. Bi-variate comparisons of characteristics of participants and different measures of adherence across treatment arms were tested using the chi-squared test or Fisher's exact test as appropriate. Time to treatment discontinuation was evaluated using Kaplan Meier analysis. The impact of treatment completion and on-treatment adherence (both PEG-IFN and ribavirin) on SVR were also evaluated.

Logistic regression analyses were used to estimate crude and adjusted odds ratios (OR) and corresponding 95% confidence intervals (95% CI) to identify predictors of HCV treatment completion and on-treatment ribavirin adherence (at least 95% of scheduled doses were taken). In unadjusted analyses, potential predictors were determined a priori and included sex, age, education, accommodation, employment, current OST treatment, social functioning, current depression, alcohol consumption, injection drug use at baseline (past month), injecting behaviours (frequency and drug injected), and treatment arm. Social functioning was calculated using a validated scale from

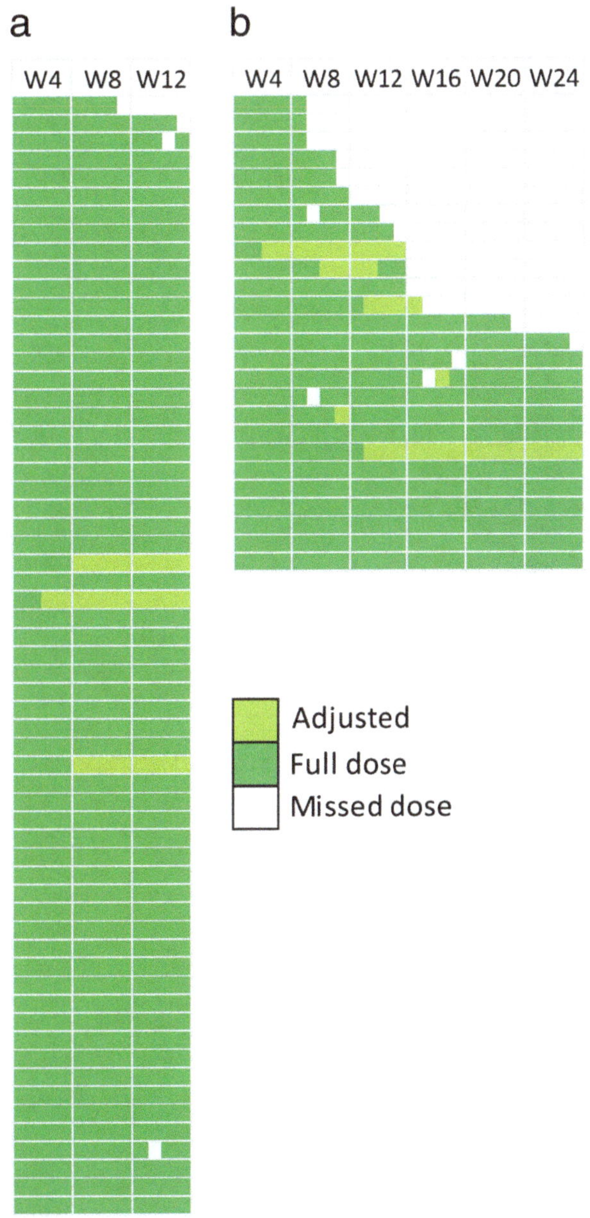

Fig. 1 Weekly PEG-IFN adherence among HCV genotype 2/3 participants on shortened (12 weeks; *n* = 61; panel **a**) and standard therapy (24 weeks; *n* = 26; panel **b**). Each row represents a study participant. Dark green boxes represent a full prescribed dose was received, light green boxes represent an adjusted dose was received, and white boxes represent a missed dose

Table 2 Adherence to PEG-IFN and RBV among the overall population, those on 12 weeks of therapy, and those on 24 weeks of therapy

Variable	Overall (*n* = 93)	12 week (*n* = 61)	24 week (*n* = 26)
Treatment completion	71 (76)	59 (97)	12 (46)
Mean on-treatment PEG-IFN adherence percent, (SD)	98.2 (4.5)	98.5 (3.1)	98.7 (3.0)
Mean on-treatment ribavirin adherence percent, (SD)	94.6 (8.8)	94.8 (8.1)	94.1 (10.8)
Missed doses of PEG-IFN, n (%)			
No missed doses	87 (94)	59 (97)	22 (85)
1 missed dose	6 (6)	2 (3)	4 (15)
2–5 missed doses	0 (0)	0 (0)	0 (0)
> 5 missed doses	0 (0)	0 (0)	0 (0)
Missed doses of ribavirin, n (%)			
100% of doses taken	22 (25)	16 (26)	5 (20)
95%- < 100% of doses taken	38 (44)	25 (41)	13 (52)
90%- < 95% of doses taken	15 (17)	11 (18)	4 (16)
80%- < 90% of doses taken	7 (8)	6 (10)	1 (4)
< 80% of doses taken	5 (6)	3 (5)	2 (8)
Number of weeks of PEG-IFN therapy, n (%)			
24 weeks	12 (13)	NA	12 (46)
13 to 23 weeks	3 (3)	NA	3 (3)
7 to 12 weeks	69 (74)	61 (100)	8 (31)
0 to 6 weeks	9 (10)	0 (0)	3 (12)
Weeks on PEG-IFN therapy			
Mean, n (SD)	NA	11.9 (0.65)	16.8 (7.8)
Median, n (IQR)	NA	12 (12–12)	21 (10–24)
PEG-IFN dose-modification	9 (10)	3 (5)	6 (23)
Ribavirin dose-modification	21 (23)	12 (20)	9 (35)

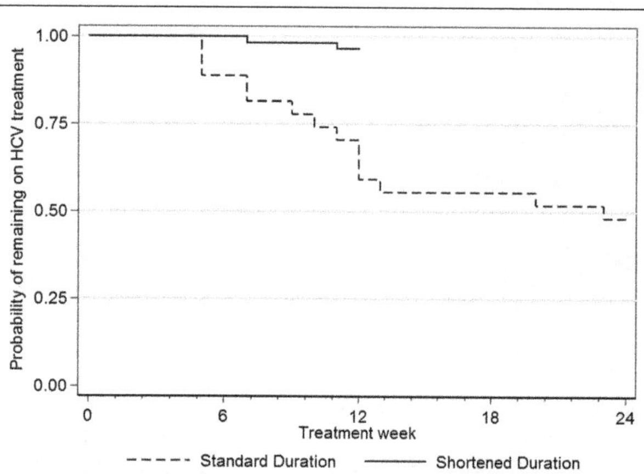

Fig. 2 Time to treatment discontinuation among study participants who were in the shortened (12 week; *n* = 61) and standard (24 week; *n* = 26) arm

the Opiate Treatment Index [27] that addresses employment, residential stability, and inter-personal conflict as well as social support. A higher score reflects poorer social functioning. This scale has been validated among opiate users in Australia (range, 0–48) [27]. All variables with $p < 0.20$ in the bivariate analysis were considered for multivariate logistic regression models using a backward stepwise approach, sequentially eliminated and subject to the result of a likelihood ratio test. Statistically significant differences were assessed at $p < 0.05$; p values are two-sided. Adjusted models for factors associated with SVR were adjusted for all variables found to be associated with SVR in the primary analysis (fibrosis stage and treatment group) as well as by study site using cluster-robust standard errors [11].

Finally, to determine whether later study visits were associated with RBV adherence, generalized estimating equation (GEE) methods were used. Unadjusted and adjusted GEE models were specified using a gaussian family function. Odds ratios (ORs) with corresponding 95% confidence intervals (CIs) and p-values were calculated. All analyses were performed using the statistical package Stata v13.1 (College Station, TX, United States).

Results

Participant characteristics

A full description of the participant characteristics is described in the primary paper [11]. In summary, 93 patients were enrolled in the study between May 2012 and August 2014 and initiated PEG-IFN/ribavirin therapy: median age 41, 83% male, 77% on OST, 59% injecting in the past month (Table 1).

PEG-IFN and RBV adherence and early treatment discontinuation

Of the 93 participants who initiated therapy, six participants discontinued therapy before week 4. Reasons for discontinuing therapy prior to week 4 include side effects (n = 3), unwillingness to continue treatment (n = 1), loss to follow up (n = 1), and imprisonment (n = 1). Among the remaining 87 participants, 70% (n = 61) were HCV RNA undetectable at week 4 (rapid virological response, RVR) and were scheduled to receive 12 weeks of therapy (shortened duration) and 30% (n = 26) did not have an RVR at week 4 and were scheduled to receive 24 weeks of therapy (standard duration).

An abbreviated description of participant adherence is described in the primary paper [11]. Weekly PEG-IFN adherence among those receiving 12 weeks of therapy and 24 weeks of therapy is shown in Fig. 1. Among the entire study population, 76% (n = 71) completed HCV therapy (Table 2). Time to discontinuation stratified by duration of therapy is shown in Fig. 2. The median time to discontinuation was 12 weeks and 23 weeks in the 12 week and 24 week groups respectively. Mean on-treatment adherence to PEG-IFN and ribavirin were 98% and 95% (Table 2). Overall, 6% of participants missed >1 dose of PEG-IFN and 31% missed >5% of their doses of ribavirin.

Completion of treatment was more frequent in the 12 week group compared to the 24 week group (97% vs. 46%, P < 0.001). In the 12 week group, completion of 0–4, 5–8, and 9–12 weeks of therapy was demonstrated by 0% (n = 0), 2% (n = 1), and 98% (n = 60), respectively. In the 24 week arm, completion of 0–4, 5–8, 9–12, 13–23, and 24 weeks was demonstrated by 0% (n = 0), 19% (n = 5), 23% (n = 6), 3% (n = 3) and 46% (n = 12) respectively. Reasons for discontinuing prior to the planned end of therapy include side effects (overall, n = 11; 12 week, n = 1; 24 week, n = 7), patient unwillingness (overall, n = 5; 12 week, n = 1; 24 week, n = 3), patient lost to follow-up (overall, n = 4; 12 week, n = 0; 24 week, n = 3), and virological failure (overall, n = 1; 12 week, n = 0; 24 week, n = 1). The mean number of weeks of PEG-IFN therapy was 11.9 and 16.8 weeks in the 12 week and 24 week groups respectively.

The mean on-treatment PEG-IFN adherence was similar between those receiving 12 and 24 weeks of therapy (98.5% vs. 98.7%, P = 0.811). The proportion of participants missing at least one dose of PEG-IFN while on therapy was 3% in those receiving 12 weeks of therapy

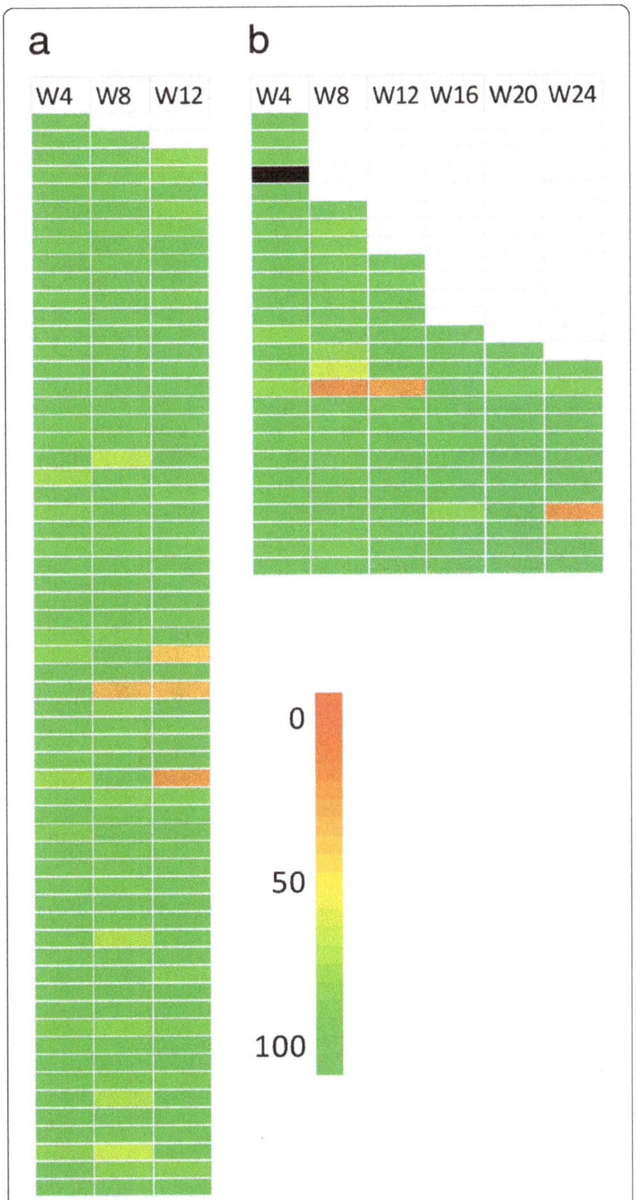

Fig. 3 Four-weekly RBV adherence among HCV genotype 2/3 participants on shortened (12 weeks; n = 61; panel **a**) and standard therapy (24 weeks; n = 26; panel **b**). Each row represents a study participant. Colours represent each participant's RBV adherence during each four-week period with dark green representing 100% adherence and red representing 0% adherence. White represents discontinuation before completion of the corresponding time-point while black represents missing data for both retuned pill counts and patient reported adherence before treatment discontinuation

Table 3 Unadjusted potential predictors of treatment completion among the study population (n = 93)

	Number completed treatment (%; n = 71	Number not completing treatment (%; n = 22)	Unadjusted OR	95% CI	P
Age (years)					
≤ 41	38 (83)	8 (17)	1.00	-	-
> 41	33 (70)	14 (30)	0.50	0.19–1.33	0.164
Gender					
Female	13 (81)	3 (19)	1.00	-	-
Male	58 (75)	19 (25)	0.70	0.18–2.74	0.613
Education[a]					
< Tertiary	52 (79)	14 (21)	1.00	-	-
Tertiary or greater	18 (75)	6 (25)	0.81	0.27–2.42	0.703
Social functioning score					
< 17	31 (78)	9 (23)	1.00	-	-
≥ 17	40 (75)	13 (25)	0.89	0.34–2.36	0.820
Stable housing					
No	17 (77)	5 (23)	1.00	-	-
Yes	54 (76)	17 (24)	0.93	0.30–2.91	0.907
Current depression[b]					
No	30 (75)	10 (25)	1.00	-	-
Yes	37 (80)	9 (20)	1.37	0.49–3.80	0.545
Hazardous alcohol consumption[c]					
No	58 (81)	14 (19)	1.00	-	-
Yes	11 (83)	2 (15)	1.71	0.35–8.43	0.512
Current OST					
No	19 (70)	8 (30)	1.00	-	-
Yes	52 (79)	14 (21)	1.56	0.57–4.32	0.388
Injecting (last month)					
No	26 (68)	12 (32)	1.00	-	-
Yes	45 (82)	10 (18)	2.08	0.79–5.47	0.139
Frequency of injecting (last month)					
Never	26 (68)	12 (32)	1.00	-	-
Less than weekly	17 (77)	5 (23)	1.57	0.47–5.26	0.465
Weekly or greater	28 (85)	5 (15)	2.58	0.80–8.34	0.112
Heroin injecting (last month)					
No	43 (72)	17 (28)	1.00	-	-
Yes	28 (85)	5 (15)	2.21	0.73–6.68	0.159
Cocaine injecting (last month)					
No	63 (76)	20 (24)	1.00	-	-
Yes	8 (80)	2 (20)	1.27	0.25–6.48	0.774
Amphetamine injecting (last month)					
No	63 (80)	16 (20)	1.00	-	-
Yes	8 (57)	6 (43)	0.34	0.10–1.12	0.075

Table 3 Unadjusted potential predictors of treatment completion among the study population (*n* = 93) *(Continued)*

Injecting on therapy					
No	30 (83)	6 (17)	1.00	-	-
Yes	41 (79)	11 (21)	0.75	0.25–2.24	0.601
Therapy duration*					
24 weeks	13 (50)	13 (50)	1.00	-	-
12 weeks	58 (95)	3 (5)	19.33	4.81–77.78	<0.001

*Among participants who attended study week 4
[a]Missing data for three participants
[b]Missing data for seven participants
[c]Missing data for eight participants; percentages refer to row percentages

compared to 15% in those receiving 24 weeks of therapy (P = 0.072).

Four-weekly RBV adherence among those receiving 12 weeks of therapy and 24 weeks of therapy is shown in Fig. 3. Returned pill counts were used in 276 of the 284 on treatment visits in Fig. 3 (97%). In the case of missing pill counts (n = 8) participant completed questionnaire data was used where available (n = 7). Data was not available, either from pill counts or patient completed questionnaires for one study visit. The mean overall on-treatment RBV adherence was similar between those receiving 12 and 24 weeks of therapy (94.8% vs. 94.1%, P = 0.751). The mean on-treatment adherence to RBV in the 12 week arm during weeks 1–4, 5–8, and 9–12 was 96.9%, 93.8% and 93.5% respectively. The mean on-treatment adherence to RBV in the 24 week arm during weeks 1–4, 5–8, and 9–12 was 96.6%, 88.3% and 95.2% respectively. Overall 65% of participants had >95% on-treatment RBV adherence.

Factors associated with treatment completion and on-treatment RBV adherence

In unadjusted analyses, treatment completion occurred more frequently in those with recent injecting at baseline, recent heroin injecting at baseline, injecting weekly or more in the past month, and those in the 12 week arm but less often in people with recent amphetamine injecting at baseline and those who were >41 years of age (Table 3). The only factor that remained independently associated with treatment completion was shortened treatment arm (aOR 31.2, P = <0.001).

In unadjusted analyses, no factors were associated with >95% on-treatment RBV adherence (Table 4). In GEE analyses, later study visit was not associated with adherence to RBV (OR 1.00, P = 0.489).

Impact of missed doses of PEG-IFN and RBV, and treatment completion on SVR

In unadjusted analyses, SVR occurred more frequently among those who completed treatment (OR 34.4, P = <0.001). Neither 100% PEG-IFN adherence, nor >95% RBV adherence were associated with SVR in unadjusted analyses and were therefore not included in the adjusted model. In adjusted analyses, when adjusted for all factors found to be associated with SVR in the primary analysis [11], treatment completion remained as being associated with SVR (aOR 23.86, P = 0.003; Table 5).

Discussion

This study investigated treatment completion and the adherence to response-guided directly observed PEG-IFN and self-administered ribavirin treatment for chronic HCV genotypes 2/3 among PWID with ongoing drug use and those receiving OST. The results demonstrated high adherence to directly observed PEG-IFN and self-administered RBV therapy, particularly among participants receiving 12 weeks, as opposed to 24 weeks, of therapy. Being scheduled to receive 12 weeks of therapy was an independent predictor of treatment completion. There were no independent predictors of >95% RBV adherence in the population. Neither recent injection drug use prior to treatment, nor injection drug use while on treatment, were associated with treatment completion or >95% on-treatment RBV adherence. Further, the majority of the sub-optimal treatment exposure was due to early discontinuation of therapy rather than missed doses while on therapy. Finally, while neither PEG-IFN nor RBV adherence was an independent predictor of SVR, treatment completion was found to be an independent predictor of SVR. These data have important clinical implications informing HCV management among PWID with ongoing drug use and those receiving OST in the DAA era, given that the majority of licensed regimens require only 12 weeks of therapy.

Overall, adherence to PEG-IFN/RBV therapy was high with few participants (6%) missing ≥1 dose of PEG-IFN while on therapy, with no one missing more than one dose for a high on-treatment adherence of 98%. This is consistent with previous studies of PEG-IFN adherence where on-treatment adherence ranged from 74% to 99% [3, 14–17]. While slightly lower than PEG-IFN adherence, a similarly high on-treatment RBV adherence was observed (94.6%) with 71% of participants taking at least 95% of their RBV doses. The proportion of the

Table 4 Unadjusted potential predictors of RBV adherence among the study population with available RBV adherence data (*n* = 86)

	RBV adherence of 95% (%; *n* = 59)	RBV adherence of < 95% (%; *n* = 27)	Unadjusted OR	95% CI	*P*
Age (years)					
≤ 41	29 (66)	15 (34)	1.00	-	-
> 41	30 (71)	12 (29)	1.25	0.50–3.11	0.632
Gender					
Female	49 (69)	22 (31)	1.00	-	-
Male	10 (67)	5 (33)	1.14	0.35–3.72	0.833
Education[a]					
< Tertiary	43 (69)	19 (31)	1.00	-	-
Tertiary or greater	15 (71)	6 (29)	1.18	0.40–3.48	0.766
Social functioning score					
< 17	29 (76)	9 (24)	1.00	-	-
≥ 17	30 (63)	18 (38)	0.53	0.21–1.38	0.195
Current depression[b]					
No	24 (65)	13 (35)	1.00	-	-
Yes	30 (68)	14 (32)	1.11	0.44–2.80	0.818
Hazardous alcohol consumption[c]					
No	48 (68)	23 (32)	1.00	-	-
Yes	8 (67)	4 (33)	0.94	0.26–3.44	0.924
Current OST					
No	16 (64)	9 (36)	1.00	-	-
Yes	43 (70)	18 (30)	1.26	0.48–3.36	0.638
Injecting (last month)					
No	22 (69)	10 (31)	1.00	-	-
Yes	37 (69)	17 (31)	0.95	0.37–2.42	0.908
Frequency of injecting (last month)					
Never	22 (69)	10 (31)	1.00	-	-
Less than weekly	14 (67)	7 (33)	0.87	0.27–2.81	0.815
Weekly or greater	23 (70)	10 (30)	1.00	0.35–2.86	1.000
Heroin injecting (last month)					
No	35 (66)	18 (34)	1.00	-	-
Yes	24 (73)	9 (27)	1.33	0.51–3.46	0.554
Cocaine injecting (last month)					
No	52 (68)	24 (32)	1.00	-	-
Yes	7 (70)	3 (30)	0.77	0.25–4.44	0.940
Amphetamine injecting (last month)					
No	51 (69)	23 (31)	1.00	-	-
Yes	8 (67)	4 (33)	0.88	0.24–3.24	0.853
Injecting on therapy					
No	25 (74)	9 (26)	1.00	-	-
Yes	34 (65)	18 (35)	0.65	0.25–1.69	0.380
Therapy duration					
24 weeks	18 (72)	7 (28)	1.00	-	-
12 weeks	41 (67)	20 (33)	0.80	0.29–2.22	0.664

[a]Missing data for three participants
[b]Missing data for five participants
[c]Missing data for three participants; percentages refer to row percentages

Table 5 Unadjusted and adjusted models of adherence-related predictors of SVR among the study population

	SVR (%)	Unadjusted OR	95% CI	*P*	Adjusted OR	95% CI	*P*
95% ribavirin adherence*							
No	17 (63)	1.00	-	-	-	-	-
Yes	44 (73)	1.62	0.61–4.26	0.330	-	-	-
100% PEG-IFN adherence*							
No	58 (67)	1.00	-	-	-	-	-
Yes	3 (50)	2.00	0.38–10.53	0.413	-	-	-
Completed therapy							
No	2 (9)	1.00	-	-	1.00	-	-
Yes	59 (83)	34.41	6.90–171.55	0.000	23.86	2.94–193.84	0.003

The adjusted model is adjusted for all factors associated with SVR from the primary analysis [11]
*On-treatment adherence

population with >95% adherence is lower than was reported in the C-EDGE CO-STAR trial (96%), a randomized controlled trial of elbasvir-grazoprevir in people receiving stable opioid agonist therapy [18]. This is potentially due to the higher toxicity of PEG-IFN/RBV therapy or the increased pill burden due to the inclusion of RBV. Also, the C-EDGE CO-STAR trial likely represents a more stable population given the inclusion of only those on stable OST and the exclusion of those actively using drugs of potential abuse. As such, it is difficult to directly compare these results.

Participants who were allocated 12 weeks of therapy demonstrated a higher proportion completing therapy than those allocated 24 weeks of therapy. Recent injection drug use prior to and during treatment was not associated with PEG-IFN adherence, RBV adherence, or treatment completion, consistent with previous data [3, 10, 19–22].

While PEG-IFN based therapies have recently been replaced by new DAA therapies in many settings, data on the adherence to HCV therapies among PWID is still needed. In many countries, concerns still exist regarding the adherence to therapy among active PWID [10, 23]. As a result many countries have restricted the use of DAA therapies to those without current injecting [23–25]. A better understanding of adherence among active injectors is therefore needed to inform policy and remove the restrictions placed on DAA therapies. This data also highlights the positive effect of shortened therapy on treatment completion in this population as pushes to further shorten HCV therapy continue. This study includes data on adherence to self-administered ribavirin, providing some insight into adherence of an oral twice-daily antiviral therapy. Given the increased tolerability and simplicity DAA regimens compared to PEG-IFN and ribavirin-based therapies, adherence should be comparable, if not better, than that observed with twice-daily ribavirin, Further data is needed to assess adherence to DAA-based therapy among people with ongoing injecting drug use.

There are some limitations to this study. Adherence to RBV was determined based on returned pill counts where available and patient surveys where pill counts were unavailable. While pill counts are generally a better estimate of the true adherence as compared to patient reported adherence [26], there is still the potential for overestimation through lost pills. The measurement of adherence to PEG-IFN was more robust, given that this was a directly observed dose in the presence of the study nurse who recorded when the dose was taken. Further, adherence is a very complex phenomenon and may be influenced by a number of unmeasured factors (e.g. past experience with adherence to other medications, patient-doctor relationships). Lastly, the small sample size of this study is a limitation. With a larger sample size, it would be possible to more accurately estimate the true effects of various factors on HCV treatment adherence and the true effect of treatment adherence on SVR. In addition, while the international nature of this study increases the generalizability to globally diverse PWID populations, the participants recruited into this study may represent a somewhat selected group, based on improved engagement in care. Irrespective of these limitations, this is the first international study to evaluate adherence to HCV therapy among PWID and those receiving OST.

Conclusions

This study demonstrates high adherence to response-guided directly observed pegylated-interferon and self-administered ribavirin therapy for chronic HCV genotypes 2/3 infection among people with ongoing injecting drug use or receiving OST. These data suggest that shortening HCV therapy has the potential to increase treatment completion among PWID. This is of particular importance given the interest in evaluating shorter durations of DAA therapy. Further, injecting drug use both prior to and during treatment was not associated with reduced adherence to therapy or treatment completions.

These data suggest that adherence to HCV therapy among HCV infected PWID is not compromised by ongoing injection drug use and supports guidelines which suggest that active PWID should not be excluded from therapy; rather decisions should be made on a case-by-case basis [27–30]. Further studies are needed to characterize adherence to interferon-free DAA therapies among PWID and those receiving OST to better understand whether adherence is actually a problem in this population in the DAA era.

Abbreviations
aOR: Adjusted odds ratio; DAA: Direct acting antiviral; HCV: Hepatitis C virus; HIV: Human immunodeficiency virus; OR: Odds ratio; OST: Opioid substitution therapy; PEG-IFN: Pegylated-interferon alfa-2b; PWID: People who inject drugs; RBV: Ribavirin; RVR: Rapid virological response; SVR: Sustained virological response

Acknowledgements
The authors would like to thank the study participants for their contribution to the research, as well as current and past researchers and staff. They would like to acknowledge members of the study group:
Protocol Steering Committee – Gregory Dore (Chair, UNSW Australia, Sydney, Australia), Jason Grebely (UNSW Australia, Sydney, Australia), Philip Bruggmann (Arud Centres for Addiction Medicine, Zurich, Switzerland), Philippa Marks (UNSW Australia, Sydney, Australia), Brian Conway (Vancouver Infectious Diseases Center, Vancouver, Canada), Geert Robaeys (Department of Gastroenterology and Hepatology, Ziekenhuis Oost Limburg, Genk, Belgium), Tracy Swan (Treatment Action Group, New York, United States), Graham Foster (The Liver Unit, Queen Mary University of London, London, United Kingdom), Markus Backmund (Ludwig Maximilians-University Munich, Munich, Germany) and Olav Dalgard (Akershus University Hospital, Oslo, Norway).
Coordinating Centre – Sophie Quiene (Study Co-ordinator), Evan Cunningham (PhD Student), Behzad Hajarizadeh (Associate Lecturer), Gregory Dore (Principal Investigator), Jason Grebely (Co-investigator), Pip Marks (Clinical Trials Manager), Ineke Shaw (Systems Manager), Sharmila Siriragavan (Data Manager) and Janaki Amin (Statistician).
Site Principal Investigators – Markus Backmund (PIT Munich, Munich, Germany), Stefan Bourgeois (ZNA Stuivenberg, Antwerp, Belgium), Philip Bruggmann (Arud Centres for Addiction Medicine, Zurich, Switzerland), Julie Bruneau (Centre Hôspitalier de l'Université de Montréal, Montréal, Canada), Brian Conway (Vancouver Infectious Diseases Center, Vancouver, Canada), Olav Dalgard (Akershus University Hospital, Oslo, Norway), Gregory Dore (St Vincent's Hospital, Sydney Australia), Adrian Dunlop (Newcastle Pharmacotherapy Service, Newcastle, Australia), Graham Foster (Tower Hamlets Specialist Addiction Unit, London, United Kingdom), Margaret Hellard (The Alfred Hospital, Melbourne, Australia), Jeff Powis (South Riverdale Community Health Centre, Toronto, Canada), Geert Robaeys (Department of Gastroenterology and Hepatology, Ziekenhuis Oost Limburg, Genk, Belgium), Stephen Ryder (Nottingham University Hospital, Nottingham, United Kingdom), Claude Scheidegger (Zentrum für Suchtmedizin, Basel, Switzerland), David Shaw (Royal Adelaide Hospital, Adelaide, Australia), Cornelia Staehelin (Poliklinik für Infektiologie, Inselspital, Bern, Switzerland) and Martin Weltman (Nepean Hospital, Penrith, Australia).
Site Co-ordinators – David Axten (Tower Hamlets Specialist Addiction Unit, London, United Kingdom), Jessica Andreassen and Ingunn Melkeraaen (Akershus University Hospital, Oslo, Norway), Anita Eevers (Department of Gastroenterology and Hepatology, Ziekenhuis Oost Limburg, Genk, Belgium), Catherine Ferguson (Royal Adelaide Hospital, Adelaide, Australia), Vincenzo Fragomeli (Nepean Hospital, Penrith, Australia), Susan Hazelwood and Rohan Holland (Newcastle Pharmacotherapy Service, Newcastle, Australia), Tina Horschik (Arud Centres for Addiction Medicine, Zurich, Switzerland), Christine Huber (Zentrum für Suchtmedizin, Basel, Switzerland), Kate Jack (Nottingham University Hospital, Nottingham, United Kingdom), Barbara Kotsoros (Centre Hôspitalier de l'Université de Montréal, Montréal, Canada), Melanie Lacalamita (Poliklinik für Infektiologie, Inselspital, Bern, Switzerland), Kristof Lesneuck (ZNA Stuivenberg, Antwerp, Belgium), Kate Mason (South Riverdale Community Health Centre, Toronto, Canada), Alison Sevehon (St Vincent's Hospital, Sydney, Australia), Shawn Sharma (Vancouver Infectious Diseases Center, Vancouver, Canada), Sally Von Bibra (The Alfred Hospital, Melbourne, Australia), Nicole Widder (PIT Munich, Munich, Germany).

Funding
Supported in part by a research grant from the Investigator Initiated Studies Program of Merck Sharp & Dohme Corp. The opinions expressed in this paper are those of the authors and do not necessarily represent those of Merck Sharp & Dohme Corp. The Kirby Institute is funded by the Australian Government Department of Health and Ageing. The views expressed in this publication do not necessarily represent the position of the Australian Government. JG is supported by a National Health and Medical Research Council Career Development Fellowship. BH is supported by a National Health and Medical Research Council Early Career Fellowship. MH is supported by a National Health and Medical Research Council Principal Research Fellowship. GD is supported by a National Health and Medical Research Council Practitioner Research Fellowships.

Availability of data and materials
The data in this study are available upon request. The data cannot be publicly available because they contain confidential and potentially identifying information. Data will be made available to all interested researchers upon request. Data requests should be submitted to ACTIVATE Steering Committee (Professor Greg Dore, the chair: gdore@kirby.unsw.edu.au).

Authors' contributions
OD, JA, MH, GRF, PB, BC, MB, GR, TS, PSM, SQ, TLA, MW, DS, AD, JB, SB, MCT, GJD, JG were responsible for design and implementation of the study. JG and EBC were responsible for conception of this analysis. EBC, JG, JA, BH, HM were responsible for analysis of the data. EBC was responsible for writing the manuscript. All authors reviewed the manuscript and gave approval for publication.

Competing interests
JG is a consultant/advisor and has received research grants from Abbvie, Bristol Myers Squibb, Cepheid, Gilead Sciences and Merck/MSD and is an associate editor for BMC Infectious Diseases. OD is a consultant/advisor and has received research grants from Abbvie, Gilead Sciences and Merck/MSD. GRF is a consultant/advisor and has received research grants from Abbvie, Bristol Myers Squibb, Gilead Sciences, Janssen, Roche and Merck/MSD. PB is consultant/advisor and has received research grants from Abbvie, Bristol Myers Squibb, Gilead, Janssen and Merck. BC is consultant/advisor and has received research grants from AbbVie, Gilead and Merck. GR has received research grants from Merck Sharp & Dohme, AbbVie, Janssen Pharmaceuticals, and has acted as a consultant/advisor and for Gilead Sciences, Abbvie, Merck Sharp & Dohme, and Bristol Myers-Squibb. MW is a consultant/advisor for Abbvie, Bristol Myers Squibb, Gilead, Merck, Janssen, Novartis and Roche. MH has received funding from Gilead Sciences, Abbvie and Bristol Myers Squibb for investigator initiated independent research. JB is a consultant/advisor and has received research grants from Gilead Sciences and Merck/MSD. SB is a consultant/advisor and has received research grants from AbbVie, MSD, BMS, Gilead, Janssen. CS has received travel grants through her institution sponsored by Gilead Sciences, Janssen and Merck/MSD. GD is a consultant/advisor and has received research grants from Abbvie, Bristol Myers Squibb, Gilead, Merck, Janssen and Roche.

Ethics approval and consent to participate
All study participants provided written informed consent before study procedures. The study protocol was approved by St. Vincent's Hospital, Sydney Human Research Ethics Committee (primary study committee), as well as through local ethics committees (Additional file 1) at all study sites, and was conducted according to the Declaration of Helsinki and International Conference on Harmonization Good Clinical Practice (ICH/GCP) guidelines. The study was registered with clinicaltrials.gov registry

(NCT01364090). The sponsor (The Kirby Institute, UNSW Australia) collected the data, monitored study conduct and performed the statistical analysis. An independant data and safety monitoring board reviewed the progress of the study.

Consent for publication

Not applicable.

Author details

[1]The Kirby Institute, UNSW Sydney, Sydney, NSW, Australia. [2]Akershus University Hospital, Oslo, Norway. [3]The Liver Unit, Queen Mary University of London, London, UK. [4]Arud Centres for Addiction Medicine, Zurich, Switzerland. [5]Vancouver Infectious Diseases Center, Vancouver, BC, Canada. [6]Ludwig Maximilians-University Munich, Munich, Germany. [7]Department of Gastroenterology and Hepatology, Ziekenhuis Oost Limburg, Genk, Belgium. [8]Department of Hepatology, UZ Leuven, Leuven, Belgium. [9]UHasselt, Hasselt, Belgium. [10]Treatment Action Group, New York, NY, USA. [11]Nepean Hospital, Sydney, NSW, Australia. [12]Royal Adelaide Hospital, Adelaide, South Australia, Australia. [13]School of Medicine and Public Health, University of Newcastle, Newcastle, NSW, Australia. [14]Burnet Institute, Melbourne, VIC, Australia. [15]Research Center, Centre Hospitalier de l'Universite de Montreal (CRCHUM), Montreal, Quebec, Canada. [16]Stuivenberg ZNA, Antwerp, Belgium. [17]Department of Infectious Diseases, Bern University Hospital, University of Bern, Bern, Switzerland.

References

1. Nelson PK, Mathers BM, Cowie B, Hagan H, Des Jarlais D, Horyniak D, et al. Global epidemiology of hepatitis B and hepatitis C in people who inject drugs: results of systematic reviews. Lancet. 2011;378(9791):571–83.
2. Hajarizadeh B, Grebely J, Dore GJ. Epidemiology and natural history of HCV infection. Nat Rev Gastroenterol Hepatol. 2013;10(9):553–62.
3. Grebely J, Matthews GV, Hellard M, Shaw D, van Beek I, Petoumenos K, et al. Adherence to treatment for recently acquired hepatitis C virus (HCV) infection among injecting drug users. J Hepatol. 2011;55(1):76–85.
4. Sylvestre DL, Clements BJ. Adherence to hepatitis C treatment in recovering heroin users maintained on methadone. Eur J Gastroenterol Hepatol. 2007; 19(9):741–7.
5. Manolakopoulos S, Deutsch MJ, Anagnostou O, Karatapanis S, Tiniakou E, Papatheodoridis GV, et al. Substitution treatment or active intravenous drug use should not be contraindications for antiviral treatment in drug users with chronic hepatitis C. Liver Int. 2010;30(10):1454–60.
6. Sasadeusz JJ, Dore G, Kronborg I, Barton D, Yoshihara M, Weltman M. Clinical experience with the treatment of hepatitis C infection in patients on opioid pharmacotherapy. Addiction. 2011;106(5):977–84.
7. Weiss JJ, Brau N, Stivala A, Swan T, Fishbein D. Review article: adherence to medication for chronic hepatitis C - building on the model of human immunodeficiency virus antiretroviral adherence research. Aliment Pharmacol Ther. 2009;30(1):14–27.
8. Burkhart PV, Sabate E. Adherence to long-term therapies: evidence for action. J Nurs Scholarship. 2003;35(3):207.
9. Cramer JA, Roy A, Burrell A, Fairchild CJ, Fuldeore MJ, Ollendorf DA, et al. Medication compliance and persistence: terminology and definitions. Value Health. 2008;11(1):44–7.
10. Grebely J, Tyndall MW. Management of HCV and HIV infections among people who inject drugs. Curr Opin HIV AIDS. 2011;6(6):501–7.
11. Grebely J, Dalgard O, Cunningham EB, Hajarizadeh B, Foster GR, Bruggmann P. Efficacy of response-guided directly observed pegylated interferon and self-administered ribavirin for people who inject drugs with hepatitis C virus genotype 2/3 infection: the ACTIVATE study. IJDP. 2016. In Press.
12. Maher L, Li J, Jalaludin B, Chant KG, Kaldor JM. High hepatitis C incidence in new injecting drug users: a policy failure? Aust N Z J Public Health. 2007; 31(1):30–5.
13. Bush K, Kivlahan DR, McDonell MB, Fihn SD, Bradley KA. The AUDIT alcohol consumption questions (AUDIT-C): an effective brief screening test for problem drinking. Ambulatory care quality improvement project (ACQUIP). Alcohol use disorders identification test. Arch Intern Med. 1998;158(16):1789–95.
14. Fumaz CR, Muñoz-Moreno JA, Ballesteros AL, Paredes R, Ferrer MJ, Salas A, et al. Influence of the type of pegylated interferon on the onset of depressive and neuropsychiatric symptoms in HIV-HCV coinfected patients. AIDS Care. 2007;19(1):138–45.
15. Smith SR, Wahed AS, Kelley SS, Conjeevaram HS, Robuck PR, Fried MW. Assessing the validity of self-reported medication adherence in hepatitis C treatment. Ann Pharmacother. 2007;41(7):1116–23.
16. Weiss JJ, Bhatti L, Dieterich DT, Edlin BR, Fishbein DA, Goetz MB, et al. Hepatitis C patients' self-reported adherence to treatment with pegylated interferon and ribavirin. Aliment Pharmacol Ther. 2008;28(3):289–93.
17. Cacoub P, Melin P, Ouzan D, Cattan L, Chousterman M, Varastet M, et al. 776 patient education improves adherence to PEGINTERFERON and ribavirin in chronic genotype 2 or 3 hepatitis c virus (HCV) infection in the real-Life. J Hepatol. 2008;48:S289–90.
18. Dore G, Altice F, Litwin AH, Dalgard O, Gane EJ, Shibolet O, Luetkemeyer A, Nahass R, Peng CY, Conway B *et al*:C-EDGE CO-STAR: Efficacy of Grazoprevir and Elbasvir in Persons who Inject Drugs (PWID) Receiving Opioid Agonist Therapy.Hepatology 2015, 62:227a-228a.
19. Marcellin P, Chousterman M, Fontanges T, Ouzan D, Rotily M, Varastet M, et al. Adherence to treatment and quality of life during hepatitis C therapy: a prospective, real-life, observational study. Liver Int. 2011;31(4):516–24.
20. Manolakopoulos S, Deutsch MJ, Anagnostou O, Karatapanis S, Tiniakou E, Papatheodoridis GV, et al. Substitution treatment or active intravenous drug use should not be contraindications for antiviral treatment in drug users with chronic hepatitis C. Liver Int. 2010;30(10):1454–60.
21. Wilkinson M, Crawford V, Tippet A, Jolly F, Turton J, Sims E, et al. Community-based treatment for chronic hepatitis C in drug users: high rates of compliance with therapy despite ongoing drug use. Aliment Pharmacol Ther. 2009;29(1):29–37.
22. Sylvestre DL, Clements BJ. Adherence to hepatitis C treatment in recovering heroin users maintained on methadone. Eur J Gastroenterol Hepatol. 2007;19(9):741–7.
23. Marshall AD, Nielsen S, Cunningham EB, Aghemo A, Alho H, Backmund M, Bruggmann P, Dalgard O: Restrictions for reimbursement of interferon-free direct acting antiviral therapies for HCV infection in Europe. ILC 2017 - LBP-505 2017.
24. Barua S, Greenwald R, Grebely J, Dore GJ, Swan T, Taylor LE. Restrictions for Medicaid Reimbursement of Sofosbuvir for the Treatment of Hepatitis C Virus Infection in the United States. Annals of Internal Medicine. 2015;163(3):215.
25. Marshall AD, Saeed S, Barrett L, Cooper CL, Treloar C, Bruneau J, et al. Restrictions for reimbursement of direct-acting antiviral treatment for hepatitis C virus infection in Canada: a descriptive study. CMAJ open. 2016; 4(4):E605–14.
26. Weiss JJ, BrÄU N, Stivala A, Swan T, Fishbein D. Review article: adherence to medication for chronic hepatitis C - building on the model of human immunodeficiency virus antiretroviral adherence research. Aliment Pharmacol Ther. 2009;30(1):14–27.
27. Swan T, Curry J. Comment on the updated AASLD practice guidelines for the diagnosis, management, and treatment of hepatitis C: treating active drug users. Hepatology. 2009;50(1):323–4.
28. Ghany MG, Strader DB, Thomas DL, Seeff LB. Diagnosis, management, and treatment of hepatitis C: an update. Hepatology. 2008;49(4):1335–74.
29. Grebely J, Haire B, Taylor LE, Macneill P, Litwin AH, Swan T, et al. Excluding people who use drugs or alcohol from access to hepatitis C treatments - is this fair, given the available data? J Hepatol. 2015;63(4):779–82.
30. Grebely J, Robaeys G, Bruggmann P, Aghemo A, Backmund M, Bruneau J, et al. Recommendations for the management of hepatitis C virus infection among people who inject drugs. The International journal on drug policy. 2015;26(10):1028–38.

Estimates of state-level chronic hepatitis C virus infection, stratified by race and sex, United States, 2010

Eric W. Hall[1*], Eli S. Rosenberg[2] and Patrick S. Sullivan[1]

Abstract

Background: Hepatitis C virus (HCV) is the most common blood-borne viral infection in the United States. Previously, we used data from the National Health and Nutrition Examination Survey (NHANES) and mortality data from the National Vital Statistics System (NVSS) to estimate the prevalence of HCV antibodies (anti-HCV) and HCV RNA among all U.S. states. However, demographic differences in HCV burden at the state-level have not been systematically described. This analysis quantified the HCV burden stratified by sex and race (and associated disparities) for each U.S. state.

Methods: Building on our previous method, we used three publicly available data sources to estimate HCV RNA prevalence among noninstitutionalized adults stratified by sex and race group. We used a small-area estimation approach that included direct standardization of NHANES demographic data with logistic regression modeling of HCV-related mortality data as an adjustment factor to estimate the state-level prevalence and total persons with chronic HCV infection for sex and race groups in all U.S. states.

Results: Nationally, males had an estimated HCV RNA prevalence of 1.56% (95% CI: 1.37–1.84%) and females had a prevalence of 0.75% (95% CI: 0.63–0.96%). Stratified by race, national estimated prevalence of HCV RNA was highest among non-Hispanic black (2.43, 95% CI: 2.10–2.90%), followed by non-Hispanic white (1.05, 95% CI: 0.90–1.27%) and Hispanic/other (0.74, 95% CI: 0.59–1.04%). Males in most jurisdictions (41/51) have an HCV RNA prevalence that is between 1.5 and 2.5 times higher than their female counterparts.

Conclusions: HCV infection disparities by sex are mostly consistent across the country. However, race differences in HCV infection differ by state and tailored prevention and treatment efforts specific to the local HCV epidemic are needed to reduce race disparities.

Keywords: Hepatitis C, Prevalence, NHANES, Mortality, Small-area

Background

Hepatitis C virus (HCV) infection is the most common blood-borne infection in the United States [1]. In 2010, an estimated 3.9 million adults had antibodies to HCV (anti-HCV), indicating a previous or current acute infection [2]. Approximately 26% of individuals with acute HCV spontaneously clear infection within 6 months of exposure, but the remaining persons develop a chronic infection [3]. Despite the recent development of curative therapies, chronic HCV remains a leading cause of hepatocellular carcinoma, cirrhosis and liver failure requiring a transplant [4, 5]. Chronic HCV infection has been associated with an increase in HCV-related mortality and in 2007, chronic HCV surpassed HIV as a cause of death in the United States [6, 7].

Current national surveillance efforts provide an incomplete picture of the burden of both HCV infection and diagnoses in the United States. Both acute and chronic HCV infection diagnoses are reportable conditions in the Centers for Disease Control and Prevention (CDC) National Notifiable Disease Surveillance System (NNDSS) [8]. However, many HCV infections are not

* Correspondence: eric.w.hall@emory.edu
[1]Department of Epidemiology, Emory University Rollins School of Public Health, 1518 Clifton Road, GCR 432, Atlanta, GA 30322, USA
Full list of author information is available at the end of the article

captured and surveillance data do not accurately represent the burden of hepatitis C in the United States [9]. Chronic HCV is often asymptomatic and about half of infected persons are unaware of their infection, and therefore could not be reported to surveillance systems [10]. Furthermore, some states do not submit viral hepatitis reports to NNDSS (only 37 states reported HCV cases in 2014) and some states report implausibly low numbers [9]. In 2015, CDC directly funded enhanced case surveillance activities in 8 jurisdictions [11]. Both the O'Neill Institute and the US National Viral Hepatitis Action Plan (Goals 4.2 and 4.3) calls for improvements in mechanisms and timeliness of data to monitor the epidemic [12, 13]. In the absence of complete surveillance data, probability-based surveys, such as the National Health and Nutrition Examination Survey (NHANES), can be used to fill this gap, for estimating HCV prevalence on a national level and for the incorporation into our recent model that estimated HCV prevalence at the state-level using a small-area estimation approach [2, 14, 15].

Nationally, the prevalence and risk of new HCV infection differs across several key demographic groups. About 70% of all chronic infections are among individuals who were born between 1945 and 1965 [1]. Overall, the prevalence of anti-HCV among adults from the 1945–1965 birth cohort was estimated to be 3.5% in 2010 [1]. NHANES analyses have demonstrated a national prevalence of anti-HCV that is higher in men (1.9% compared vs. 1.1% in women) and non-Hispanic blacks (2.2% vs. 1.3% among non-Hispanic whites) [1]. Disparities by race have been demonstrated repeatedly in programmatic data and in jurisdiction-specific epidemiologic profiles [16], which collectively form the basis for national goals of reducing HCV-related mortality among African-Americans and American Indians/Alaska Natives [12]. However, extant published demographic differences in HCV burden at local levels are not typically described by prevalence indicators (anti-HCV or HCV RNA) and have not been systematically described for all states. This analysis extends our earlier method for state-level prevalence estimation to quantify the burden of chronic hepatitis C infection, stratified by race and by sex in each U.S. state.

Methods

Data sources

We extended a previously-described small-area estimation approach that synthesizes NHANES national estimates of HCV infection with state-level data on HCV-related mortality from the National Vital Statistics System [2]. The data sources and analytic methods are briefly described below.

NHANES uses a complex, multistage sampling design to collect nationally representative questionnaire and laboratory data on the health of the non-institutionalized United States population [17]. Data and corresponding sampling weights are released every 2 years. Data from seven NHANES release cycles (1999–2012) were pooled in order to ensure sufficient data for all demographic groups. All analyses were restricted to respondents aged ≥18 years of age at time of survey. Race/ethnicity was categorized into non-Hispanic black, non-Hispanic white and Hispanic/other. Similar to previous analyses, birth year was classified into three cohorts: before 1945, 1945–1965 and after 1965 [18, 19].

NHANES tested lab samples for anti-HCV using an anti-HCV screening chemiluminescence immunoassay and a confirmatory recombinant immunoblot assay (RIBA) [20]. Samples with positive results on RIBA were tested for HCV RNA using an in vitro nucleic acid amplification test. Participants with a positive or indeterminate anti-HCV test and positive HCV RNA test were considered to represent chronic HCV infection. As done in previous analyses, participants who tested positive for anti-HCV but negative for HCV RNA (resolved infections; $n = 112$) and those who tested positive for anti-HCV but did not have a HCV RNA test ($n = 160$) were not included in this analysis [14].

The National Vital Statistics System (NVSS) collects demographic, geographic and cause of death data from all death certificates in the United States [21]. Mortality Multiple Cause Microdata files (from 1999 to 2012) were used and data were categorized into the same sex, race and birth cohort categories described above. Any death records that listed the ICD-10 code for acute viral hepatitis C (B17.1) or chronic viral hepatitis C (B18.2) as the underlying or a multiple cause of death were considered to indicate HCV-related mortality.

Annual intercensal population estimates (1999–2012) from the US Vintage 2000, 2009 and 2014 data sets were used as denominators for HCV-related mortality rates within each demographic strata [22]. Microdata from the 2010 5-year American Community Survey (ACS, years 2006–2010) were used to generate estimates of the non-institutionalized population [23, 24], which were combined with our estimated number of HCV cases to estimate HCV prevalence rates for each state. The incorporation of ACS population totals into this analysis is an update to our previously published approach and reflect current NHANES guidance [25]. Estimated population total for each sex and race group are reported in Additional file 1: Table S1.

Analysis

The number of persons with chronic hepatitis C in each state were estimated using a standardization-based estimator described in detail earlier [2]. Briefly, we used NHANES data to calculate weighted estimates for national HCV RNA prevalence for 18 strata of sex (2),

Table 1 Estimated total and prevalence rate with chronic hepatitis C infection by sex, US States and District of Columbia, 2010[a]

	Female				Male					
	HCV RNA prevalence rate (per 100)		Total persons[b] with HCV RNA		HCV RNA Prevalence rate (per 100)		Total persons with HCV RNA		Rate ratio (ref = Female)	
State	Rate	(95% CI)	n	(95% CI)	Rate	(95% CI)	n	(95% CI)	Ratio	(95% CI)
ALABAMA	0.69	(0.57 0.89)	12,720	(10,481 16,461)	1.36	(1.17 1.62)	22,615	(19,448 26,975)	1.98	(1.48 2.57)
ALASKA	1.21	(0.89 1.87)	2915	(2,133 4,502)	1.49	(1.22 1.92)	3,859	(3,164 4,968)	1.23	(0.79 1.81)
ARIZONA	0.75	(0.60 1.02)	17,505	(14,091 23,769)	1.75	(1.49 2.10)	38,770	(33,121 46,690)	2.33	(1.65 3.10)
ARKANSAS	0.69	(0.55 0.94)	7645	(6,094 10,384)	1.64	(1.38 1.99)	16,652	(14,001 20,215)	2.36	(1.67 3.20)
CALIFORNIA	1.04	(0.86 1.39)	143,193	(118,480 190,894)	2.04	(1.78 2.42)	268,277	(234,254 318,754)	1.96	(1.42 2.54)
COLORADO	0.75	(0.61 1.01)	13,846	(11,246 18,633)	1.59	(1.37 1.90)	28,476	(24,518 34,108)	2.11	(1.51 2.78)
CONNECTICUT	0.57	(0.48 0.75)	7974	(6,681 10,408)	1.30	(1.13 1.55)	16,562	(14,390 19,681)	2.28	(1.70 2.91)
DELAWARE	0.94	(0.76 1.25)	3,279	(2,664 4,375)	1.93	(1.65 2.36)	6,086	(5,197 7,437)	2.05	(1.49 2.75)
DISTRICT OF COLUMBIA	2.40	(1.87 3.20)	6,116	(4,771 8,163)	3.12	(2.58 3.92)	6,844	(5,651 8,590)	1.30	(0.92 1.81)
FLORIDA	0.73	(0.60 0.96)	54,329	(44,975 71,090)	1.57	(1.35 1.87)	107,089	(92,016 127,575)	2.15	(1.58 2.79)
GEORGIA	0.55	(0.46 0.71)	19,954	(16,645 25,475)	1.16	(1.00 1.37)	37,754	(32,655 44,598)	2.09	(1.58 2.67)
HAWAII	0.49	(0.37 0.76)	2513	(1,894 3,933)	1.37	(1.16 1.68)	6,937	(5,861 8,524)	2.81	(1.75 3.99)
IDAHO	0.62	(0.47 0.91)	3441	(2,586 5,025)	1.22	(1.00 1.53)	6,572	(5,411 8,257)	1.96	(1.28 2.83)
ILLINOIS	0.36	(0.31 0.47)	17,719	(14,973 22,752)	0.65	(0.57 0.77)	29,683	(25,847 35,021)	1.81	(1.36 2.29)
INDIANA	0.54	(0.44 0.72)	13,275	(10,800 17,573)	1.12	(0.95 1.35)	25,482	(21,695 30,652)	2.06	(1.49 2.73)
IOWA	0.39	(0.30 0.56)	4483	(3,460 6,418)	1.02	(0.86 1.26)	11,227	(9,425 13,871)	2.63	(1.76 3.69)
KANSAS	0.58	(0.46 0.80)	6118	(4,869 8,406)	1.31	(1.10 1.60)	13,131	(11,043 16,037)	2.25	(1.58 3.07)
KENTUCKY	0.66	(0.52 0.92)	11,040	(8,643 15,204)	1.50	(1.25 1.86)	23,080	(19,226 28,571)	2.26	(1.56 3.13)
LOUISIANA	1.10	(0.92 1.40)	18,743	(15,656 23,771)	2.18	(1.90 2.57)	33,463	(29,151 39,519)	1.98	(1.51 2.53)
MAINE	0.33	(0.24 0.51)	1762	(1,262 2,717)	1.12	(0.91 1.44)	5,602	(4,527 7,177)	3.42[c]	(2.11 5.22)
MARYLAND	1.05	(0.87 1.34)	23,576	(19,653 30,142)	1.72	(1.50 2.02)	34,714	(30,318 40,706)	1.65	(1.25 2.10)
MASSACHUSETTS	0.60	(0.49 0.81)	15,784	(12,882 21,165)	1.35	(1.16 1.61)	31,749	(27,376 38,029)	2.22	(1.60 2.92)
MICHIGAN	0.65	(0.54 0.82)	25,033	(20,984 31,617)	1.28	(1.11 1.51)	45,682	(39,723 53,804)	1.97	(1.50 2.50)
MINNESOTA	0.42	(0.35 0.55)	8333	(6,876 10,999)	0.99	(0.85 1.18)	18,974	(16,364 22,647)	2.36	(1.74 3.08)
MISSISSIPPI	0.71	(0.58 0.93)	8034	(6,574 10,554)	1.56	(1.33 1.89)	15,610	(13,332 18,890)	2.19	(1.60 2.87)
MISSOURI	0.72	(0.59 0.95)	16,628	(13,620 21,803)	1.62	(1.39 1.93)	34,139	(29,234 40,812)	2.23	(1.64 2.93)
MONTANA	0.88	(0.66 1.30)	3298	(2,476 4,860)	1.46	(1.21 1.85)	5,361	(4,433 6,798)	1.65	(1.08 2.40)
NEBRASKA	0.52	(0.42 0.72)	3535	(2,827 4,895)	1.06	(0.90 1.31)	6,883	(5,833 8,491)	2.03	(1.42 2.77)
NEVADA	0.69	(0.55 0.94)	6725	(5,392 9,135)	1.74	(1.47 2.11)	16,979	(14,362 20,621)	2.52	(1.77 3.38)
NEW HAMPSHIRE	0.38	(0.28 0.59)	1970	(1,421 3,026)	1.06	(0.86 1.35)	5,168	(4,193 6,630)	2.76	(1.71 4.19)
NEW JERSEY	0.65	(0.55 0.83)	22,188	(18,789 28,416)	1.26	(1.10 1.48)	39,331	(34,413 46,239)	1.95	(1.48 2.46)

Table 1 Estimated total and prevalence rate with chronic hepatitis C infection by sex, US States and District of Columbia, 2010[a] *(Continued)*

	Female				Male					
	HCV RNA prevalence rate (per 100)		Total persons[b] with HCV RNA		HCV RNA Prevalence rate (per 100)		Total persons with HCV RNA		Rate ratio (ref = Female)	
State	Rate	(95% CI)	n	(95% CI)	Rate	(95% CI)	n	(95% CI)	Ratio	(95% CI)
NEW MEXICO	1.11	(0.85 1.65)	8457	(6,473 12,632)	2.48	(2.07 3.15)	17,671	(14,799 22,460)	2.23	(1.44 3.20)
NEW YORK	0.74	(0.63 0.95)	57,238	(48,850 73,330)	1.42	(1.26 1.66)	98,479	(87,408 114,701)	1.92	(1.46 2.38)
NORTH CAROLINA	0.71	(0.59 0.90)	25,610	(21,296 32,564)	1.62	(1.41 1.91)	53,569	(46,585 63,012)	2.30	(1.74 2.94)
NORTH DAKOTA	0.29[c]	(0.20 0.51)	719[c]	(509 1,273)	0.74	(0.60 1.01)	1,864	(1,503 2,545)	2.57[c]	(1.40 4.05)
OHIO	0.60	(0.50 0.77)	26,886	(22,401 34,365)	1.33	(1.15 1.57)	54,497	(47,135 64,214)	2.21	(1.67 2.84)
OKLAHOMA	1.51	(1.19 2.07)	21,062	(16,592 28,918)	2.73	(2.31 3.30)	35,554	(30,068 43,031)	1.81	(1.26 2.46)
OREGON	1.27	(0.97 1.76)	18,567	(14,291 25,838)	2.71	(2.27 3.32)	37,859	(31,612 46,314)	2.15	(1.48 3.02)
PENNSYLVANIA	0.62	(0.52 0.78)	31,075	(26,101 39,459)	1.41	(1.22 1.66)	64,388	(55,988 75,877)	2.28	(1.73 2.90)
RHODE ISLAND	0.95	(0.76 1.32)	4052	(3,234 5,641)	1.88	(1.60 2.30)	7,240	(6,149 8,853)	1.98	(1.38 2.69)
SOUTH CAROLINA	0.79	(0.66 1.02)	14,076	(11,646 18,121)	1.73	(1.49 2.05)	27,740	(23,940 32,864)	2.18	(1.63 2.82)
SOUTH DAKOTA	0.39	(0.28 0.63)	1155	(847 1,889)	0.87	(0.70 1.15)	2,502	(2,036 3,317)	2.23[c]	(1.32 3.37)
TENNESSEE	1.05	(0.85 1.38)	25,633	(20,703 33,783)	2.43	(2.06 2.92)	53,969	(45,855 65,023)	2.31	(1.68 3.07)
TEXAS	0.95	(0.80 1.22)	84,617	(71,627 109,034)	1.93	(1.69 2.27)	161,293	(141,235 190,237)	2.03	(1.52 2.58)
UTAH	0.39	(0.30 0.56)	3541	(2,739 5,073)	0.84	(0.70 1.05)	7,497	(6,254 9,351)	2.17	(1.45 3.08)
VERMONT	0.53	(0.37 0.86)	1335	(934 2,136)	1.41	(1.12 1.85)	3,335	(2,640 4,383)	2.64[c]	(1.57 4.16)
VIRGINIA	0.47	(0.40 0.61)	14,500	(12,153 18,560)	1.10	(0.96 1.30)	31,281	(27,183 36,821)	2.33	(1.77 2.96)
WASHINGTON	0.98	(0.78 1.32)	24,627	(19,593 33,172)	2.08	(1.76 2.51)	50,526	(42,851 60,918)	2.12	(1.51 2.88)
WEST VIRGINIA	0.60	(0.45 0.89)	4450	(3,326 6,579)	1.55	(1.27 1.96)	10,674	(8,745 13,462)	2.57	(1.66 3.73)
WISCONSIN	0.31	(0.25 0.40)	6628	(5,467 8,715)	0.70	(0.60 0.83)	14,320	(12,291 17,191)	2.26	(1.66 2.95)
WYOMING	0.83	(0.60 1.31)	1684	(1,220 2,653)	1.44	(1.15 1.92)	2,981	(2,370 3,969)	1.74[c]	(1.04 2.67)
U.S. STATES & WASHINGTON D.C.	0.75	(0.63 0.96)	879,589	(743,338 1,128,362)	1.56	(1.37 1.84)	1,699,989	(1,486,193 2,001,396)	2.08	(1.57 2.63)

Abbreviations: CI confidence interval, HCV RNA hepatitis C virus ribonucleic acid
[a]Defined as persons with HCV RNA
[b]Represents the non-institutionalized population
[c]Coefficient of variation is ≥ 23%; estimate is unreliable

Table 2 Estimated total and prevalence rate with chronic hepatitis C infection among non-Hispanic white persons, US States and District of Columbia, 2010[a]

	HCV RNA prevalence rate (per 100)		Total persons with HCV RNA[b]	
State	Rate	(95% CI)	n	(95% CI)
ALABAMA	0.94	(0.80 1.14)	23,139	(19,654 28,258)
ALASKA	1.54	(1.27 2.01)	5285	(4,332 6,869)
ARIZONA	1.35	(1.15 1.64)	39,779	(33,842 48,151)
ARKANSAS	1.15	(0.97 1.41)	19,102	(16,089 23,463)
CALIFORNIA	1.88	(1.61 2.27)	231,304	(197,678 278,733)
COLORADO	1.02	(0.86 1.24)	27,578	(23,299 33,469)
CONNECTICUT	0.72	(0.61 0.88)	14,426	(12,215 17,645)
DELAWARE	1.09	(0.91 1.37)	5078	(4,232 6,410)
DISTRICT OF COLUMBIA	0.43	(0.34 0.61)	770	(605 1,073)
FLORIDA	1.29	(1.10 1.56)	115,222	(98,297 139,057)
GEORGIA	0.82	(0.70 1.00)	34,005	(28,820 41,321)
HAWAII	2.29	(1.90 2.87)	6043	(5,014 7,568)
IDAHO	0.93	(0.78 1.16)	8838	(7,399 11,049)
ILLINOIS	0.44	(0.37 0.53)	28,061	(23,875 34,244)
INDIANA	0.72	(0.61 0.88)	28,747	(24,444 35,069)
IOWA	0.64	(0.54 0.80)	13,279	(11,198 16,460)
KANSAS	0.89	(0.75 1.10)	15,080	(12,680 18,563)
KENTUCKY	1.00	(0.83 1.23)	28,246	(23,690 34,890)
LOUISIANA	1.30	(1.10 1.58)	27,096	(23,024 33,040)
MAINE	0.71	(0.59 0.90)	7033	(5,856 8,877)
MARYLAND	0.92	(0.78 1.13)	22,931	(19,392 28,097)
MASSACHUSETTS	0.85	(0.72 1.03)	33,610	(28,529 40,907)
MICHIGAN	0.69	(0.59 0.84)	41,050	(34,774 49,679)
MINNESOTA	0.54	(0.45 0.65)	18,190	(15,369 22,162)
MISSISSIPPI	1.20	(1.01 1.48)	15,857	(13,373 19,566)
MISSOURI	0.98	(0.84 1.20)	36,273	(30,840 44,098)
MONTANA	1.07	(0.88 1.35)	7135	(5,907 9,051)
NEBRASKA	0.66	(0.55 0.82)	7474	(6,231 9,366)
NEVADA	1.54	(1.30 1.89)	18,219	(15,334 22,295)
NEW HAMPSHIRE	0.71	(0.59 0.90)	6719	(5,600 8,491)
NEW JERSEY	0.86	(0.73 1.04)	35,420	(30,164 43,063)
NEW MEXICO	1.69	(1.43 2.07)	11,576	(9,752 14,142)
NEW YORK	0.73	(0.62 0.88)	65,307	(55,785 78,812)
NORTH CAROLINA	0.99	(0.84 1.19)	47,365	(40,211 57,252)
NORTH DAKOTA	0.45	(0.36 0.63)	2084	(1,671 2,883)
OHIO	0.72	(0.61 0.87)	51,804	(43,989 62,811)
OKLAHOMA	2.31	(1.96 2.82)	46,062	(39,054 56,331)
OREGON	2.11	(1.79 2.56)	50,091	(42,511 60,837)
PENNSYLVANIA	0.74	(0.63 0.89)	58,578	(49,866 70,820)
RHODE ISLAND	1.21	(1.01 1.52)	7,962	(6,652 9,982)
SOUTH CAROLINA	1.15	(0.97 1.40)	26,141	(22,134 31,835)
SOUTH DAKOTA	0.54	(0.43 0.72)	2793	(2,243 3,768)

Table 2 Estimated total and prevalence rate with chronic hepatitis C infection among non-Hispanic white persons, US States and District of Columbia, 2010[a] *(Continued)*

	HCV RNA prevalence rate (per 100)		Total persons with HCV RNA[b]	
State	Rate	(95% CI)	n	(95% CI)
TENNESSEE	1.63	(1.38 1.99)	59,986	(50,921 73,192)
TEXAS	1.51	(1.29 1.82)	132,698	(113,228 160,163)
UTAH	0.60	(0.50 0.75)	9051	(7,587 11,269)
VERMONT	0.96	(0.79 1.25)	4460	(3,664 5,782)
VIRGINIA	0.65	(0.55 0.79)	26,111	(22,183 31,786)
WASHINGTON	1.58	(1.34 1.91)	60,245	(51,196 72,808)
WEST VIRGINIA	1.01	(0.84 1.27)	13,625	(11,335 17,068)
WISCONSIN	0.39	(0.33 0.47)	14,229	(12,029 17,463)
WYOMING	1.12	(0.91 1.48)	4041	(3,287 5,336)
U.S. STATES & WASHINGTON D.C.	1.05	(0.90 1.27)	1,615,202	(1,380,727 1,947,882)

Abbreviations: *CI* confidence interval, *HCV RNA* hepatitis C virus ribonucleic acid
[a]Defined as persons with HCV RNA
[b]Represents the non-institutionalized population

race/ethnicity (3) and birth cohort (3) [25]. We multiplied these weighted estimates by 2010 ACS 5-year population estimates for the corresponding demographic stratum for each state to generate crude state-by-stratum totals. We used NVSS mortality data and intercensal population totals to fit a high-order logistic regression model the average HCV-related death rates in the corresponding 12 strata over the 14-year period. We compared observed state-by-strata HCV-related mortality totals to model predictions to assess collinearity and model fit [26, 27]. A ratio of state-by-demographic stratum effects were calculated by comparing state specific HCV-related death rates to national HCV-related death rates (within the same strata). The crude state-by-stratum HCV RNA totals were adjusted by the state-by-stratum effects to calculate mortality-adjusted HCV RNA prevalence totals in each strata in each state. Totals were summed within single strata of race (white non-Hispanic, black non-Hispanic and Hispanic/other race) or sex and divided by corresponding population totals. This yielded HCV RNA prevalence rate estimates by sex and race for each state. Prevalence rate ratios were generated to compare HCV RNA prevalence for men vs women and non-Hispanic black vs non-Hispanic white. An analogous approach and model was used to estimate the prevalence rate and number of persons with HCV antibodies (anti-HCV), which is often used as an indicator of past or current infection [14]. The results for anti-HCV prevalence by race and sex in each state are presented in Additional file 1: Tables S2-S5.

We calculated 95% confidence intervals (CI) for state-level estimates to account for the joint statistical uncertainty in the NHANES prevalence estimates and HCV-related mortality rate estimates from the logistic regression model. Confidence intervals were calculated using a Monte Carlo simulation that sampled from logit-normal and normal distributions, respectively ($k = 10{,}000$). We calculated the coefficient of variation for all prevalence rate and ratio estimates. Similar to the guidelines used by NVSS, any estimates with a coefficient of variation of 23% or greater are potentially unreliable and marked accordingly [28].

Results

There were an estimated 2,583,986 (95% CI: 2,338,079–2,978,150) non-institutionalized US adults with chronic HCV infection in 2010, which corresponds to a prevalence of 1.14% (95% CI: 1.03–1.32%). Nationally, males had an HCV RNA prevalence of 1.56% (95% CI: 1.37–1.84%) and females had a prevalence of 0.75% (95% CI: 0.63–0.96%) (Table 1). Stratified by race, prevalence of HCV RNA was highest among non-Hispanic black (2.43, 95% CI: 2.10–2.90%), followed by non-Hispanic white (1.05, 95% CI: 0.90–1.27%) and Hispanic/other (0.74, 95% CI: 0.59–1.04%) (Tables 2, 3 and 4).

Among males, estimated HCV RNA prevalence ranged from 0.65% (Illinois) to 3.12% (District of Columbia, Table 1). Among females, reliable prevalence estimates ranged from 0.31% (Wisconsin) to 2.40% (District of Columbia). In all 51 jurisdictions, estimated HCV RNA prevalence was higher in males compared to females (Rate Ratio (RR) > 1, Fig. 1). In all but two jurisdictions (Alaska and District of Columbia) the corresponding rate ratio 95% confidence interval did not include the null value (RR = 1). Of the 51 jurisdictions, 41 have an estimated male-to-female prevalence ratio between 1.5 and 2.5.

State-level HCV RNA prevalence among non-Hispanic white persons ranged from 0.39% (Wisconsin) to 2.31%

Table 3 Estimated total and prevalence rate with chronic hepatitis C infection among non-Hispanic black persons, US States and District of Columbia, 2010[a]

State	HCV RNA prevalence rate (per 100)		Total persons with HCV RNA[b]		Rate ratio (ref = white)	
	Rate	(95% CI)	n	(95% CI)	Ratio	(95% CI)
ALABAMA	1.39	(1.19 1.69)	11,817	(10,098 14,362)	1.48	(1.15 1.90)
ALASKA	2.27	(1.64 3.72)	352	(255 579)	1.47	(1.06 2.32)
ARIZONA	2.42	(2.03 2.99)	3732	(3,129 4,606)	1.79	(1.39 2.33)
ARKANSAS	1.65	(1.39 2.03)	4863	(4,113 6,010)	1.43	(1.10 1.87)
CALIFORNIA	4.12	(3.56 4.91)	63,293	(54,696 75,368)	2.19	(1.73 2.75)
COLORADO	3.70	(3.14 4.51)	4604	(3,897 5,599)	3.64	(2.81 4.69)
CONNECTICUT	2.65	(2.24 3.24)	6003	(5,086 7,339)	3.70	(2.86 4.78)
DELAWARE	3.21	(2.69 4.03)	4009	(3,354 5,036)	2.95	(2.21 3.95)
DISTRICT OF COLUMBIA	5.23	(4.45 6.41)	11,997	(10,209 14,709)	12.03	(8.36 16.51)
FLORIDA	1.54	(1.33 1.85)	29,046	(25,019 34,879)	1.20	(0.94 1.52)
GEORGIA	1.17	(1.00 1.41)	22,519	(19,281 27,139)	1.42	(1.11 1.81)
HAWAII	2.29	(1.73 3.32)	352	(266 510)	1.00	(0.70 1.49)
IDAHO	1.37[c]	(0.77 3.41)	70[c]	(40 174)	1.48[c]	(0.79 3.71)
ILLINOIS	1.28	(1.10 1.54)	15,988	(13,747 19,242)	2.91	(2.28 3.70)
INDIANA	2.43	(2.08 2.94)	9022	(7,728 10,951)	3.38	(2.63 4.33)
IOWA	3.31	(2.70 4.26)	1644	(1,343 2,116)	5.13	(3.85 6.93)
KANSAS	2.62	(2.20 3.26)	2790	(2,334 3,465)	2.94	(2.25 3.86)
KENTUCKY	2.46	(2.07 3.07)	5442	(4,573 6,771)	2.48	(1.89 3.25)
LOUISIANA	2.60	(2.23 3.14)	24,261	(20,834 29,291)	2.00	(1.562.56)
MAINE	2.30[c]	(1.55 3.95)	169[c]	(114 291)	3.24[c]	(2.02 5.70)
MARYLAND	2.90	(2.48 3.50)	33,960	(29,082 41,053)	3.15	(2.45 4.05)
MASSACHUSETTS	2.84	(2.42 3.47)	7788	(6,626 9,510)	3.36	(2.60 4.32)
MICHIGAN	2.82	(2.43 3.38)	26,795	(23,037 32,127)	4.06	(3.18 5.15)
MINNESOTA	4.10	(3.46 5.03)	6371	(5,367 7,809)	7.66	(5.91 9.89)
MISSISSIPPI	1.03	(0.88 1.27)	7470	(6,358 9,183)	0.86	(0.66 1.12)
MISSOURI	2.94	(2.52 3.54)	13,252	(11,367 15,967)	2.98	(2.33 3.82)
MONTANA	5.04[c]	(3.29 9.29)	127[c]	(83 235)	4.72[c]	(2.87 8.82)
NEBRASKA	4.16	(3.44 5.34)	2132	(1,763 2,733)	6.36	(4.74 8.63)
NEVADA	1.90	(1.59 2.35)	2626	(2,200 3,245)	1.23	(0.94 1.60)
NEW HAMPSHIRE	2.07[c]	(1.39 3.49)	186[c]	(126 315)	2.90[c]	(1.82 5.00)
NEW JERSEY	2.44	(2.11 2.94)	19,250	(16,610 23,150)	2.85	(2.23 3.62)
NEW MEXICO	2.66	(2.12 3.54)	685	(545 911)	1.57	(1.16 2.18)
NEW YORK	2.76	(2.39 3.29)	55,406	(47,847 65,884)	3.80	(3.00 4.80)
NORTH CAROLINA	2.14	(1.84 2.57)	29,472	(25,328 35,455)	2.17	(1.70 2.76)
NORTH DAKOTA	0.83[c]	(0.44 2.67)	39[c]	(20 125)	1.82[c]	(0.87 5.93)
OHIO	2.99	(2.58 3.58)	27,791	(23,967 33,281)	4.16	(3.26 5.27)
OKLAHOMA	2.61	(2.21 3.21)	4594	(3,883 5,637)	1.13	(0.87 1.47)
OREGON	4.93	(4.10 6.13)	2092	(1,742 2,603)	2.33	(1.78 3.05)
PENNSYLVANIA	3.51	(3.02 4.21)	30,986	(26,683 37,175)	4.77	(3.75 6.04)
RHODE ISLAND	5.32	(4.39 6.83)	1979	(1,634 2,540)	4.39	(3.27 5.90)
SOUTH CAROLINA	1.69	(1.45 2.04)	14,899	(12,752 17,960)	1.48	(1.15 1.88)
SOUTH DAKOTA	3.16[c]	(2.10 5.85)	147[c]	(97 272)	5.89[c]	(3.50 11.16)

Table 3 Estimated total and prevalence rate with chronic hepatitis C infection among non-Hispanic black persons, US States and District of Columbia, 2010[a] *(Continued)*

State	HCV RNA prevalence rate (per 100)		Total persons with HCV RNA[b]		Rate ratio (ref = white)	
	Rate	(95% CI)	n	(95% CI)	Ratio	(95% CI)
TENNESSEE	2.66	(2.27 3.22)	18,656	(15,900 22,622)	1.63	(1.26 2.10)
TEXAS	3.10	(2.66 3.72)	58,916	(50,662 70,870)	2.05	(1.61 2.60)
UTAH	2.60	(1.92 3.80)	386	(286 564)	4.32	(2.97 6.49)
VERMONT	2.61[c]	(1.70 4.95)	90[c]	(58 170)	2.72[c]	(1.64 5.26)
VIRGINIA	1.66	(1.42 2.00)	17,734	(15,209 21,337)	2.56	(2.00 3.27)
WASHINGTON	4.41	(3.77 5.34)	6780	(5,794 8,214)	2.79	(2.19 3.58)
WEST VIRGINIA	3.60	(2.95 4.62)	1434	(1,175 1,840)	3.55	(2.63 4.82)
WISCONSIN	2.55	(2.16 3.11)	5372	(4,555 6,568)	6.59	(5.07 8.52)
WYOMING	1.88[c]	(1.12 4.47)	53[c]	(32 126)	1.68[c]	(0.92 4.01)
U.S. STATES & WASHINGTON D.C.	2.43	(2.10 2.90)	619,438	(536,458 739,838)	2.31	(1.83 2.91)

Abbreviations: *CI* confidence interval, *HCV RNA* hepatitis C virus ribonucleic acid
[a]Defined as persons with HCV RNA
[b]Represents the non-institutionalized population
[c]Coefficient of variation is ≥ 23%; estimate is unreliable

(Oklahoma, Table 2). Prevalence ranged from 0.83% (North Dakota, unreliable estimate) to 5.32 (Rhode Island) among non-Hispanic black persons and from 0.15% (Georgia) to 2.03% (Montana) among Hispanic/ other persons (Tables 3 and 4). In all jurisdictions except for Mississippi and Hawaii, the estimated HCV RNA prevalence was higher among non-Hispanic black compared to non-Hispanic white (RR range from 1.13 to 12.03, Fig. 2). The District of Columbia had the largest relative difference in prevalence between non-Hispanic black and non-Hispanic white (RR = 12.03, 95% CI: 8.36–16.51). Race stratified prevalence estimates are displayed geographically in Fig. 3. Among all state-level race-stratified HCV RNA prevalence estimates, the entire top two deciles are from the non-Hispanic black race (Fig. 3).

Discussion

These results are consistent with previous analysis of chronic HCV infection across demographic groups and provide a more detailed picture of the HCV burden in each US state. Using and NHANES based approach, Denniston et al. estimated a higher prevalence of chronic HCV in men compared to women, which is consistent with all our individual state-level estimates [14]. In general, these results indicate a homogeneity in disparity of HCV prevalence in males and females across the country; with males having roughly double the prevalence as females. This consistency across states is not seen when comparing prevalence of HCV infection by race.

Differences in chronic HCV prevalence by subgroups can be a result of differences in risk behaviors, biological mechanisms, and access to screening and treatment. A higher proportion of men report having ever injected drugs (3.6% vs. 1.6% for women), which is a risk factor for infection [29]. However, female injection drug users have a higher risk of HCV infection than male counterparts [30]. Additionally, the consistent difference in HCV prevalence in men and women is likely the result of a biological mechanism in HCV infection and viral clearance. Spontaneous acute HCV resolution has been shown to be higher in females (40%) compared to males (19%) [3, 31]. The exact mechanism for higher viral clearance in women is unknown, but has been hypothesized to be due to the estrogen hormone [3].

In contrast to the homogeneity seen in the stratified sex estimates, these results indicate racial disparities in HCV infection differ by state. For example, while the estimated HCV RNA prevalence among non-Hispanic whites is similar in Rhode Island (1.21%) and Arkansas (1.15%), the estimated prevalence among non-Hispanic blacks differs greatly between the two states (5.32 and 1.65%, respectively). Even areas with similar relative disparities may have largely different epidemics. California and North Carolina have similar estimated prevalence rate ratios (2.19 and 2.17, respectively) even though prevalence rates are higher across all three race groups in California.

Racial differences in HCV prevalence could result from a variety of societal and biological factors that lead to differences in exposure to risk factors and disease progression. While difficult to assess, state-level differences in racial disparities of transmission risk factors (such as injection drug use) could contribute to differences in HCV prevalence. While the risk of HCV infection during incarceration is not well-know, several surveys indicate that incarcerated individuals have a higher HCV prevalence than the general population [32]. State-level

Table 4 Estimated total and prevalence rate with chronic hepatitis C infection among Hispanic persons, US States and District of Columbia, 2010[a]

State	HCV RNA prevalence rate (per 100)		Total persons with HCV RNA[b]		Rate ratio (ref = white)	
	Rate	(95% CI)	n	(95% CI)	Ratio	(95% CI)
ALABAMA	0.20	(0.15 0.30)	379	(286 573)	0.21	(0.15 0.33)
ALASKA	0.80	(0.59 1.27)	1137	(838 1,805)	0.52	(0.38 0.79)
ARIZONA	0.88	(0.69 1.22)	12,765	(10,112 17,836)	0.65	(0.48 0.94)
ARKANSAS	0.20	(0.15 0.31)	332	(246 512)	0.18	(0.12 0.28)
CALIFORNIA	0.89	(0.71 1.26)	116,873	(92,893 165,162)	0.47	(0.35 0.69)
COLORADO	1.28	(1.02 1.78)	10,139	(8,066 14,121)	1.25	(0.93 1.83)
CONNECTICUT	0.96	(0.75 1.37)	4107	(3,220 5,862)	1.34	(0.99 1.98)
DELAWARE	0.38	(0.28 0.62)	279	(203 446)	0.35[c]	(0.24 0.58)
DISTRICT OF COLUMBIA	0.29	(0.21 0.47)	193	(140 315)	0.66[c]	(0.42 1.13)
FLORIDA	0.50	(0.39 0.71)	17,151	(13,604 24,428)	0.39	(0.29 0.56)
GEORGIA	0.15	(0.11 0.21)	1185	(918 1,718)	0.18	(0.13 0.27)
HAWAII	0.41	(0.32 0.61)	3055	(2,359 4,502)	0.18	(0.13 0.28)
IDAHO	0.83	(0.65 1.21)	1106	(858 1,612)	0.90	(0.65 1.37)
ILLINOIS	0.19	(0.15 0.28)	3352	(2,623 4,950)	0.43	(0.32 0.65)
INDIANA	0.28	(0.22 0.42)	988	(765 1,447)	0.40	(0.29 0.59)
IOWA	0.56	(0.43 0.85)	787	(596 1,190)	0.88	(0.62 1.37)
KANSAS	0.53	(0.41 0.78)	1379	(1,063 2,012)	0.60	(0.43 0.90)
KENTUCKY	0.31	(0.23 0.50)	432	(315 692)	0.31	(0.21 0.51)
LOUISIANA	0.39	(0.30 0.57)	849	(659 1,245)	0.30	(0.22 0.45)
MAINE	0.46	(0.32 0.75)	161	(114 265)	0.64[c]	(0.42 1.09)
MARYLAND	0.23	(0.18 0.34)	1399	(1,091 2,045)	0.25	(0.18 0.38)
MASSACHUSETTS	0.84	(0.66 1.20)	6134	(4,814 8,734)	0.99	(0.73 1.47)
MICHIGAN	0.51	(0.41 0.72)	2869	(2,270 4,036)	0.74	(0.54 1.09)
MINNESOTA	0.77	(0.60 1.09)	2746	(2,154 3,874)	1.44	(1.06 2.10)
MISSISSIPPI	0.37	(0.27 0.57)	318	(237 499)	0.30	(0.21 0.49)
MISSOURI	0.46	(0.36 0.66)	1242	(969 1,780)	0.47	(0.34 0.70)
MONTANA	2.03	(1.56 3.00)	1397	(1,076 2,064)	1.90	(1.35 2.92)
NEBRASKA	0.62	(0.47 0.95)	812	(615 1,243)	0.95	(0.66 1.49)
NEVADA	0.45	(0.36 0.64)	2859	(2,248 4,039)	0.29	(0.22 0.43)
NEW HAMPSHIRE	0.45	(0.32 0.72)	233	(168 373)	0.63[c]	(0.42 1.04)
NEW JERSEY	0.42	(0.33 0.60)	6848	(5,440 9,714)	0.49	(0.37 0.72)
NEW MEXICO	1.81	(1.43 2.56)	13,867	(10,982 19,648)	1.07	(0.79 1.57)
NEW YORK	0.96	(0.77 1.37)	35,004	(27,847 49,662)	1.33	(0.99 1.94)
NORTH CAROLINA	0.32	(0.25 0.46)	2343	(1,812 3,362)	0.32	(0.24 0.48)
NORTH DAKOTA	1.21	(0.89 2.01)	459	(337 766)	2.66[c]	(1.72 4.57)
OHIO	0.40	(0.32 0.57)	1788	(1,413 2,518)	0.56	(0.41 0.81)
OKLAHOMA	1.13	(0.89 1.60)	5960	(4,690 8,439)	0.49	(0.36 0.72)
OREGON	0.95	(0.75 1.32)	4244	(3,343 5,896)	0.45	(0.33 0.65)
PENNSYLVANIA	0.79	(0.62 1.11)	5899	(4,660 8,303)	1.07	(0.79 1.56)
RHODE ISLAND	1.14	(0.88 1.69)	1351	(1,043 2,000)	0.94	(0.67 1.44)
SOUTH CAROLINA	0.36	(0.28 0.52)	775	(600 1,138)	0.31	(0.23 0.47)
SOUTH DAKOTA	1.18	(0.88 1.87)	718	(534 1,140)	2.19[c]	(1.45 3.64)

Table 4 Estimated total and prevalence rate with chronic hepatitis C infection among Hispanic persons, US States and District of Columbia, 2010[a] *(Continued)*

State	HCV RNA prevalence rate (per 100)		Total persons with HCV RNA[b]		Rate ratio (ref = white)	
	Rate	(95% CI)	n	(95% CI)	Ratio	(95% CI)
TENNESSEE	0.34	(0.26 0.51)	960	(727 1,453)	0.21	(0.15 0.32)
TEXAS	0.83	(0.65 1.16)	54,296	(43,036 76,317)	0.55	(0.41 0.80)
UTAH	0.56	(0.44 0.82)	1601	(1,244 2,328)	0.94	(0.68 1.43)
VERMONT	0.64[c]	(0.44 1.13)	120[c]	(83 211)	0.67[c]	(0.42 1.20)
VIRGINIA	0.24	(0.19 0.34)	1935	(1,519 2,749)	0.37	(0.27 0.55)
WASHINGTON	0.84	(0.67 1.18)	8127	(6,478 11,442)	0.53	(0.39 0.77)
WEST VIRGINIA	0.17[c]	(0.11 0.34)	66[c]	(42 134)	0.17[c]	(0.10 0.35)
WISCONSIN	0.41	(0.32 0.59)	1346	(1,047 1,943)	1.05	(0.76 1.57)
WYOMING	1.27	(0.94 2.01)	571	(422 906)	1.13[c]	(0.76 1.86)
U.S. STATES & WASHINGTON D.C.	0.74	(0.59 1.04)	344,938	(275,446 485,020)	0.70	(0.53 1.03)

Abbreviations: *CI* confidence interval, *HCV RNA* hepatitis C virus ribonucleic acid
[a]Defined as persons with HCV RNA
[b]Represents the non-institutionalized population
[c]Coefficient of variation is ≥ 23%; estimate is unreliable

differences in incarceration rates by race might also track with local differences in HCV prevalence. Acute HCV clearance has been hypothesized to be lower in African Americans compared to Hispanic and white counterparts [33–35]. This is supported by viral clearance being lower in genotype 1 infections, which occur more frequently in African Americans. African-Americans are also more likely to be screened for HCV, leading to higher rates of diagnosis [36]. Furthermore, African-Americans, Hispanics and Asians are all less likely to receive traditional treatment (interferon-based) than Caucasians [37, 38]. This is partially because of a higher rate of treatment ineligibility (due to comorbidities) [37, 39] and a lower efficacy for viral genotype 1, which is more common in African Americans

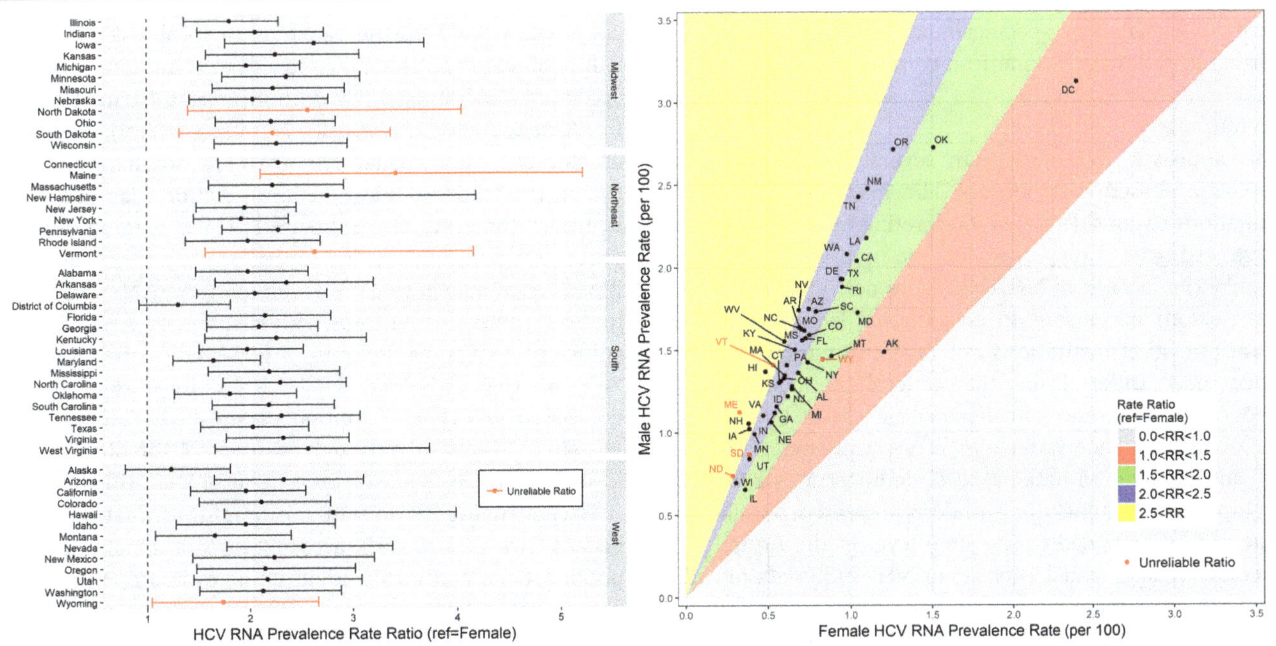

Fig. 1 Estimated Prevalence Rate and Rate Ratios of Chronic HCV Infection by Sex, US States and District of Columbia, 2010[a,b]. Abbreviations: HCV RNA, hepatitis C virus ribonucleic acid; RR, rate ratio. [a]Defined as persons with HCV RNA. [b]Using estimates of the non-institutionalized population from the 2006–2010 American Community Survey (ACS) 5-year dataset. *Coefficient of variation is ≥ 23%; estimate is unreliable

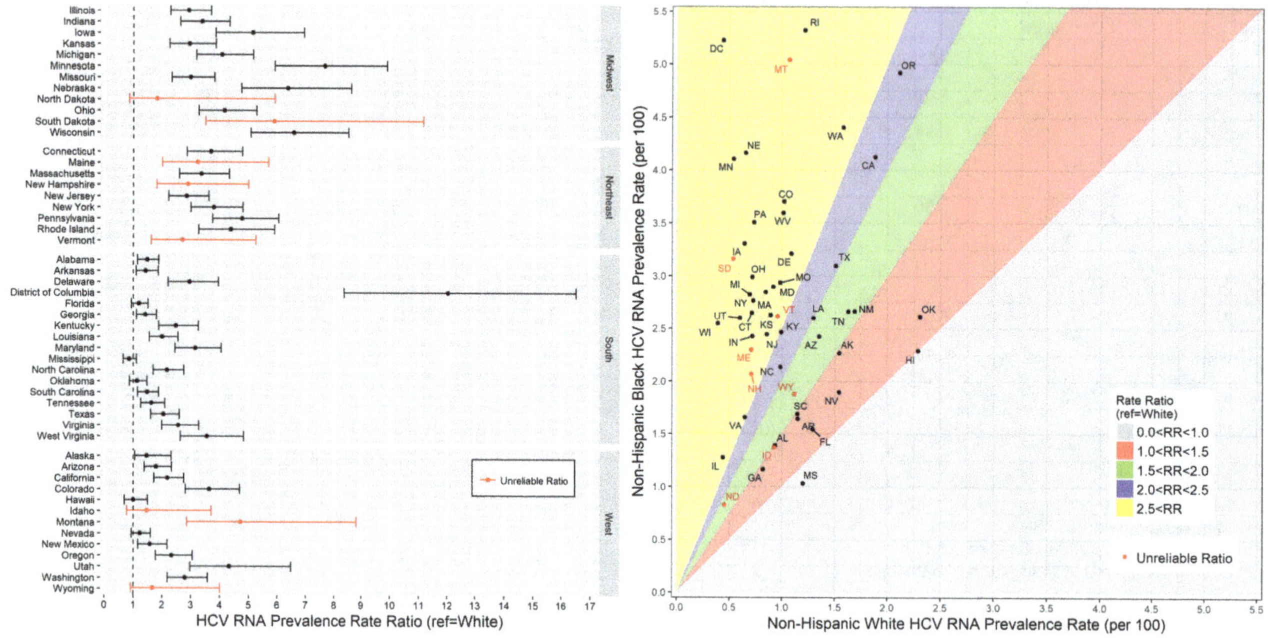

Fig. 2 Estimated Prevalence Rate and Rate Ratios of Chronic HCV Infection by non-Hispanic Black and non-Hispanic White Race, US States and District of Columbia, 2010[a,b]. Abbreviations: HCV RNA, hepatitis C virus ribonucleic acid; RR, rate ratio. [a]Defined as persons with HCV RNA. [b]Using estimates of the non-institutionalized population from the 2006–2010 American Community Survey (ACS) 5-year dataset. *Coefficient of variation is ≥ 23%; estimate is unreliable

[40, 41]. African-Americans are also more likely to defer interferon-based treatment [42–44] and receive direct activing antiretroviral treatment [45]. To address this disparity, CDC has generated a set of materials and public health messages that specifically aim to reduce the HCV burden in the African-American community [46].

Limitations

This approach uses data from several large, public and population-based data sources. However, there are some limitations to consider when interpreting these results. First, these estimates only represent the non-institutionalized population. Data from NHANES does not represent homeless persons or persons in correctional facilities, nursing homes or other institutions in which chronic HCV prevalence may differ from the general population [47]. Geographic differences in incarceration rates by race and sex could influence statewide HCV prevalence. However, previous work on a national level demonstrates a promising approach for including underrepresented populations that can be extended to the state level in the future [47]. Second, we aggregated 14 years of NHANES data in order to have a sufficient sample size to produce reliable estimates. Slight changes in local HCV incidence over that time period might not be captured in this approach. In the NHANES data, the national overall prevalence of HCV RNA changes slightly from 1999 to 2006 (1.26%; 95% CI: 1.06–1.48%) to 2007–2012 (1.05%; 95%: 0.82–1.34%). However, there is not enough data to reliably determine if there are temporal changes in prevalence within subgroups. Interpreting these results in conjunction with further analysis of local risk behaviors will help state health departments better understand their epidemic. Additionally, we do not present separate results for American Indians/Alaska Natives (AI/AN), who face an elevated HCV burden and are a key population identified in the National Viral Hepatitis Action Plan [12]. Due to under sampling and sparse NHANES data within this group, we are not able to separate AI/AN into an additional race category. We combined AI/AN and other under sampled race groups with Hispanic in order to have sufficient data in each strata of NHANES data. However, 76% of the estimated HCV RNA infections in this combined group were among persons who identified as Hispanic. Similarly, although we control for birth cohort in our model, we do not present results stratified by age. It is challenging to present meaningful estimates for age because we pooled data across 14 years. Finally, despite pooling data, some individual point estimates might still be unreliable. However, those values have been indicated as potentially unreliable, and confidence intervals have been provided for all estimates. Improved direct surveillance data or additional model input data are needed to overcome the demographic limitations of using NHANES data.

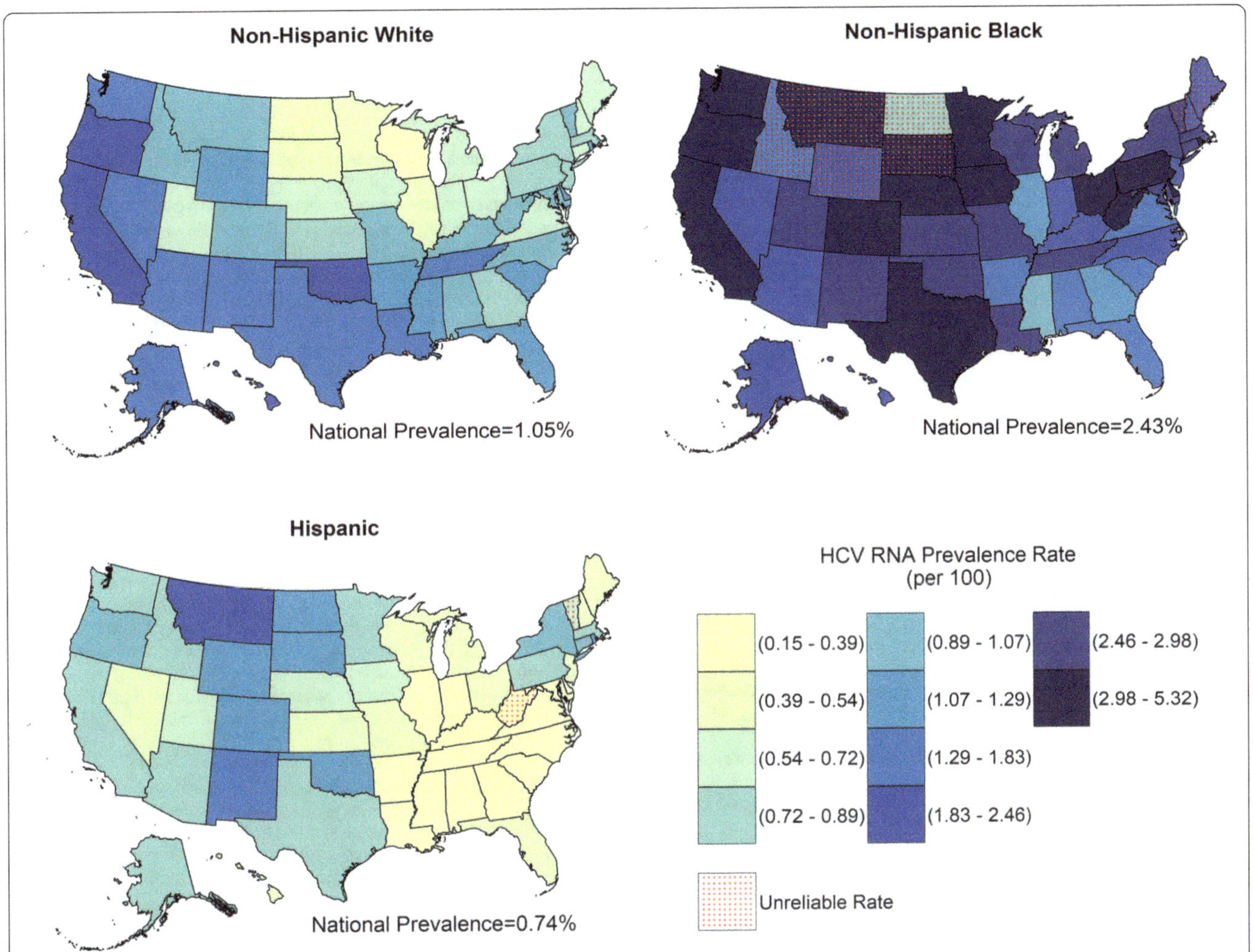

Fig. 3 Estimated Prevalence Rate of Chronic HCV Infection by Race, US States and District of Columbia, 2010[a,b]. Abbreviations: HCV RNA, hepatitis C virus ribonucleic acid. [a]Defined as persons with HCV RNA. [b]Using estimates of the non-institutionalized population from the 2006–2010 American Community Survey (ACS) 5-year dataset. *Coefficient of variation is ≥ 23%; estimate is unreliable

Conclusions

Our approach synthesizes large scale, population based data systems to provide comprehensive state-level estimates that can be used to compare the HCV burden across different states and demographic groups. As the expanded availability of curative therapies continues to increase and acute infection rates rise, this method of prevalence estimation will need to be updated in the future. In the meantime, these data shine an important light on the intersection of geographic and demographic differences of chronic HCV infection. Estimates of chronic HCV prevalence by race and sex can help state health departments understand their local epidemic and assist with their development of targeted prevention and treatment programs. Utilizing these population-based systematic results with local knowledge of HCV risk behaviors and treatment practices provide more granular insight into the chronic hepatitis C epidemic.

Abbreviations

ACS: American Community Survey; AI/AN: American Indians/Alaska Natives; anti-HCV: Hepatitis C virus antibodies; CDC: Centers for Disease Control and Prevention; CI: Confidence interval; HCV RNA: Hepatitis C virus ribonucleic acid; HCV: Hepatitis C virus; NHANES: National Health and Nutrition Examination Survey; NNDSS: National Notifiable Disease Surveillance System; NVSS: National Vital Statistics Systems; RIBA: Recombinant immunoblot assay; RR: Rate ratio; U.S.: United States

Funding

This work was supported by funding from the CDC National Center for HIV/AIDS, Viral Hepatitis, STD, and TB Prevention Epidemic and Economic Modeling Agreement (NEEMA) (U38 PS004646).

Authors' contributions
EWH conducted the statistical analysis and drafted the manuscript. ESR conceived of the analysis, participated in the design and coordination of the study and reviewed the manuscript. PSS participated in the design and coordination of the study and reviewed the manuscript. All authors read and approved the final manuscript.

Competing interests
The authors declare that they have no competing interests.

Author details
[1]Department of Epidemiology, Emory University Rollins School of Public Health, 1518 Clifton Road, GCR 432, Atlanta, GA 30322, USA. [2]Department of Epidemiology and Biostatistics, University at Albany School of Public Health, 1 University Place, rm 123, Rensselaer, NY 12144, USA.

References
1. Ditah I, Ditah F, Devaki P, Ewelukwa O, Ditah C, Njei B, Luma HN, Charlton M. The changing epidemiology of hepatitis C virus infection in the United States: National Health and nutrition examination survey 2001 through 2010. J Hepatol. 2014;60(4):691–8.
2. Rosenberg ES, Hall EW, Sullivan PS, Sanchez TH, Workowski KA, Ward JW, Holtzman D. Estimation of state-level prevalence of hepatitis C virus infection, US states and District of Columbia, 2010. In: Clinical infectious diseases: an official publication of the Infectious Diseases Society of America; 2017.
3. Micallef JM, Kaldor JM, Dore GJ. Spontaneous viral clearance following acute hepatitis C infection: a systematic review of longitudinal studies. J Viral Hepat. 2006;13(1):34–41.
4. Lingala S, Ghany MG. Natural history of hepatitis C. Gastroenterol Clin N Am. 2015;44(4):717–34.
5. Liver Transplantation [http://www.niddk.nih.gov/health-information/health-topics/liver-disease/liver-transplant/Pages/facts.aspx]. Accessed 11 Nov 2016.
6. Ly KN, Xing J, Klevens RM, Jiles RB, Ward JW, Holmberg SD. The increasing burden of mortality from viral hepatitis in the United States between 1999 and 2007. Ann Intern Med. 2012;156(4):271–8.
7. Razavi H, Elkhoury AC, Elbasha E, Estes C, Pasini K, Poynard T, Kumar R. Chronic hepatitis C virus (HCV) disease burden and cost in the United States. Hepatology (Baltimore, Md). 2013;57(6):2164–70.
8. National Notifiable Disease Surveillance System (NNDSS) [http://wwwn.cdc.gov/nndss/]. Accessed 11 Nov 2016.
9. Viral Hepatitis Surveillance, United States, 2014 [http://www.cdc.gov/hepatitis/statistics/2014surveillance/pdfs/2014hepsurveillancerpt.pdf]. Accessed 11 Nov 2016.
10. Spradling PR, Rupp L, Moorman AC, Lu M, Teshale EH, Gordon SC, Nakasato C, Boscarino JA, Henkle EM, Nerenz DR, et al. Hepatitis B and C virus infection among 1.2 million persons with access to care: factors associated with testing and infection prevalence. Clin Infect Dis. 2012;55(8):1047–55.
11. Surveillance for Viral Hepatitis - United States, 2015: Summary [https://www.cdc.gov/hepatitis/statistics/2015surveillance/commentary.htm]. Accessed 11 Nov 2016.
12. National Viral Hepatitis Action Plan 2017–2020 [https://www.hhs.gov/sites/default/files/National%20Viral%20Hepatitis%20Action%20Plan%202017-2020.pdf]. Accessed 11 Nov 2016.
13. Monitoring the Hepatitis C Epidemic in the United States: What Tools Are Needed to Achieve Elimination [https://www.law.georgetown.edu/oneillinstitute/research/documents/HEPC_Brief_1_PF.pdf]. Accessed 11 Nov 2016.
14. Denniston MM, Jiles RB, Drobeniuc J, Klevens RM, Ward JW, McQuillan GM, Holmberg SD. Chronic hepatitis C virus infection in the United States, National Health and nutrition examination survey 2003 to 2010. Ann Intern Med. 2014;160(5):293–300.
15. Armstrong GL, Wasley A, Simard EP, McQuillan GM, Kuhnert WL, Alter MJ. The prevalence of hepatitis C virus infection in the United States, 1999 through 2002. Ann Intern Med. 2006;144(10):705–14.
16. Hepatitis C Infections in Oregon [http://www.oregon.gov/oha/PH/DISEASESCONDITIONS/HIVSTDVIRALHEPATITIS/ADULTVIRALHEPATITIS/Documents/Hepatitis-C-in-Oregon.pdf]. Accessed 11 Nov 2016.
17. National Health and Nutrition Examination Survey (NHANES) [http://www.cdc.gov/nchs/nhanes.htm]. Accessed 11 Nov 2016.
18. Fishman EI, Stokes A, Preston SH. The dynamics of diabetes among birth cohorts in the U.S. Diabetes Care. 2014;37(4):1052–9.
19. Holmberg SD, Spradling PR, Moorman AC, Denniston MM. Hepatitis C in the United States. N Engl J Med. 2013;368(20):1859–61.
20. Centers for Disease Control and Prevention: National Health and nutrition examination survey: laboratory procedures manual. 2011.
21. Recommendations for Prevention and Control of Hepatitis C Virus (HCV) Infection and HCV-Related Chronic Disease [http://www.cdc.gov/hepatitis/hcv/management.htm]. Accessed 11 Nov 2016.
22. Population Estimates [https://www.census.gov/programs-surveys/popest/data/data-sets.html]. Accessed 11 Nov 2016.
23. Ruggles S, Genadek K, Goeken R, Grover J, Sobek M. Integrated public use microdata series: version 6.0. Minneapolis: University of Minnesota; 2015.
24. American Community Survey (ACS) [https://www.census.gov/programs-surveys/acs/]. Accessed 11 Nov 2016.
25. National Health and Nutrition Examination Survey: Analytic Guidelines, 2011–2012 [https://wwwn.cdc.gov/nchs/data/nhanes/2011-2012/analytic_guidelines_11_12.pdf]. Accessed 11 Nov 2016.
26. Rao JNK, Molina I. Small Area Estimation. Hoboken: Wiley; 2015.
27. Kleinbaum DG, Kupper LL, Nizam A, Rosenberg ES: Applied regression analysis and other multivariable methods: Nelson education; 2013.
28. Klein RJ, Proctor SE, Boudreault MA, Turczyn KM. Healthy people 2010 criteria for data suppression. Healthy People 2010 Stat Notes. 2002;(24):1–12.
29. Lansky A, Finlayson T, Johnson C, Holtzman D, Wejnert C, Mitsch A, Gust D, Chen R, Mizuno Y, Crepaz N. Estimating the number of persons who inject drugs in the United States by meta-analysis to calculate national rates of HIV and hepatitis C virus infections. PLoS One. 2014;9(5):e97596.
30. Esmaeili A, Mirzazadeh A, Carter GM, Esmaeili A, Hajarizadeh B, Sacks HS, Page KA. Higher incidence of HCV in females compared to males who inject drugs: a systematic review and meta-analysis. J Viral Hepat. 2017;24(2):117–27.
31. Page K, Hahn JA, Evans J, Shiboski S, Lum P, Delwart E, Tobler L, Andrews W, Avanesyan L, Cooper S, et al. Acute hepatitis C virus infection in young adult injection drug users: a prospective study of incident infection, resolution, and reinfection. J Infect Dis. 2009;200(8):1216–26.
32. Varan AK, Mercer DW, Stein MS, Spaulding AC. Hepatitis C seroprevalence among prison inmates since 2001: still high but declining. Public Health Reports (Washington, DC : 1974). 2014;129(2):187–95.
33. Thomas DL, Astemborski J, Rai RM, Anania FA, Schaeffer M, Galai N, Nolt K, Nelson KE, Strathdee SA, Johnson L, et al. The natural history of hepatitis C virus infection: host, viral, and environmental factors. JAMA. 2000;284(4):450–6.
34. Villano SA, Vlahov D, Nelson KE, Cohn S, Thomas DL. Persistence of viremia and the importance of long-term follow-up after acute hepatitis C infection. Hepatology (Baltimore, Md). 1999;29(3):908–14.
35. Sarkar M, Bacchetti P, Tien P, Mileti E, French AL, Edlin BR, Keller M, Seaberg E, Nowicki MJ, Young M, et al. Racial/ethnic differences in spontaneous HCV clearance in HIV infected and uninfected women. Dig Dis Sci. 2013;58(5):1341–8.
36. Bourgi K, Brar I, Baker-Genaw K. Health disparities in hepatitis C screening and linkage to Care at an Integrated Health System in Southeast Michigan. PLoS One. 2016;11(8):e0161241.
37. Melia MT, Muir AJ, McCone J, Shiffman ML, King JW, Herrine SK, Galler GW, Bloomer JR, Nunes FA, Brown KA, et al. Racial differences in hepatitis C treatment eligibility. Hepatology (Baltimore, Md). 2011;54(1):70–8.
38. Vutien P, Hoang J, Brooks L, Jr., Nguyen NH, Nguyen MH. Racial disparities in treatment rates for chronic hepatitis C: analysis of a population-based cohort of 73,665 patients in the United States. Medicine 2016, 95(22):e3719.
39. Schaeffer S, Khalili M. Reasons for HCV non-treatment in underserved African Americans: implications for treatment with new therapeutics. Ann Hepatol. 2015;14(2):234–42.
40. Fried MW, Shiffman ML, Reddy KR, Smith C, Marinos G, Goncales FL Jr, Haussinger D, Diago M, Carosi G, Dhumeaux D, et al. Peginterferon alfa-2a plus ribavirin for chronic hepatitis C virus infection. N Engl J Med. 2002;347(13):975–82.
41. Manns MP, McHutchison JG, Gordon SC, Rustgi VK, Shiffman M, Reindollar R, Goodman ZD, Koury K, Ling M, Albrecht JK. Peginterferon alfa-2b plus ribavirin compared with interferon alfa-2b plus ribavirin for initial treatment of chronic hepatitis C: a randomised trial. Lancet (London England). 2001;358(9286):958–65.

42. Khokhar OS, Lewis JH. Reasons why patients infected with chronic hepatitis C virus choose to defer treatment: do they alter their decision with time? Dig Dis Sci. 2007;52(5):1168–76.
43. Borum ML, Igiehon E, Shafa S. African Americans may differ in their reasons for declining hepatitis C therapy compared to non-African Americans. Dig Dis Sci. 2009;54(7):1604. author reply 1604-1605
44. Rousseau CM, Ioannou GN, Todd-Stenberg JA, Sloan KL, Larson MF, Forsberg CW, Dominitz JA. Racial differences in the evaluation and treatment of hepatitis C among veterans: a retrospective cohort study. Am J Public Health. 2008;98(5):846–52.
45. Kanwal F, Kramer JR, El-Serag HB, Frayne S, Clark J, Cao Y, Taylor T, Smith D, White D, Asch SM. Race and gender differences in the use of direct acting antiviral agents for hepatitis C virus. Clin Infect Dis. 2016;63(3):291–9.
46. Hepatitis C Disproportionately Affects the African American Community [https://www.cdc.gov/hepatitis/blackhistmnth-hepc.htm]. Accessed 11 Nov 2016.
47. Edlin BR, Eckhardt BJ, Shu MA, Holmberg SD, Swan T. Toward a more accurate estimate of the prevalence of hepatitis C in the United States. Hepatology (Baltimore, Md). 2015;62(5):1353–63.

14

Future complications of chronic hepatitis C in a low-risk area: projections from the hepatitis c study in Northern Norway

H. Kileng[1,3*], L. Bernfort[2], T. Gutteberg[4,5], O.S. Moen[1], M.G. Kristiansen[6], E.J. Paulssen[1,3], L.K. Berg[7], J. Florholmen[1,3] and R. Goll[1,3]

Abstract

Background: Hepatitis C (HCV) infection causes an asymptomatic chronic hepatitis in most affected individuals, which often remains undetected until cirrhosis and cirrhosis-related complications occur. Screening of high-risk subjects in Northern Norway has revealed a relatively low prevalence in the general population (0.24%). Despite this, late complications of HCV infection are increasing. Our object was to estimate the future prevalence and complications of chronic HCV infection in the period 2013–2050 in a low-risk area.

Methods: We have entered available data into a prognostic Markov model to project future complications to HCV infection.

Results: The model extrapolates the prevalence in the present cohort of HCV-infected individuals, and assumes a stable low incidence in the projection period. We predict an almost three-fold increase in the incidence of cirrhosis (68 per 100,000), of decompensated cirrhosis (21 per 100,000) and of hepatocellular carcinoma (4 per 100,000) by 2050, as well as a six-fold increase in the cumulated number of deaths from HCV-related liver disease (170 per 100,000 inhabitants). All estimates are made assuming an unchanged treatment coverage of approximately 15%. The estimated numbers can be reduced by approximately 50% for cirrhosis, and by approximately one third for the other endpoints if treatment coverage is raised to 50%.

Conclusion: These projections from a low-prevalence area indicate a substantial rise in HCV-related morbidity and mortality in the coming years. The global HCV epidemic is of great concern and increased treatment coverage is necessary to reduce the burden of the disease.

Keywords: Disease burden, Fibrosis development, Hepatitis C, Markov modelling, Natural course

Background

Chronic hepatitis C virus (HCV) infection is a major cause of chronic liver disease and the burden of the disease is expected to increase [1–3]. Worldwide, 64–103 million people are persistently infected with HCV [4]. After acute HCV infection, between 75% and 85% of the patients establish a chronic infection [5]. In industrial countries, most of the patients infected with HCV will have contracted the disease in the 1970s and 1980s. Thus, at the beginning of the twenty-first century, a large pool of infected patients exists, and in many countries, the cohorts of patients with chronic HCV infection have come of age. Most infected individuals are asymptomatic, but the number of patients with liver cirrhosis and hepatocellular carcinoma (HCC) is increasing [6, 7]. Thus, 30–40 years after the start of the epidemic, the disease is a growing burden on the health care system in many countries.

The natural course of late-stage HCV infection is so far unsettled. The disease increases the risk of developing liver cirrhosis and its complications such as liver cancer and liver failure. The prognosis is highly dependent on the rate of progression of liver fibrosis

* Correspondence: hege.kileng@unn.no
[1]Gastroenterology and Nutrition Research Group, Department of Clinical Medicine, UiT The Arctic University of Norway, Tromsø, Norway
[3]Department of Internal Medicine, Section of Gastroenterology, University Hospital of North Norway, Tromsø, Norway

towards cirrhosis. Most studies have shown that the rate of fibrosis is slow the first two decades. However, the estimated risk of cirrhosis varies as much as 3–30% in different populations [5, 8–10], suggesting that the progression of the disease may not be universal but rather depend on additional risk factors [11]. Beyond the two first decades, the rate of fibrosis progression is sparsely documented. One study reported that fibrosis progression is non-linear with an estimated a risk of cirrhosis of 41% after 30 years [8], whereas an autopsy study reported septal fibrosis or cirrhosis in 35% of cases with disease duration of 25 years or longer [12].

Among patients with liver cirrhosis the annual rate of progression to hepatic decompensation and HCC has been described to be in the range 4–8% and 2.4–3.4%, respectively [13–15]. In the absence of retrospective as well as prospective data for the long-term progression of the disease (>20 years), various mathematical models have been used to reconstruct the natural course and estimate future complications of HCV infection [1, 13, 16–18]. Even with a decline in the incidence rate after 1990, an increase in the number of patients with complicated disease and deaths from chronic HCV is expected in the coming decades [1–3, 19, 20].

Norway is a country with a low prevalence of HCV [21, 22]. Drug abuse is the primary transmission route, and low age at transmission indicates a low risk for rapid disease progression. Despite this, late complications of HCV infection is a growing problem [23] and health costs are expected to increase. Markov models are well suited for simulation of chronic diseases [24], and we have used a Markov model to estimate the future prevalence and complications of chronic HCV infection in the period 2013–2050 in a low-risk area.

Methods

The study population consists of individuals included in the Hepatitis C study in Northern Norway between 1992 and 2011 [21, 23]. In addition, we performed a registration study to assess the number of newly diagnosed individuals with HCV each year between 1998 and 2012 at the two microbiological departments in our region.

The Hepatitis C study in Northern Norway

In 1992, a screening and medical follow-up programme of patients with HCV infection was established in the Health Region of Northern Norway (460.000 inhabitants). In brief, general practitioners were encouraged to screen patients with former or present risk behavior for HCV infection. If chronic HCV infection was detected, the general practitioners were encouraged to refer the patient for follow-up at one of the 11 medical centers in the region. An estimate of the year of transmission was made for all referred patients based on either the year of acute HCV infection or the first year of high-risk behaviour [23]. Liver biopsies were performed, and fibrosis was graded (0–6) according to Ishak et al. [25]. Presence of concomitant alcoholic liver disease was assessed by clinical judgment.

The registry study

Individuals with a positive anti-HCV test registered at the two microbiological departments in Northern Norway between 1998 and 2012 were included. The year of diagnosis was defined as the first year of a positive anti-HCV test (ARCHITECT Anti-HCV Reagens kit. Abbott System, Wiesbaden, Germany). Until 2004, a positive anti-HCV test was directly confirmed with a recombinant immunoblot assay (RIBA HCV 3.0 SIA test, Chiron Cooperation, Emeryville, CA, USA). Individuals with a positive RIBA (two or more positive bands) or indeterminate RIBA (one band) were included, while individuals with a negative RIBA (no bands) were excluded. The result of the HCV RNA test was recorded if available: an in-house reverse transcriptase polymerase chain reaction (RT-PCR) until 2004, where after the ROCHE RT-PCR (Cobas Amplicor Hepatitis C Viral Polymerase Chain Reaction, Roche Molecular System Inc., Branchburg NJ, USA) was used. The ROCHE PCR test replaced the RIBA test for confirmation of HCV infection from 2005. HCV genotyping was performed as a hybridization assay on products from the HCV RNA PCR according to the manufacturers' instructions (INNO-LIPA HCV II kit, INNOGENETICS, Ghent, Belgium). Individuals without a registered residence in Norway were excluded. The results of HBsAg (hepatitis B surface antigen) and anti-HIV (human immunodeficiency virus) were recorded if available.

Markov model

In order to predict HCV-related morbidity and mortality an open Markov model was constructed (Fig. 1). Of infected patients, 20% were assumed to recover spontaneously during the first year of infection [26]. Yearly transitions between categories were done according to probability estimates generated from different sources. The effect of medical treatment was modelled in three scenarios where 0%, 15% and 50% of all patients were assumed to receive medical treatment. Before the introduction of direct acting antivirals (DAAs), treatment was offered to eligible patients irrespective of fibrosis stage, i.e. patients with Metavir fibrosis score F0/F1 were also treated. The treatment coverage at this time was approximately 15%. When the highly expensive DAAs became available, the Norwegian national guidelines restricted treatment to patients with fibrosis score ≥ F2. However, since DAAs offer a simple, tolerable, short-term and highly effective therapy, we consider an

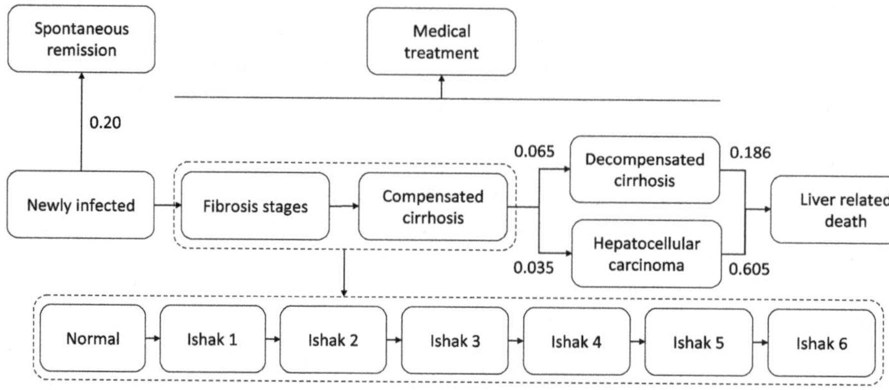

Fig. 1 The natural course of hepatitis C. The Markov model is based on simulation of transition from a given category to the next based on probability estimates. The progression of fibrosis towards cirrhosis is based on local data, whereas most of the remaining estimated probabilities are previously published from other cohorts. In all states of HCV, there is also an annual risk of dying from natural courses, which is implicitly included in the model

increased treatment coverage to 50% as possible. Recently (March 2017), updated national guidelines recommend treatment for all patients with genotype 1, irrespective of fibrosis grade. Treatment of genotype 2 and 3 is still restricted to patients with fibrosis score ≥ F2.

To estimate the rate of fibrosis progression in the cohort, 237 records with a positive HCV RNA test, known duration of infection, and available liver biopsy results were entered into an ordinal regression analysis, which can be described as a multilayer logistic regression. This method estimates points of transition on an ordinal scale (like the Ishak fibrosis scale). Sex, time after contraction of the disease and HCV genotype were included as predictors of Ishak fibrosis grade. Non-significant terms were removed from the model leaving time after contraction and genotype as significant predictors. Genotype 1 and 4 were analyzed as a single group due to few observations of genotype 4. The model predicted 70% of the observed fibrosis grades correctly within a margin of error of one Ishak grade, but overestimated fibrosis grade in 13% and underestimated in 17%. From this model, a matrix of estimated probabilities of transition to a higher fibrosis grade versus staying in the present grade for each year of infection could be constructed. It was assumed that fibrosis development during ongoing HCV infection could only either stay the same or change to a higher stage each year of infection. Additional file 1 shows the regression model in more detail. The Markov model was adjusted for genotypes in the estimation of fibrosis progression, according to the prevalence of the different genotypes in our population. For transitions from Ishak 6 (compensated cirrhosis) to more severe states, fixed probabilities were used. We did not have exact data from Northern Norway for the various transitions, and have thus used data from a Scottish HCV population of drug-injecting abusers (as in our study), as described by Hutchinson et al. [13], with transition probabilities similar to that reported by others [14, 27], as shown in Table 1. The model was corrected for standardized mortality rate according to Norwegian population characteristics. Non-cirrhotic subjects successfully treated for HCV with achieved sustained virological response (SVR) were removed from the model. Subjects with cirrhosis remain in risk of liver complications in spite of SVR, and of those, 50% were retained in the model [28]. All successfully treated subjects with decompensated cirrhosis and HCC were kept in the model.

The overall SVR rate until 2015 was 71.3%, based on the response of interferon-based treatment in our own

Table 1 Transition rates between different states of hepatitis C

Transition rates			
From state	To state	Yearly transition rate	Reference
Infection time	Spontaneous remission	0.200	Thomas Clin Liver Dis 2005 [26]
Compensated cirrhosis	Decompensated cirrhosis	0.065	Hutchinson Hepatol 2005 [13]
Decompensated cirrhosis	Liver-related death	0.186	Hutchinson Hepatol 2005 [13]
Cirrhosis	Hepatocellular carcinoma	0.035	Hutchinson Hepatol 2005 [13]
Hepatocellular carcinoma	Death	0.605	Hutchinson Hepatol 2005 [13]

The table shows the estimated rates of transition between different states of development of hepatitis C and its complications, as used in the Markov model clinical practice. For individuals treated from 2015 onwards, the overall SVR rate was set to 90% to reflect the improved treatment response provided by DAAs.

Entering of data into the Markov model

Figure 2 shows the actual incidence of newly diagnosed HCV infection per year in the period from 1992 to 2012 (dark bars). After 2004, the incidence decreased to a stable level of approximately 90 newly diagnosed cases each year. In view of this stable number, we have projected a stable occurrence of 90 newly diagnosed cases each year from 2013 and forwards (light bars).

HCV-positive individuals were entered into the model at time of contraction. Since only a subgroup had a known time of transmission, this had to be estimated for the remaining records. First, we investigated the 402 records with known times of transmission. In 2004, all general practitioners in the area were subject to a HCV campaign encouraging screening of their patients with known risk behaviour. We found an increased amount of early diagnoses (within the first year of transmission) in the years after this campaign compared to before (35.5% vs. 21.3%). From these data, probability distributions could be derived in order to estimate time of contraction for records diagnosed before and after 2004, respectively. Records without known time of transmission were then entered into the model using these distributions as weights. From 2013 forward, the estimated number of 90 newly diagnosed cases each year were allocated due to the late probability distribution in order to estimate their time of contraction.

The registration of HCV infection revealed incomplete records regarding confirmation testing. A positive anti-HCV test normally should be followed up with a new blood sample for the confirmation with RIBA and/or HCV RNA. Not all the persons with positive anti-HCV tests had a recorded confirmation test. The starting cohort in the model thus consists of patients with confirmed HCV infection (either a positive RIBA or a positive HCV RNA test), as well as individuals with unconfirmed HCV (either only a positive anti-HCV or an indeterminate RIBA). We therefore estimated the likelihood of a true positive test in incomplete records in the following way: In a sample of 326 records with a positive anti-HCV-test where RIBA had been measured, 207 subjects (63%) had a positive RIBA test, and the probability of a true positive anti-HCV test was estimated to 0.63. Similarly, in a sample of 14 records with an inconclusive RIBA and a HCV RNA test, we found three individuals with a positive HCV RNA test, and the probability of a true positive record in case of inconclusive RIBA was estimated to 0.21. Summarized, individuals with either a positive HCV RNA or RIBA were weighted 1.0, and individuals with only a positive anti-HCV test or an inconclusive RIBA were weighted 0.63 and 0.21, respectively.

Results

Based on the registration and subsequent weighting described above, the estimated HCV cohort consists of

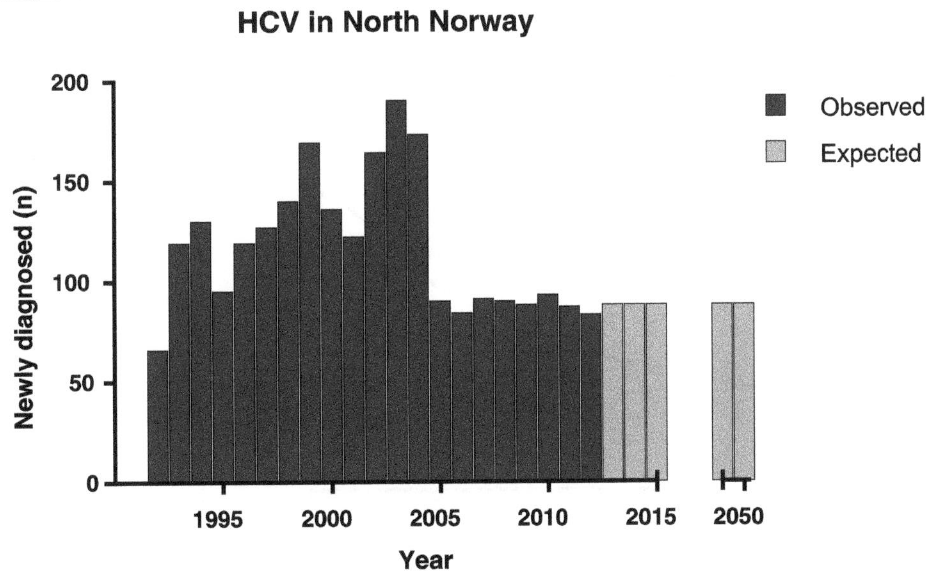

Fig. 2 Newly diagnosed hepatitis C in Northern Norway. The figure shows numbers per year of newly diagnosed individuals with hepatitis C in Northern Norway, from the first registration in 1992 to the end of 2012 (dark bars). The estimated yearly occurrence of newly diagnosed from 2013 and forward are also shown (light bars)

2589 individuals (positive HCV RNA or positive RIBA) with a sex distribution of 64% men and 36% women. Additional file 2 shows the estimation of the HCV cohort in more detail. The distribution between genotypes 1 through 4 was 45%, 8%, 46% and 1%, respectively. The prevalence of HBsAg and anti-HIV was 2.3% and 1%, respectively.

Modeled fibrosis progression

In the subgroup that was the basis for estimation of fibrosis progression ($n = 237$), the sex distribution was the same as in the total cohort and the distribution between HCV genotypes 1 through 4 were approximately equal to the total cohort, 45%, 10%, 44%, and 1%, respectively. The median duration of infection was 13 years (range 0–42 years) and the mean age at liver biopsy was 40 years. The rate of fibrosis progression was relatively slow in the first 20–25 years of infection, followed by an accelerated fibrosis progression, especially in patients with genotype 3 (Fig. 3).

Markov modelling

The Markov model projects the number of patients (per 100,000 inhabitants) in the different states of compensated cirrhosis, decompensated cirrhosis and HCC for the years 2013 to 2050, given various scenarios of HCV treatment coverage. It estimates an almost threefold increase in the incidence of cirrhosis (68 per 100,000), of decompensated cirrhosis (21 per 100,000) and of hepatocellular carcinoma (4 per 100,000) by 2050, as shown in Fig. 4a-c. Complications are expected to reach a peak around 2040. The model predicts a sixfold increase in the cumulated number of deaths from HCV-related liver disease (170 per 100,000 inhabitants), as shown in Fig. 4d. All estimates are made assuming an unchanged treatment coverage of approximately 15%. The estimated numbers can be reduced by approximately 50% for cirrhosis, and by approximately one third for the other endpoints if treatment coverage were scaled up to 50%.

Discussion

In our low-risk area of HCV infection, we have estimated the fibrosis progression in untreated hepatitis C. Fibrosis develops slowly the first 20–25 years of infection, where after an accelerated fibrosis progression, especially in genotype 3, is predicted.

Using a Markov model, we have estimated the future complications of HCV based on the actual number of infected individuals until the year 2012, followed by an estimated low and stable incidence rate. The model predicts a gradual increase in HCV-related liver cirrhosis, decompensated cirrhosis and HCC with an apparent peak around 2040, accompanied by a gradual increase in liver-related deaths.

Modelling

Precision of dynamic modelling for prognosis of prevalence, morbidity and mortality depends on the quality of the data entered and the assumptions made. We have used locally acquired data whenever possible. The critical aspect in HCV pathophysiology is the progressive development of fibrosis towards cirrhosis, and in this aspect, our model also made use of local data. The further

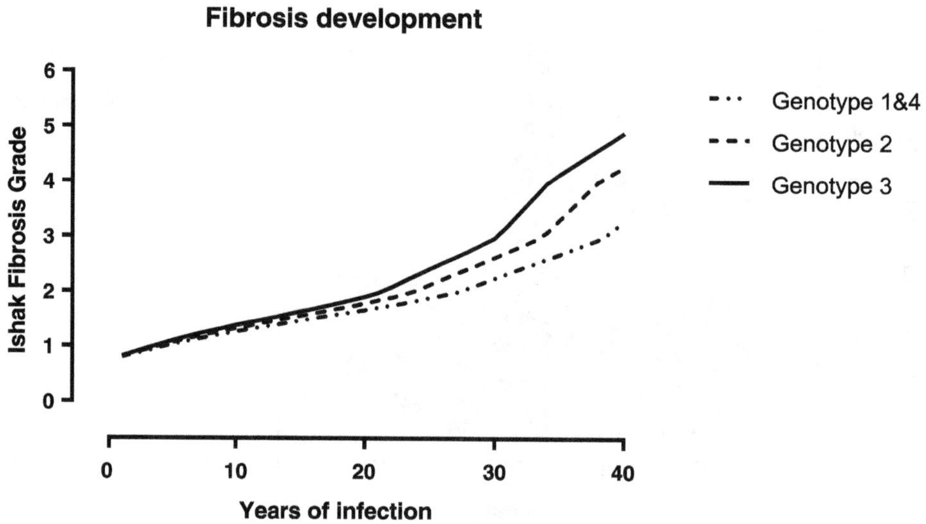

Fig. 3 Development of fibrosis in hepatitis C. The figure shows the time course of distribution of estimated median fibrosis grade according to genotype and duration of HCV disease. Estimates were derived by ordinal regression analysis of Ishak scores in 237 patients with duration of infection and genotype as independent variables

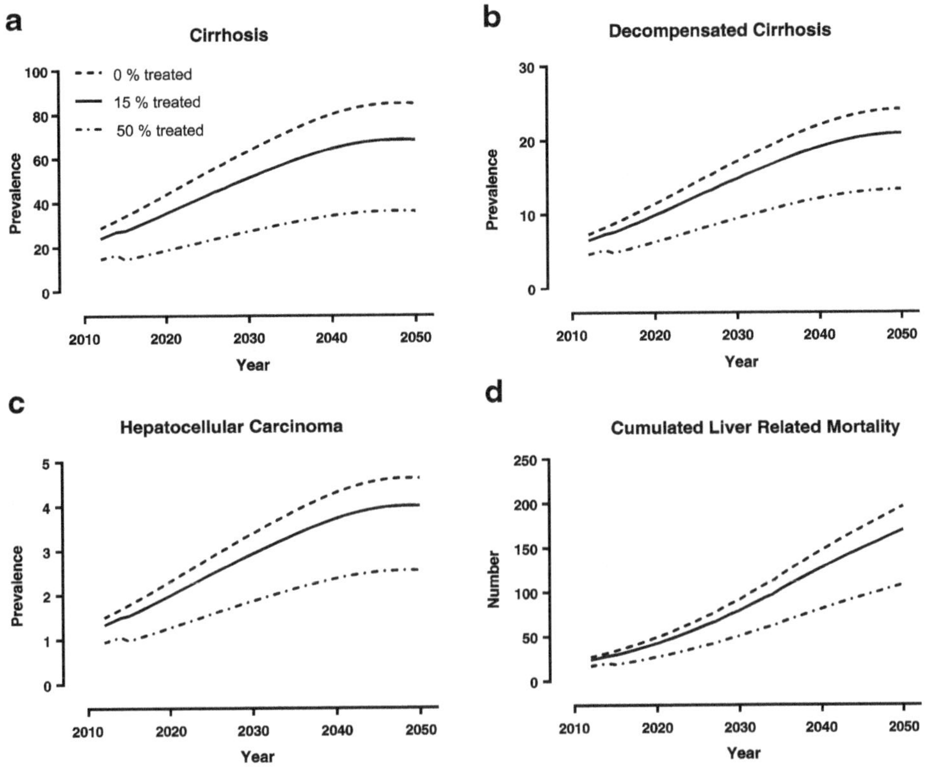

Fig. 4 Prediction of hepatitis C-related complications. The figure shows the predicted number of patients with cirrhosis, decompensated cirrhosis and hepatocellular carcinoma (panels **a**-**c**), and predicted cumulated number of deaths from liver disease (panel **d**) in the period 2013 to 2050 according to different treatment coverage. Numbers are given per 100,000 inhabitants

development from established cirrhosis is not likely to be very different from that of other cohorts, and the use of estimated transition rates from other studies [13] should not affect the prognosis measurably.

Our Markov model is based on an assumed low and stable incidence until 2050, whereas other reports estimate a declining or stable incidence [2]. The observed incidence peak in 2002–2004 in our data is probably a result of increased focus on HCV infection among general practitioners due to our encouragement of diagnosis in that period.

Our cohort is relatively young, and the liver biopsy data has a limited number of observations of severe fibrosis (Ishak grade 4–6). Hence, the estimates generated from these data are less precise regarding progression through high fibrosis stages.

Published data show variable rates of liver fibrosis progression, with 10%–40% developing cirrhosis after 20–35 years of infection [5, 8, 29]. A large systematic review supports nonlinear fibrosis progression [8] and other studies have shown that HCV genotype 3 is associated with a faster fibrosis progression [30–33]. Male sex is a reported risk factor for disease progression [5, 31]. However, we found no effect of sex in the progression of fibrosis, which is also observed in other studies [34].

Strengths and weaknesses

The strengths of this study are; first, we have reliable data on the HCV-infected subjects in our health region; second, the simulated fibrosis progression in the cohort is based on local data. However, there are apparent weaknesses. First, the number of undiagnosed HCV-infected individuals in the population is unknown. In Sweden, a comparable country regarding HCV epidemiology, it has been suggested that the rate of undiagnosed HCV infection is approximately 20% [35]. Second, incomplete records regarding confirmation testing has made it necessary to estimate the number of true positive cases, resulting in uncertainty regarding the true prevalence. However, our estimate of 63% true positives among those who only tested positive for anti-HCV is not controversial compared to another reported value of 68% true positive [36]. Moreover, the significance of RIBA-indeterminate reactions is unclear. Most individuals with indeterminate RIBA have a negative HCV RNA test, which may represent previous exposure to, but spontaneous recovery from HCV [37]. Authors have shown that approximately half of those with indeterminate RIBA have a resolved HCV infection [38, 39]. The proportion of RIBA-indeterminate records in our HCV population was low, making the contribution of these records less significant.

Third, the future incidence may be underestimated. Most likely, transmission of HCV will still be mainly by drug abuse, which is an ongoing problem in our region as is the case in the rest of Europe [40]. On the other hand, the introduction of highly effective, simple, short-term and tolerable therapies has the potential to increase treatment coverage among people who inject drugs. Thus, scaling up treatment in people with a transmission risk could reduce the future incidence and have a major impact on the HCV prevalence [41]. Fourth, it is documented that both moderate and excessive alcohol intake increase fibrosis progression in patients with HCV [42, 43]. Presence of concomitant excessive alcohol use was in our study assessed by clinical judgment, and not by a validated questionnaire of drinking habits. We have therefore chosen to omit alcohol use from the model over concerns on the quality of the data. Several other factors have been shown to accelerate the fibrosis progression, like co-infection with hepatitis B virus or HIV, diabetes and obesity [9]. The prevalence of HBV or HIV co-infections in our HCV population were low, 2.3% and 1% respectively, and therefore not included in the model. Data regarding diabetes and obesity were incomplete and neither included in the model.

Fifth, the exact time of infection is often not known. In individuals with unknown time of infection, we have used the first year of high-risk behavior as the presumed year of transmission, as others have done [30, 44, 45]. However, it has been reported that the interval between onset of drug injection and HCV infection has lengthened in recent years [46], which may indicate that the duration of infection could be shorter than estimated in our model of fibrosis progression. If so, our fibrosis model produces a spuriously slow rate of fibrosis progression, making the prognosis relatively conservative.

Sixth, the Markov model assumes that HCC only occurs when liver cirrhosis is established (Ishak 6). However, HCC can develop in lower fibrosis stages in chronic HCV infection [47, 48]. Finally, regression of fibrosis, cirrhosis and cirrhosis complications is possible after achieving SVR [49–51]. We do not have data to assess the effect of SVR on fibrosis regression, i.e. available pretreatment and post-treatment liver biopsies, and this is another limitation of the model. However, removing subjects achieving SVR from the model can mimic fibrosis regression in non-cirrhotic cases. In patients with cirrhosis, about 60% can regress after SVR [49, 50], and much less likely in decompensated cirrhosis. In patients with HCV-induced cirrhosis who attain SVR, the risk of HCC declines, but persists [52, 53]. To reflect that model cases with cirrhosis and SVR still are in risk of cirrhosis complications, we have retained 50% of these in the model.

Implications

HCV is the leading cause of chronic liver disease and cirrhosis and is the main cause of liver transplantation in the Western world [10]. Although the total number of HCV-infected individuals is estimated to be stable or decline in the future, an increase in liver cirrhosis, liver cancer, hepatic decompensation and liver-related deaths is expected in the coming years.

This assessment is underlined by the World Health Organization (WHO) statement that the burden of HCV disease has been largely ignored as a health priority, and the organization has developed the first-ever global health sector strategy for addressing the viral hepatitis pandemic [54].

To reduce the future burden of hepatitis C it is necessary to meet the challenge at three levels. First, prophylaxis measures must focus on reducing the transmission rate among active injection drug users. In addition, recent guidelines suggest that treatment should be offered to this group of individuals at high risk of transmitting HCV due to a potential prevention benefit [55]. Second, HCV infection among apparently healthy subjects must be diagnosed by screening of high-risk groups. Strategies to expand screening beyond high-risk groups should be considered since a substantial proportion of infected are unaware of their status [56]. Third, antiviral treatment has been offered only to a small percentage of patients, as treatment is hampered by the high cost of the new direct-acting antiviral drugs (DAAs). Based on the unpredictable course of liver fibrosis at the individual level, delaying treatment of patients with early fibrosis stages will increase the risk of liver complications [11]. DAAs has the potential to reduce the future burden of disease of HCV, but this is restricted by the current treatment levels [19]. In spite of the high costs of DAAs, several studies show that interferon-free regimens are cost-effective compared to interferon-based regimens [57–61].

Conclusion

Based on the registration of patients with HCV in a low risk area, we estimate a relatively slow fibrosis progression within the first 20–25 years of infection, followed by an accelerated fibrosis progression, especially in subjects with HCV genotype 3. This may have important implications in the clinical management of patients infected with genotype 3.

Furthermore, we estimate a gradual increase in future complications with an estimated peak around 2040. The projected scenario implies a substantial increase in HCV-related morbidity and mortality in the coming years. An increased number of patients need to be treated to have an impact on the future burden of HCV disease.

Abbreviations

DAA: Direct acting antiviral; HCC: Hepatocellular carcinoma; HCV: Hepatitis C virus; SVR: Sustained virological response; WHO: World Health Organization

Author's contributions

Conception and study design: RG, JF. Data collection: HK, OSM, MGK, LKB. Data analyses: LB, RG. HK and RG drafted the manuscript. Data interpretation, discussion and preparation of the final manuscript: HK, RG, JF, EP, TG, LB, OSM, MGK, LKB. All authors read and approved the final manuscript.

Competing interests

The authors declare that they have no competing interests.

Author details

[1]Gastroenterology and Nutrition Research Group, Department of Clinical Medicine, UiT The Arctic University of Norway, Tromsø, Norway. [2]Department of Medical and Health Sciences, University of Linköping, Linköping, Sweden. [3]Department of Internal Medicine, Section of Gastroenterology, University Hospital of North Norway, Tromsø, Norway. [4]Research Group for Host-Microbe Interactions, Department of Medical Biology, UiT The Arctic University of Norway, Tromsø, Norway. [5]Department of Microbiology, University Hospital of North Norway, Tromsø, Norway. [6]Department of Medicine, Nordland Hospital, Bodø, Norway. [7]Department of Medicine, Helgeland Hospital, Mo i Rana, Norway.

References

1. Davis GL, Alter MJ, El-Serag H, Poynard T, Jennings LW. Aging of hepatitis C virus (HCV)-infected persons in the United States: a multiple cohort model of HCV prevalence and disease progression. Gastroenterology. 2010;138(2):513–21.
2. Razavi H, Waked I, Sarrazin C, Myers R, Idilman R, Calinas F, Vogel W, Correa M, Hézode C, Lázaro P. The present and future disease burden of hepatitis C virus (HCV) infection with today's treatment paradigm. J Viral Hepat. 2014; 21(s1):34–59.
3. Duberg A-S, Blach S, Falconer K, Kåberg M, Razavi H, Aleman S. The future disease burden of hepatitis C virus infection in Sweden and the impact of different treatment strategies. Scand J Gastroenterol. 2015;50(2):233–44.
4. Gower E, Estes C, Blach S, Razavi-Shearer K, Razavi H. Global epidemiology and genotype distribution of the hepatitis C virus infection. J Hepatol. 2014; 61(1, Supplement):S45–57.
5. Chen SL, Morgan TR. The natural history of hepatitis C virus (HCV) infection. Int J Med Sci. 2006;3(2):47.
6. Kanwal F, Hoang T, Kramer JR, Asch SM, Goetz MB, Zeringue A, Richardson P, El-Serag HB. Increasing prevalence of HCC and cirrhosis in patients with chronic hepatitis C virus infection. Gastroenterology. 2011;140(4):1182–1188. e1181.
7. Younossi ZM, Kanwal F, Saab S, Brown KA, El-Serag HB, Kim WR, Ahmed A, Kugelmas M, Gordon SC. The impact of hepatitis C burden: an evidence-based approach. Aliment Pharmacol Ther. 2014;39(5):518–31.
8. Thein HH, Yi Q, Dore GJ, Krahn MD. Estimation of stage-specific fibrosis progression rates in chronic hepatitis C virus infection: A meta-analysis and meta-regression. Hepatology. 2008;48(2):418–31.
9. Seeff LB. The history of the "natural history" of hepatitis C (1968–2009). Liver Int. 2009;29:89–99.
10. Westbrook RH, Dusheiko G. Natural history of hepatitis C. J Hepatol. 2014; 61(1):S58–68.
11. Calvaruso V, Craxì A. Why do I treat my patients with mild hepatitis C? Liver Int. 2016;36:7–12.
12. Kielland KB, Delaveris GJM, Rogde S, Eide TJ, Amundsen EJ, Dalgard O. Liver fibrosis progression at autopsy in injecting drug users infected by hepatitis C: A longitudinal long-term cohort study. J Hepatol. 2014;60(2):260–6.
13. Hutchinson SJ, Bird SM, Goldberg DJ. Modeling the current and future disease burden of hepatitis C among injection drug users in Scotland. Hepatology. 2005;42(3):711–23.
14. Alazawi W, Cunningham M, Dearden J, Foster GR. Systematic review: outcome of compensated cirrhosis due to chronic hepatitis C infection. Aliment Pharmacol Ther. 2010;32(3):344–55.
15. Dienstag JL, Ghany MG, Morgan TR, Di Bisceglie AM, Bonkovsky HL, Kim H-Y, Seeff LB, Szabo G, Wright EC, Sterling RK, et al. A prospective study of the rate of progression in compensated, histologically advanced chronic hepatitis C. Hepatology. 2011;54(2):396–405.
16. Deuffic-Burban S, Poynard T, Valleron AJ. Quantification of fibrosis progression in patients with chronic hepatitis C using a Markov model. J Viral Hepat. 2002;9(2):114–22.
17. Krahn M, Wong JB, Heathcote J, Scully L, Seeff L. Estimating the prognosis of hepatitis C patients infected by transfusion in Canada between 1986 and 1990. Med Decis Mak. 2004;24(1):20–9.
18. Yi Q, Wang PP, Krahn M. Improving the accuracy of long-term prognostic estimates in hepatitis C virus infection. J Viral Hepat. 2004;11(2):166–74.
19. Cramp ME, Rosenberg WM, Ryder SD, Blach S, Parkes J. Modelling the impact of improving screening and treatment of chronic hepatitis C virus infection on future hepatocellular carcinoma rates and liver-related mortality. BMC Gastroenterol. 2014;14:137–7.
20. Harris RJ, Thomas B, Griffiths J, Costella A, Chapman R, Ramsay M, De Angelis D, Harris HE. Increased uptake and new therapies are needed to avert rising hepatitis C-related end stage liver disease in England: Modelling the predicted impact of treatment under different scenarios. J Hepatol. 2014;61(3):530–7.
21. Kristiansen MG, Gutteberg T, Berg LK, Sjursen H, Mortensen L, Florholmen J. Hepatitis C in Northern Norway–an 8-year material. Tidsskr Nor Laegeforen. 2002;122(20):1974–6.
22. Dalgard O, Jeansson S, Skaug K, Raknerud N, Bell H. Hepatitis C in the general adult population of Oslo: prevalence and clinical spectrum. Scand J Gastroenterol. 2003;38(8):864–70.
23. Kristiansen MG, Gutteberg TJ, Mortensen L, Berg LK, Goll R, Florholmen J. Clinical outcomes in a prospective study of community-acquired hepatitis C virus infection in Northern Norway. Scand J Gastroenterol. 2010;45(6):746–51.
24. Sonnenberg FA, Beck JR. Markov Models in Medical Decision Making: A Practical Guide. Med Decis Mak. 1993;13(4):322–38.
25. Ishak K, Baptista A, Bianchi L, Callea F, De GJ, Gudat F, Denk H, Desmet V, Korb G, MacSween RN. Histological grading and staging of chronic hepatitis. JHepatol. 1995;22(6):696–9.
26. Thomas DL, Seeff LB. Natural History of Hepatitis C. Clinics in Liver Disease. 2005;9(3):383–98.
27. Sangiovanni A, Prati GM, Fasani P, Ronchi G, Romeo R, Manini M, Del Ninno E, Morabito A, Colombo M. The natural history of compensated cirrhosis due to hepatitis C virus: A 17-year cohort study of 214 patients. Hepatology. 2006;43(6):1303–10.
28. Dahari H, Cotler SJ, Feld JJ. Cure prevents more than transmission of hepatitis C virus. Hepatology. 2016;64(3):1003–4.
29. Wiese M, Fischer J, Löbermann M, Göbel U, Grüngreiff K, Güthoff W, Kullig U, Richter F, Schiefke I, Tenckhoff H, et al. Evaluation of liver disease progression in the German hepatitis C virus (1b)-contaminated anti-D cohort at 35 years after infection. Hepatology. 2014;59(1):49–57.
30. Bochud PY, Cai T, Overbeck K, Bochud M, Dufour JF. M++llhaupt B, Borovicka J, Heim M, Moradpour D, Cerny A: Genotype 3 is associated with accelerated fibrosis progression in chronic hepatitis C. J Hepatol. 2009;51(4): 655–66.
31. Marabita F, Aghemo A, De Nicola S, Rumi MG, Cheroni C, Scavelli R, Crimi M, Soffredini R, Abrignani S, De Francesco R, et al. Genetic variation in the interleukin-28B gene is not associated with fibrosis progression in patients with chronic hepatitis C and known date of infection. Hepatology. 2011; 54(4):1127–34.

32. Probst A, Dang T, Bochud M, Egger M, Negro F, Bochud PY. Role of Hepatitis C virus genotype 3 in liver fibrosis progression – a systematic review and meta-analysis. J Viral Hepat. 2011;18(11):745–59.
33. Kanwal F, Kramer JR, Ilyas J, Duan Z, El-Serag HB. HCV genotype 3 is associated with an increased risk of cirrhosis and hepatocellular cancer in a national sample of US Veterans with HCV. Hepatology. 2014;60(1):98–105.
34. Williams MJ, Lang-Lenton M. Progression of initially mild hepatic fibrosis in patients with chronic hepatitis C infection. J Viral Hepat. 2011;18(1):17–22.
35. Cornberg M, Razavi HA, Alberti A, Bernasconi E, Buti M, Cooper C, Dalgard O, Dillion JF, Flisiak R, Forns X. A systematic review of hepatitis C virus epidemiology in Europe, Canada and Israel. Liver Int. 2011;31:30–60.
36. Moorman AC, Drobenuic J, Kamili S. Prevalence of false-positive hepatitis C antibody results, National Health and Nutrition Examination Study (NHANES) 2007–2012. J Clin Virol. 2017;89:1–4.
37. Makuria AT, Raghuraman S, Burbelo PD, Cantilena CC, Allison RD, Gibble J, Rehermann B, Alter HJ. The clinical relevance of persistent recombinant immunoblot assay–indeterminate reactions: insights into the natural history of hepatitis C virus infection and implications for donor counseling. Transfusion. 2012;52(9):1940–8.
38. Bes M, Esteban JI, Casamitjana N, Piron M, Quer J, Cubero M, Puig L, Guardia J, Sauleda S. Hepatitis C virus (HCV)-specific T-cell responses among recombinant immunoblot assay-3–indeterminate blood donors: a confirmatory evidence of HCV exposure. Transfusion. 2009;49(7):1296–305.
39. Hitziger T, Schmidt M, Schottstedt V, Hennig H, Schumann A, Ross S, Lu M, Seifried E, Roggendorf M. Cellular immune response to hepatitis C virus (HCV) in nonviremic blood donors with indeterminate anti-HCV reactivity. Transfusion. 2009;49(7):1306–13.
40. Duffell EF, van de Laar MJW, Amato-Gauci AJ. Enhanced surveillance of hepatitis C in the EU, 2006 – 2012. J Viral Hepat. 2015;22(7):590–5.
41. Martin NK, Vickerman P, Grebely J, Hellard M, Hutchinson SJ, Lima VD, Foster GR, Dillon JF, Goldberg DJ, Dore GJ, et al. Hepatitis C virus treatment for prevention among people who inject drugs: Modeling treatment scale-up in the age of direct-acting antivirals. Hepatology. 2013;58(5):1598–609.
42. Westin J, Lagging LM, Spak F, Aires N, Svensson E, Lindh M, Dhillon AP, Norkrans G, Wejstål R. Moderate alcohol intake increases fibrosis progression in untreated patients with hepatitis C virus infection. J Viral Hepat. 2002;9(3):235–41.
43. Ascione A, Tartaglione T, Di Costanzo GG. Natural history of chronic hepatitis C virus infection. DigLiver Dis. 2007;39(Suppl 1):S4–7.
44. Poynard T, Ratziu V, Charlotte F, Goodman Z, McHutchison J, Albrecht J. Rates and risk factors of liver fibrosis progression in patients with chronic hepatitis C. J Hepatol. 2001;34(5):730–9.
45. Sypsa V, Touloumi G, Tassopoulos NC, Ketikoglou I, Vafiadi I, Hatzis G, Tsantoulas D, Akriviadis E, Delladetsima J, Demonakou M, et al. Reconstructing and predicting the hepatitis C virus epidemic in Greece: increasing trends of cirrhosis and hepatocellular carcinoma despite the decline in incidence of HCV infection. J Viral Hepat. 2004;11(4):366-74.
46. Hagan H, Pouget ER, Des Jarlais DC, Lelutiu-Weinberger C. Meta-Regression of Hepatitis C Virus Infection in Relation to Time Since Onset of Illicit Drug Injection: The Influence of Time and Place. Am J Epidemiol. 2008;168(10): 1099–109.
47. Yoshida H, Shiratori Y, Moriyama M, et al. Interferon therapy reduces the risk for hepatocellular carcinoma: National surveillance program of cirrhotic and noncirrhotic patients with chronic hepatitis c in japan. Ann Intern Med. 1999;131(3):174–81.
48. Fattovich G, Stroffolini T, Zagni I, Donato F. Hepatocellular carcinoma in cirrhosis: Incidence and risk factors. Gastroenterology. 2004;127(5, Supplement 1):S35–50.
49. D'Ambrosio R, Aghemo A, Rumi MG, Ronchi G, Donato MF, Paradis V, Colombo M, Bedossa P. A morphometric and immunohistochemical study to assess the benefit of a sustained virological response in hepatitis C virus patients with cirrhosis. Hepatology. 2012;56(2):532–43.
50. Maylin S, Martinot-Peignoux M, Moucari R, Boyer N, Ripault MP, Cazals-Hatem D, Giuily N, Castelnau C, Cardoso AC, Asselah T, et al. Eradication of Hepatitis C Virus in Patients Successfully Treated for Chronic Hepatitis C. Gastroenterology. 2008;135(3):821–9.
51. Cousien A, Tran VC, Deuffic-Burban S, Jauffret-Roustide M, Dhersin J-S, Yazdanpanah Y. Hepatitis C treatment as prevention of viral transmission and liver-related morbidity in persons who inject drugs. Hepatology. 2016; 63(4):1090–101.
52. El-Serag HB, Kanwal F, Richardson P, Kramer J. Risk of hepatocellular carcinoma after sustained virological response in Veterans with hepatitis C virus infection. Hepatology. 2016;64(1):130–7.
53. van der Meer AJ, Veldt BJ, Feld JJ, et al. ASsociation between sustained virological response and all-cause mortality among patients with chronic hepatitis c and advanced hepatic fibrosis. JAMA. 2012;308(24):2584–93.
54. WHO: Global Health Sector Strategy on Viral Hepatitis, 2016–2021 2016.
55. European Association for the Study of the L: EASL Recommendations on Treatment of Hepatitis C. 2016. J Hepatol. 2017;66(1):153-94.
56. Coffin PO, Scott JD, Golden MR, Sullivan SD. Cost-effectiveness and Population Outcomes of General Population Screening for Hepatitis C. Clin Infect Dis. 2012;54(9):1259–71.
57. Hagan LM, Yang Z, Ehteshami M, Schinazi RF. All-oral, interferon-free treatment for chronic hepatitis C: cost-effectiveness analyses. J Viral Hepat. 2013;20(12):847–57.
58. Younossi ZM, Singer ME, Mir HM, Henry L, Hunt S. Impact of interferon free regimens on clinical and cost outcomes for chronic hepatitis C genotype 1 patients. J Hepatol. 2014;60(3):530–7.
59. Chhatwal J, Kanwal F, Roberts MS, Dunn MA. Cost-Effectiveness and Budget Impact of Hepatitis C Virus Treatment With Sofosbuvir and Ledipasvir in the United StatesCost-Effectiveness of HCV Treatment With Sofosbuvir and Ledipasvir. Ann Intern Med. 2015;162(6):397–406.
60. Deuffic-Burban S, Obach D, Canva V, Pol S, Roudot-Thoraval F, Dhumeaux D, Mathurin P, Yazdanpanah Y. Cost-effectiveness and budget impact of interferon-free direct-acting antiviral-based regimens for hepatitis C treatment: the French case. J Viral Hepat. 2016;23(10):767-79.
61. Gray E, O'Leary A, Kieran JA, Fogarty E, Dowling T, Norris S, Irish Hepatitis C Outcomes and Research Network (ICORN): Direct costs of interferon-based and interferon-free direct-acting antiviral regimens for the treatment of chronic hepatitis C infection. J Viral Hepat. 2016;23(9):677-86.

15

The geographic variation and spatiotemporal distribution of hepatitis C virus infection in Libya: 2007–2016

Mohamed A. Daw[1*], Lutfi A. Buktir Ali[2], Amina M. Daw[3], Nadia E. M. Sifennasr[1], Aghnyia A. Dau[4], Mohamed M. Agnan[5], Abdallah El-Bouzedi[6] and In association with the Libyan Study Group of Hepatitis & HIV

Abstract

Background: Hepatitis C Virus infection has been considered an important hidden pandemic in developing countries, particularly in Africa. It varies greatly from one region to another and even within districts of the same region. Macroscopic geospatial analysis has become an important scientific tool for identifying the density and clustering of HCV infection and provides epidemiological information for planning interventions and control strategies. The application of these parameters provides a better knowledge of the hepatitis C virus infection prevalence at the national level and can help to implement pertinent strategies to address the HCV-related burdens. This study aims to determine the geographical variability of HCV infection in Libya and to identify the hot spots within regions and districts of the country, and to analyze the population-based demographic determinants involved and outline the intervention programs needed.

Methods: Disease mapping and spatial analysis were conducted using geographic information data available on all documented cases of HCV infections in Libya between 2007 and 2016. Spatial autocorrelation was tested using Moran's Index, which determines and measures the degree of clustering and dispersion of HCV infection in a country.

Results: A total 114,928 HCV infection cases during a ten-year period with accurate geographic information were studied. Ages ranged between 16 and 50 years and the male to female ratio was 2:1. HCV infection was unevenly distributed in Libya, and its incidence increased steadily over the study period. Several hot spots and cold spots were found mainly in the southern and eastern regions of the country.

Conclusion: HCV infection in Libya was geographically variable, with several hot spots particularly in eastern and southern Libya associated with different demographic determinants. Future intervention planning should consider the geospatial variability and risk factors involved.

Keywords: HCV infection, Libya, Geospatial analysis, HCV hotspots, Spatiotemporal distribution, Geographic variation

Background

Hepatitis C virus (HCV) infection is an important burden for healthcare services worldwide. Over 32 million people are chronically infected with HCV in Southeast Asia and more than 6 million in Latin America. Also, sub-Saharan Africa houses almost 20% of world's HCV-infected individuals [1, 2]. HCV-infected individuals have a 2.4 times higher risk of all-cause mortality compared to the non-infected population, 26.5 times the risk of liver-related mortality, and 1.8 times the risk of non-liver-related mortality [3, 4].

In North and sub-Saharan African countries, where HCV is considered endemic, its prevalence varies greatly among African countries [5]. It has recently been aggravated by immigration and massive population displacements caused by economic hardship and political instability. These factors could influence the geographical status of HCV infections, particularly in North African countries, which are transited by African migrants on their way to Europe [6].

* Correspondence: mohamedadaw@gmail.com
[1]Department of Medical Microbiology &Immunology, Faculty of Medicine, University of Tripoli, CC 82668 Tripoli, Libya
Full list of author information is available at the end of the article

Libya is the second largest country in North Africa and has the longest coast on the Mediterranean basin. It is surrounded by six countries where HCV is endemic, including Egypt, which has the highest prevalence of HCV in the world. Close proximity to these countries could provide transmission arteries for HCV infection into and across Libya [7, 8]. Furthermore, Libya is an oil-rich country that has for decades performed well economically and attracted many Africans as a place to work and as a route to Europe. In Libya, HCV prevalence has been reported to be relatively moderate at 1.2%, although it varied greatly from one region to another [9, 10]. Immigration is a particularly important factor in HCV prevalence in Libya. A recent study carried out on African immigrants residing in Tripoli showed a prevalence of HCV ranging from 2 to 26%, depending on the country of origin of the immigrants. The highest rate was among those from Egypt (18.7%) and West Africa (14.1%), followed by immigrants from the Horn of Africa and sub-Saharan countries [11]. Furthermore, the geographic variation of HCV genotypes in Libya varied from one region to another [12]. Genotype 4 was predominant, with a higher level in the eastern region, followed by genotypes 1 and 2, which were common in the western part of the country [12].

The World Health Organization recommends in its new guidelines that HCV tests be offered to people with high risk behavior and to those from high risk populations [13]. However, screening programs targeting these risk groups, and particularly intravenous drug users and promiscuous individuals, have not always been effective, particularly in developing countries at least partly due to stigmatization of such behaviors. Hence, specific studies, such as geospatial analysis, should be applied to determine clustering of HCV infections associated with socio-economic characteristics, level of urbanization, and population density [14–16].

Geospatial analysis is valuable in determining the spatial distribution and quantifying the impact of socio-economic determinants on the incidence of infectious diseases. In China, Europe and USA, such information has been widely used by public health services to identify areas of high risk for HCV, HIV and other concomitant infections [17, 18]. There is little information on the spatiotemporal dynamics of HCV, particularly in North and sub-Saharan Africa, where HCV infection is endemic [19–21].

A better understanding of the distribution of these diseases would provide a rational basis for allocating medical resources and providing effective guidance for public health interventions. The aims of this study were to determine the geographic variation and spatiotemporal distribution of HCV infection in Libya and to analyze the socio-economic and demographic determinants associated with the distribution of HCV infection.

Methods

Data source

In 2006, Libya carried out one of the largest nation-based surveillance studies of hepatitis B and hepatitis C viruses using a sample of > 1% of the total Libyan population [9]. Since then, all diagnosed cases of HCV infection are being reported and officially documented. The HCV screening policy and notification system in Libya is based on mandatory, anonymous notification of newly diagnosed HCV cases by laboratories all over the country combined with epidemiological information on the mode of transmission and other clinical data reported by physicians and trained clinical epidemiologists. The national screening policy for HCV in Libya, which is uniform all over the country, includes screening of blood donors, preoperative patients, pregnant women, and kidney and liver disease patients, as well as pre-marriage screening.

The data collected so far consist of all the HCV infections newly reported throughout the country between January 2007 and December 2016 and include 114,926 individuals. The data covered all the Libyan regions and the residence of each case was localized at the city and district levels (Fig. 1).

Laboratory diagnosis was carried out according to the procedures of the Libyan Central Laboratory. HCV testing was carried out by detecting HCV antibodies using an enzyme-linked immunosorbent assay (ELISA) and confirmed by immunoblot and/or polymerase chain reaction. Any person found to be positive and confirmed by these diagnostic tests is considered to be a case of HCV infection [9, 11].

Geospatial analysis and mapping of HCV infections

Geo-data (Libya's map and the administrative municipalities' geographical borders) and patient data were used for geospatial analysis on grid maps. Overall HCV prevalence was estimated based on the number of patients found infected and the total population of Libya and of each of its municipalities during the study. The locations of the infected individuals were marked at the district level on the most recently updated map of Libya showing its districts. On the maps were indicated the spatial mean center and spatial standard distance ±2 standard deviations.

The electronic maps were made with ArcGIS 10.1 software (Environmental Systems Research Institute (ESRI), Inc., 1999; Redlands, CA, USA) and the data were processed and analyzed with SPSS18.0 software (IBM Inc., Armonk, NY, USA).

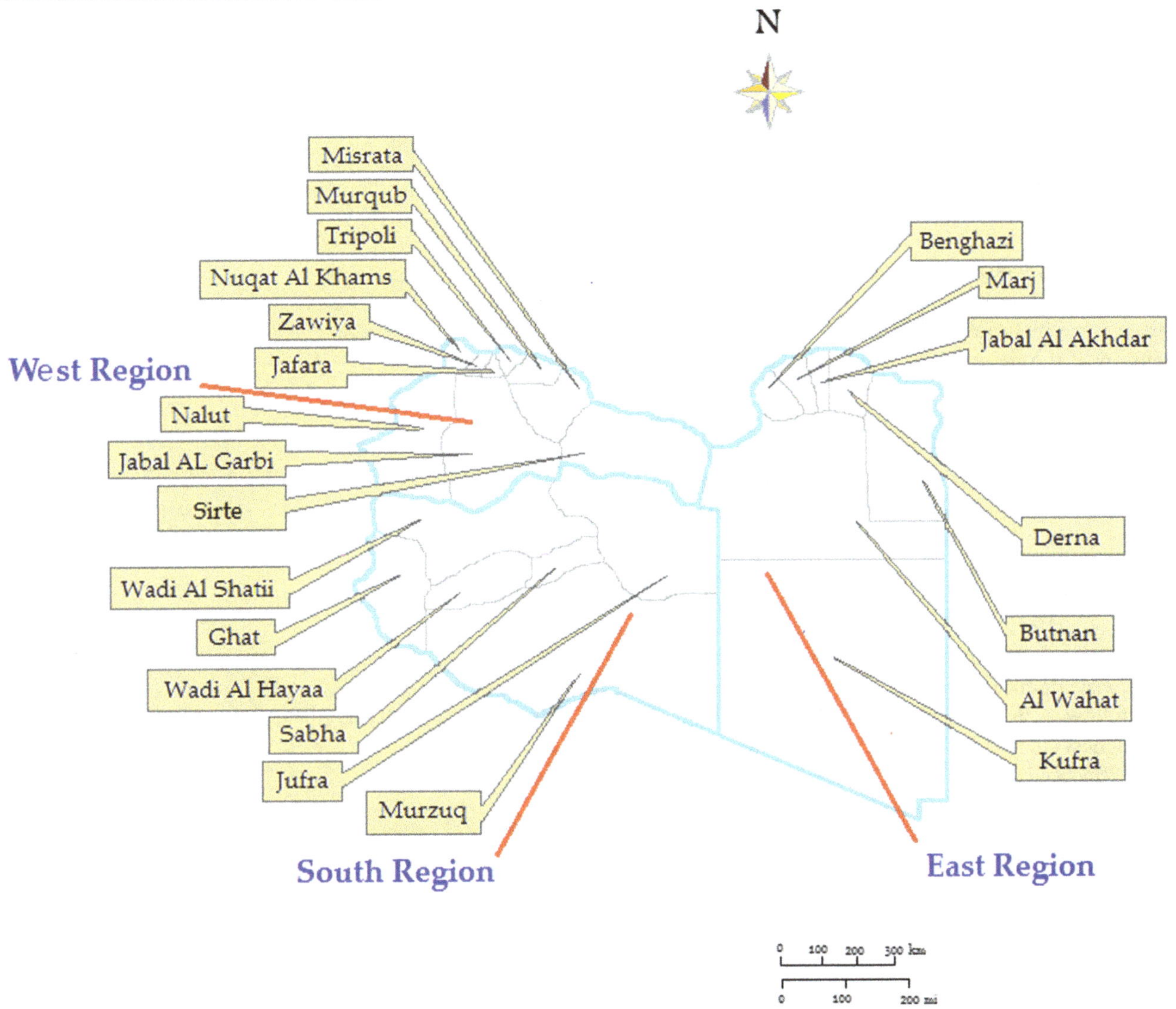

Fig. 1 The geographical locations and boundaries of the Libyan regions and districts

Spatial autocorrelation

Spatial analysis was carried out to identify the locations of HCV clusters and surrounding areas. To identify the spatial patterns of the infected cases, gobal Moran's I statistic was used to analyze the presence and nature of HCV spatial autocorrelation (or dependency) in the original 22 districts for each year between 2007 and 2016 by using Open-GeoDa 1.2.0 [22, 23]. A Moran index value of − 1 indicates perfect dispersion, + 1 perfect correlation, and zero value random spatial distribution. The measures of spatial association were used to identify the locations of clusters and outliers and to determine the importance and the type of spatial correlation.

HCV clustering, which could be inferred from the presence of spatial autocorrelation, sometimes indicates hierarchical expansion in urban areas and across districts. A high frequency area means that it contained many HCV cases and that it was surrounded by regions also with a large number of cases. Conversely, a low frequency area means that it had few cases and was surrounded by areas also with few cases.

Statistical analysis

The epidemiological data were collected using a standard registry form report, as previously described (12879_2013_2969_MOESM2_ESM.docx),(12879_2013_2969_MOESM1_ESM.doc).

The statistical analysis was performed using computer software version 11.0 (StataCorp. 2013. Stata Statistical Software: Release 13. College Station, TX: StataCorp LP). Logistic regression was conducted to identify the factors associated with HCV infection. Data were expressed as means ± standard deviation (SD), and as number and percentage with 95% confidence interval (CI), as appropriate.

The z-test was used to determine if the rate ratio was statistically significant ($p < 0.001$) [9]. The adjusted relative risk (RR) of HCV infection comparing females to males was estimated. RR calculations were adjusted for variables known to be associated with HCV infection in Libya, such as social status, living conditions or demographic characteristics (age, gender, marital status and education, etc.)

Results

A total of 114,928 newly reported HCV cases during a ten-year period with specific, accurate geographic information were included in this study. The geographic distribution of the reported HCV infection cases was found to vary between the Libyan regions and districts (Table 1). There were 53,358 cases in the western region (46%), 39,220 in the eastern region (34%) and 22,350 (19%) in the southern region. The distribution of the identified HCV cases was also found to differ between the cities in the same region. In the western region, the largest number of cases was reported in Tripoli (16,560; 31%) followed by Murqub (15,811; 30%) and Jabal al Gharbi (13,219; 25%). There were fewer cases in Sirte (3059; 6%) and Nalut (4660; 9%). In the eastern region, the largest number of cases was in Benghazi (15,932; 41%) followed by Butnan (6640; 17%). In the south, it was highest in Sebha (7493; 34%) followed by Ghat (4426; 20%) and Wadi al Shati (4309; 19%).

Analysis based on continuous images and district-level analysis showed spatiotemporal variation during the ten-year period characterized by an initial expansion and followed by a decline in HCV infection rates. During 2007–2012, the southern region consistently had the highest distribution of HCV, with 5% of the population infected during 2007–2011 (Table 1). The western region had the lowest prevalence rate, particularly in the central districts. HCV density decreased gradually from 2007 till 2011. This was followed by general intensification in the spatial patterns during 2012–2016. In addition, the district distribution of HCV showed persistently high rates in the southern region, particularly in Murzuq (bordering Algeria) and Butnan (bordering Egypt). Figure 2 shows the geographic variability and temporal distribution of HCV infection in each five-year period (Fig. 2a, 2007–2011; b, 2012–2016).

There was clear variability in HCV infection cases at the regional level during the study period. This was more evident in the southern and eastern regions, particularly Sebha, Wadi al Shati and Ghat near the south-western borders, and Murzuq in the far south. But it was less pronounced in Jufra in the middle of the country, bordering Sert. A similar trend was obvious in districts of the eastern region, with a high rate in Benghazi followed by Butnan on the North-Eastern border. In the Western region, HCV infection rates were stable and without significant variation among the districts. HCV infection rates were very low in the middle part of the country, represented by Jufra, Sirte and Musrata.

Table 1 The Distribution of HCV cases over the Libyan regions and districts 2007–2016

Regions and districts	Study period		
	2007–2011	2012–2016	Total n(%)
Eastern region			
Butnan	2520	3020	5540 (14)
Derna	975	1400	2375 (6)
Jabal al Akhdar	1832	3000	4832 (12)
Marj	1320	2100	3420 (9)
Benghazi	6100	6312	12,412 (32)
Al Wahat	2860	3158	6018 (15)
Kufra	1513	3110	4623 (12)
Total	17,120	22,100	39,220 (34)
Western region			
Sirte	699	930	1629 (3)
Misrata	841	1199	2040(4)
Murqub	3401	4059	7460 (14)
Tripoli	7160	8900	16,060 (30)
Jafara	2750	2290	5040 (9)
Zawiya	1419	2150	3569 (7)
Nuqat al Khams	1400	2330	3730 (7)
Jabal al Gharbi	4050	5020	9070 (17)
Nalut	1490	3270	4760 (9)
Total	23,210	30,148	53,358 (46)
Southern region			
Jufra	752	1020	1772 (8)
Wadi al Shati	1190	2119	3309 (15)
Sebha	3222	4011	7233 (32)
Wadi al Hayaa	1320	1860	3180 (14)
Ghat	1316	2150	3466 (16)
Murzuq	1400	1990	3390 (15)
Total	9200	13,150	22,350 (19)
All regions	49,530 (43)	65,398 (57)	114,928

Between 2007 and 2016, Moran's Index generally increased, meaning that the strength of clustering of HCV cases became more prominent. This allowed us to classify the geospatial areas either as a high prevalence area (HPA) or a low prevalence area (LPA) (Fig. 3a, 2007–2011; b, 2012–2016; c, 2007–2016). The high prevalence areas are in districts with a large number of HCV infections with a prevalence rate higher than 1.2% and low prevalence area (LPA-HC) are those of HCV prevalence rate 1–1.2%). This is clearly seen in the eastern region in two districts (Batnan and Benghazi), in four districts in the

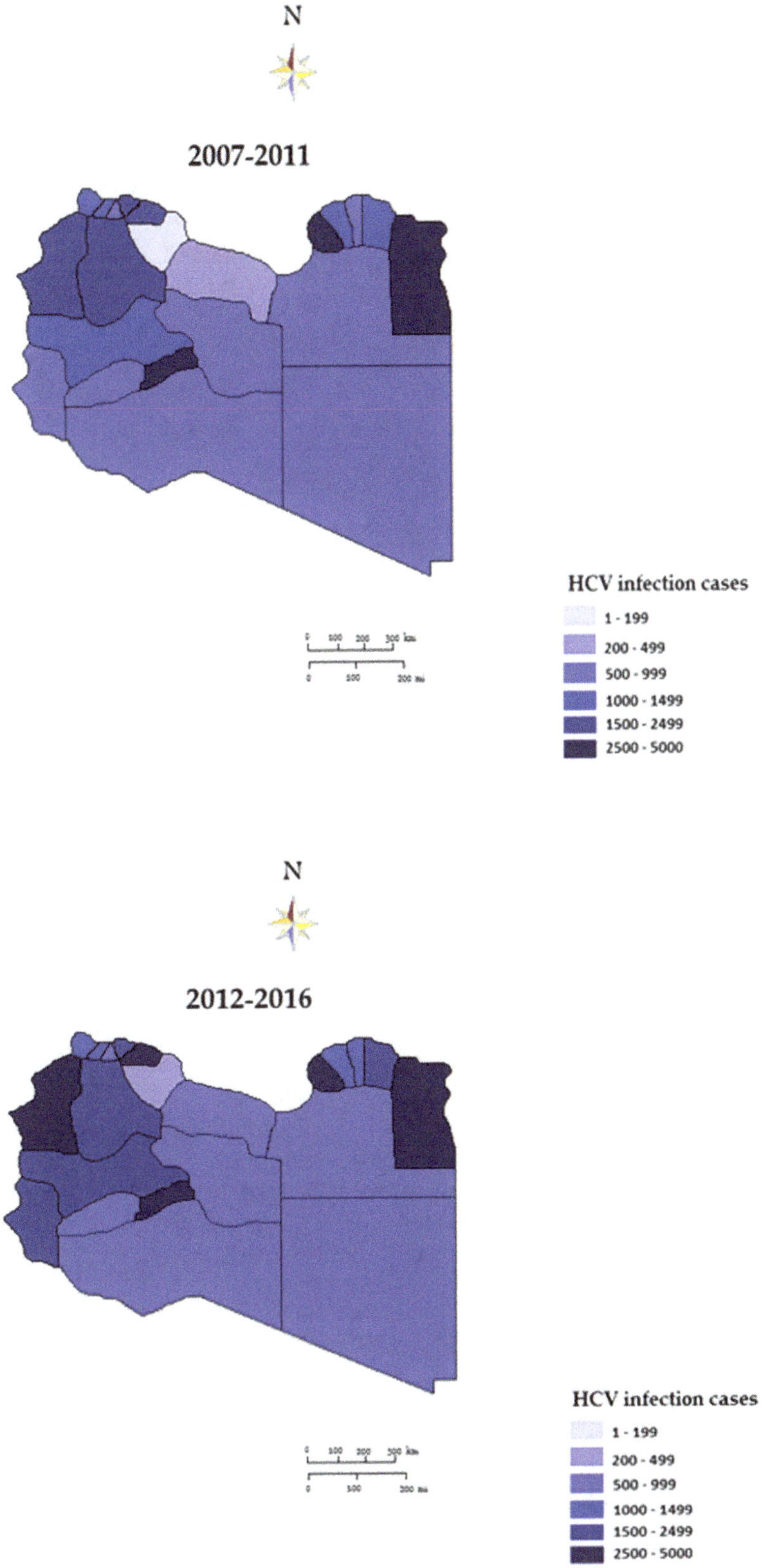

Fig. 2 Geo-spatial distributions of identified cases of HCV infection in Libya at district level

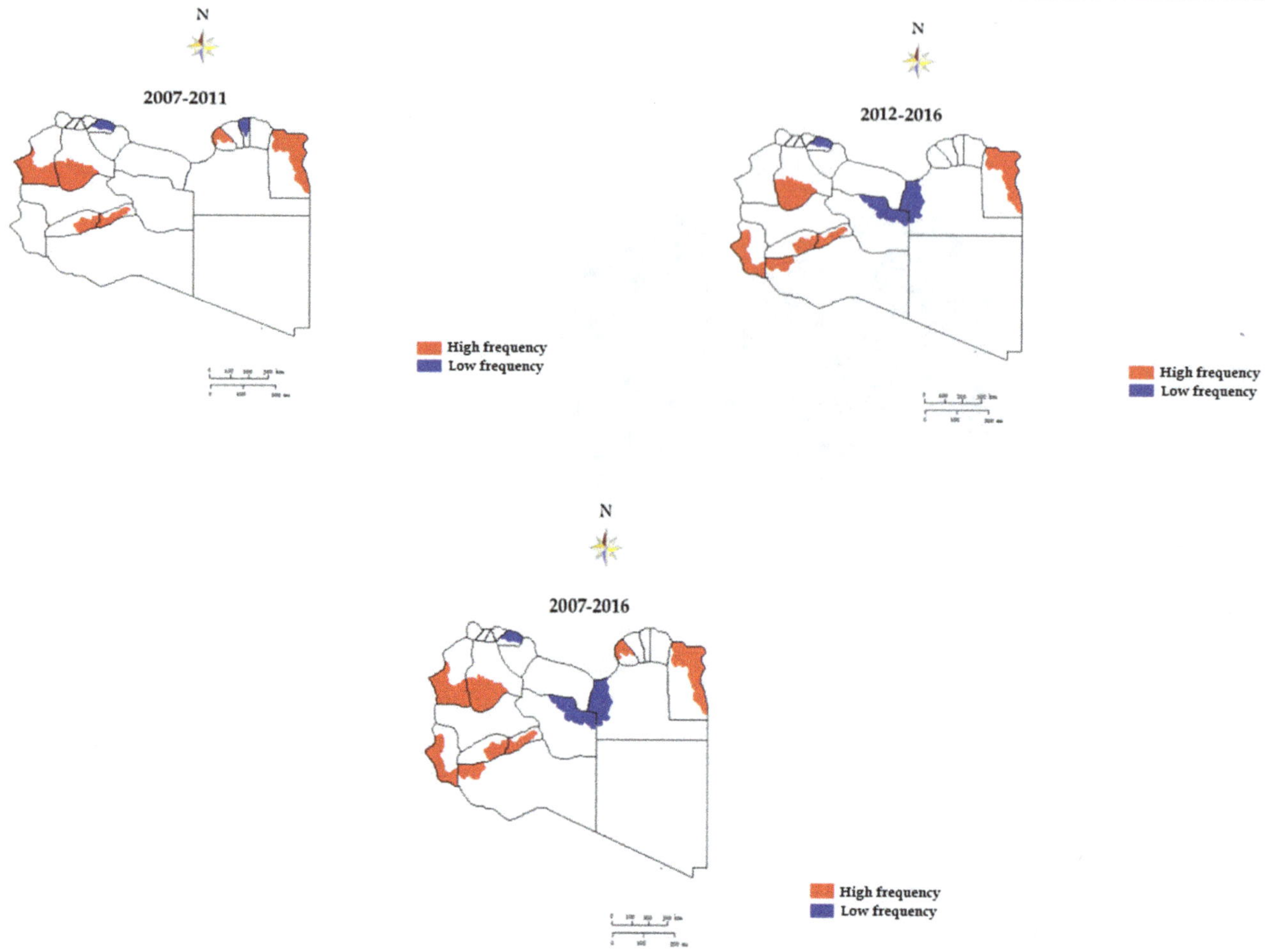

Fig. 3 Spatiotemporal patterns of high and low prevalence areas of HCV infection reported during a ten-year study period. **a**, 2007–2011; **b**, 2012–2016; **c**, 2007–2016

southern region (Sebha, Wadi al Shati and Ghat) and in Nalout and Al-Jabel Gharbi in western Libya. Table 2 shows the distribution of high prevalence areas (HPA) and low prevalence areas (LPA) of HCV infection between 2007 and 2016. High prevalence areas were observed in Benghazi, Butnan, Sebha, Nalut, Jabal al Gharbi in the first 5 years (2007–2011) and in Butnan, Murzuq, Wadi al Shati, Ghat and Nalut during 2012–2016.

We also studied the population characteristics and demographics of HCV-infected patients. During 2007–2016, the overall male-to-female ratio was 1:1.33, the mean age of all patients was 47.31 years (95% CI: 47.27–47.35); 39% of them were < 35 years

Table 2 Distribution of reported high prevalence areas (HPA) and low prevalence area (LPA) of HCV infection in Libya from 2007 to 2016

Year	High frequency area		Low frequency area	
	No.	Location	No.	Location
2007–2008	12	Benghazi, Butnan, Sebha, Jabal al Gharbi	1	Murqub
2009–2010	10	Benghazi, Butnan, Sebha, Nalut, Jabal al Gharbi	1	Murqub, Jabal Alakhdar
2011–2012	9	Benghazi, Butnan, Sebha, Nalut, Jabal al Gharbi	2	Murqub, Al Wahat
2013–2014	14	Butnan, Sebha, Ghat, Jabal al Gharbi	2	Murqub,
2015–2016	17	Butnan, Kufra, Wadi al Shati, Ghat, Nalut	3	Murqub, Al Wahat, Jufra
Total	13	Benghazi, Butnan, Sebha, Nalut, Jabal al Gharbi, Wadi al Shati, Ghat, Kufra	3	Murqub, Al Wahat, Jufra

old, and 32% were over 50 years. The relative risk (RR) of HCV infection was compared between males and females. The RR in females compared to males was 1.03 (95% CI: 1.01–1.21) in 2007 and 1.83 (95% CI: 1.42–2.24) in 2016, which is relatively higher during 2012–2016.

Table 3 shows the different demographic factors that could have been involved in HCV infection in the Libyan population during 2007–2016. The socio-demographic determinants included age, sex, education, population density and place of residence. The HCV prevalence rate increased with age. Those aged below 24 years had the lowest prevalence, followed by those 25–35 years old. The reported prevalence was higher among those 36–49 years old but highest in those over 50 years ($P < 0.001$). HCV infection was also higher among males than females aged between 25 and 39 years. The prevalence of HCV was also higher among the illiterate group (37%), in which it ranged from 6 to 25%, depending on the level of education. The place of residence had a significant impact on HCV infection: over 60% of the infections were in urbanized areas ($p < 0.001$). Moreover, the infection rate was higher among unmarried people (39%), those whose living conditions were of a low standard (41%), and those with a minimum income (47%). The impact of the socio-demographic factors on the HCV infection varied from one district to another according to population density, family members and annual income. The high prevalence areas in Benghazi and Tripoli were associated with a high population density, with a population rate over 60 persons/km^2 with 95%CI 52.95 (51.55–54.34). Although the high prevalence areas in rural districts was contributed with large families size (> 5 members) and low annual income of less than 6500$/year.

Table 3 Analysis of demographic characteristics associated with HCV infection in the Libyan population2007–2016

Variables	HCV infection n (%)	Z-test	95% CI	*P* value
Gender				
Male	49,419 (43)	31.23	42.56–43.44	< 0.001
Female	65,509 (57)	35.833	56.62–57.38	0.001
Age (years)				
< 24	13,791 (12)	35.26	11.46–12.55	0.001
25–35	31,031 (27)	8.136	26.51–27.50	0.001
36–49	33,329 (29)	16.818	26.51–29.49	< 0.001
> 50	36,777 (32)	30.916	31.52–32.48	0.001
Marital status				
Below age	11,493 (10)	26.801	9.46–10.56	0.001
Married	44,822 (39)	100.536	35.55–39.45	0.001
Single	32,180 (28)	35.878	27.51–28.49	< 0.001
Divorced	10,344 (9)	27.969	8.46–9.57	0.001
Unknown	16,090 (14)	19.027	13.47–14.55	0.001
Education				
Illiterate	42,523 (37)	87.64	35.54–37.46	0.001
Primary	28,732 (25)	21.188	24.5–25.00	0.001
Secondary	20,687 (18)	18.62	21.7–24.91	< 0.001
Tertiary	6896 (6)	29.065	5.45–6.59	0.001
Unknown	16,090 (14)	19.027	13.47–14.55	0.001
Place of residence				
Urban	70,106 (61)	58.251	60.64–61.36	< 0.001
Rural	44,822(39)	46.577	38.55–39.45	0.001
Population density				
Low	54,016(47)	13.907	46.58–47.42	0.001
High	60,912(53)	4.398	51.55–54.34	< 0.001

Discussion

Medical geospatial analysis has become an important tool for making accurate estimates of the trends in HCV infection epidemics. The number of sero-epidemiological studies of HCV has been increasing, but spatiotemporal studies to detect geographical clusters of the disease are few, particularly in African countries [24]. This study used this technique to analyze the spatiotemporal variation of HCV infection in Libya from 2007 to 2016. The distribution of HCV infections in Libya varied geographically from one region to another and between districts in the same region. The highest prevalence of cases was reported in Sebha, Wadi al Shati, Ghat and Murzuq in the southern region, followed by Benghazi and Butnan in the eastern region, and then Tripoli, Nalut and Jabal al Gharbi in in the western region. A previous national surveillance study has also shown that the sero-prevalence of HCV in Libya varied from 1.2 to 2.2%. The highest prevalence was reported in Sebha (Fezzan) close to sub-Saharan African countries, as well as in Butnan, bordering Egypt [9]. Our results correspond with the findings of a spatial analysis of HCV in China and the Republic of Korea [25, 26], which showed the emergence of an HCV infection epidemic in these countries concentrated in certain provinces and cities. Therefore, HCV prevalence varies not only between countries but also on smaller geographic scales within the same country.

Demographic factors have been found to influence the distribution of HCV infection worldwide. A recent study carried out in Tripoli has shown that the prevalence of HCV, HBV and HIV was associated with intravenous drug use, promiscuity, unemployment, large families and low incomes [27]. Our study is in agreement with this observation: HCV infection rate was higher in the western districts, including Nalut and Jabal al Gharbi, which had large families with poor economic conditions. Further studies are needed to clarify associations with other determinants, including unemployment and drug use.

Butnan and Benghazi in the northeast of Libya had concentrations of HCV cases because they are closer to the Egyptian borders. This is also evident in Murzuq, Wadi al Shati, Sebha and Ghat, which border the sub-Saharan countries of Chad and Niger and have large concentrations of African immigrants. Egypt is the most heavily populated North African nation and has the highest prevalence of HCV in the world. It acts as a main source of labor for the region. Before the 2011 uprising in Libya, there are about two million Egyptians working in Libya, but now there are only about half a million [28]. The prevalence of HCV among these Egyptians reached up to 19% [11]. A recent study carried out in sub-Saharan countries showed that people in that region can move easily around the continent, particularly after the introduction of new regulations by the African Union. Nowadays, there is a massive population exodus from these regions and into Libya, as migrants seek work locally or strive for an expected better life in Europe. Further studies are needed to shed light on the integration and inter-location of HCV infection within neighboring countries of North and sub-Saharan Africa.

These demographic and socio-economic determinants could be used in planning and prevention strategies. Districts where these determinants could point to higher HCV prevalence could be targeted for screening and intervention policies. Similar spatial analyses were carried out in other African countries, such as Malawi, were it was found to be valuable in improving access to healthcare services for HIV and tuberculosis patients [29, 30].

Spatial analysis indicated that hotspots and cold spots existed and were unevenly distributed all over the country. The elevated HCV clusters were located in Benghazi, Butnan, Sebha, Nalut, Jabal al Gharbi, Wadi al Shati, and Ghat. They accounted for over 63% of the identified HCV infection cases during the study period.

In contrast to the changing status of the hotspots and the cold-spots, they were confined to Murqub, Al Wahat and Jufra during the study period. Due to drug-trafficking, the eastern districts bordering Egypt, the western districts bordering Tunisia and Algeria, and the southern districts bordering sub-Saharan countries are considered endemic as a result of HCV. However, drug trafficking poses specific problems for North African countries, and it is exacerbated by the geographical location and the vast area of the region. Morocco is the world's foremost producer of cannabis resin and remains the main source of the drug for the consumer markets in North Africa and Europe. Studies carried out in North America by Oliveira-Filho et al. have shown that non-injecting drug users have a high HCV infection rate, particularly those who use cannabis and cocaine paste. Hence, this may have an impact on HCV infection in these countries. Further studies are needed to highlight the integration of HCV within North and sub-Saharan countries [31–34]".

Similar results of local clustering of HCV and other associated infections such as HIV have been reported in South Africa and Italy [35, 36]. Our detection of HCV clusters could be used by healthcare planners in Libya to plan screening and treatment policies. However, it should be noted that not all HCV cases were detected in these clusters. The other cases showed a more random distribution over the whole country. Hence, policies are needed on a national level to cover all the regions and districts [37].

The large sample size and the analysis of geographical distribution and hotspots and cold-spots of the HCV epidemic could be considered important strengths of this study. Uniquely, it goes beyond clustering analysis to map the spatiotemporal variation of HCV risk driven by population-based determinants. It identifies the areas at high risk of HCV infections and thus its consequent complications where public health measures for prevention and treatment could be applied. A modeling system has recently been constructed to predict the prevalence of HCV among risk groups, such as blood donors, in order to propose a preventive strategy in Libya [38]. However, further analysis performed randomly may be needed [5, 39].

Limitations

Though this study makes an important contribution to advancing the spatiotemporal analysis of HCV infections in Libya, the African continent and developing countries in general, it has some limitations that might have affected the results.

1. Like other studies based on case records and using spatial analysis, some districts may under-report HCV infection cases. Hence, further studies are needed, particularly in the regions of high prevalence of HCV infection.
2. Data collection was based on certain surveillance studies and preserving the confidentiality of the individuals was important. Therefore, it is not always easy to give an accurate timing of HCV infection cases and the precise geographical locations of the patients.
3. Other determinants that were not included in this study may also explain inequalities in HCV infections, such as environmental, social and cultural factors, and access to health care facilities and HCV testing.

4. Data analysis did not take into account the movement of individuals from one region to another within the country, the impact of the variability and the extent of exposure to risk determinants, and the time lag between exposure and detection of HIV infection.

Conclusion

To the best of our knowledge, this is the first study in North Africa and Arab countries to describe the epidemiological characteristics of HCV infection using geospatial analysis at the country level. We used geospatial analysis to determine geographic and spatiotemporal trends of HCV infection in Libya and highlighted the associated population-based determinants. The results show a distinct variation in the prevalence of HCV infection at regional and district levels in Libya during 2007–2016. This indicates that intervention strategies for HCV prevention should take into account both individual and geographic-area variation. A homogenous national policy may not be effective due to inequalities in HCV prevalence. Understanding the impact of region and district on HCV infection can ensure that intervention is effective in areas with higher infection rates [40, 41]. HCV infections are particularly more prevalent in the southern and eastern districts, but this could have been due to the increasing number of African immigrants in these regions. Hence, further studies are needed at the regional level within North and sub-Saharan countries bordering Libya, particularly Egypt, Sudan, Chad and Niger to shed light on the population-related determinants that may play a role in the upsurge of HCV and other concomitant infections in North Africa [42, 43].

Abbreviations

HCV: hepatitis C virus; HPA: High prevalence areas; LPA: Low prevalence areas; MI: Moran's Index; RR: adjusted relative risk; SD: standard deviation

Acknowledgements

We are deeply grateful to the Libyan Study Group of Hepatitis & HIV, the Department of Medical Microbiology, Faculty of Medicine and the Department of Infectious Diseases, Tripoli Medical Centre, for their help and support.

Funding

No funding was received for this study.

Authors' contributions

MD conceived and designed the study. MD and LA contributed to the analysis tools,. MD and AMD designed the analysis, analyzed the data, and performed cartography. MD wrote the paper. AE and NS; made substantial contributions to conception and design, or acquisition of data, or analysis and interpretation of data MD, MA, and AD provided advice and critically reviewed the manuscript. All authors read and approved the final manuscript.

Consent for publication

Not applicable.

Competing interests

The authors declare that they have no competing interests.

Author details

[1]Department of Medical Microbiology &Immunology, Faculty of Medicine, University of Tripoli, CC 82668 Tripoli, Libya. [2]Department of Infectious Disease, Tripoli Medical Centre, Tripoli, CC 82668 Tripoli, Libya. [3]Department of General Medicine, Faculty of Medicine, University of Tripoli, CC 82668 Tripoli, Libya. [4]Department of Surgery, Tripoli Medical Centre, Faculty of Medicine, University of Tripoli, CC 82668 Tripoli, Libya. [5]Department of Toxicology, Faculty of Medical Technology, AlgabalAl-garbi University, Nalut, Libya. [6]Department of Laboratory Medicine, Faculty of Biotechnology, Tripoli University, CC 82668 Tripoli, Libya.

References

1. Petruzziello A, Marigliano S, Loquercio G, Cozzolino A, Cacciapuoti C. Global epidemiology of hepatitis C virus infection: an up-date of the distribution and circulation of hepatitis C virus genotypes. World J Gastroenterol. 2016; 22(34):7824–40.
2. Mohd Hanafiah K, Groeger J, Flaxman AD, Wiersma ST. Global epidemiology of hepatitis C virus infection: new estimates of age-specific antibody to HCV seroprevalence. Hepatology. 2013;57(4):1333–42.
3. Daw MA, El-Bouzedi A, Ahmed MO, et al. Geographic integration of hepatitis C virus: a global threat. WorldJVirol. 2016;12:170–82. https://doi.org/10.5501/wjv.v5.i4.170 PMID: 27878104.
4. Deuffic-Burban S, Mohamed MK, Larouze B, et al. Expected increase in hepatitis C-related mortality in Egypt due to pre-2000 infections. J Hepatol. 2006;44:455–61 [PMID: 16310281. https://doi.org/10.1016/j.jhep.2005.08.008.
5. Daw MA, El-Bouzedi A, Ahmed MO, et al. Hepatitis C virus in North Africa: an emerging threat. Sci World J. 2016;2016:11. https://doi.org/10.1155/2016/7370524 Article ID 7370524. PMID: 27610403.
6. Daw MA, El-Bouzedi A, Ahmed MO, et al. Epidemiology of hepatitis C virus and genotype distribution in immigrants crossing to Europe from North and Sub-Saharan Africa. Travel Med Infect Dis. 2016;15. https://doi.org/10.1016/j.tmaid.2016.05.020 PMID: 2C7502972.
7. Kalipeni E, Zulu L. HIV and AIDS in Africa: a geographic analysis at multiple spatial scales. GeoJournal. 2012;77:505–23.
8. Messina JP, Emch M, Muwonga J, Mwandagalirwa K, Edidi SB, Mama N, Okenge A, Meshnick SR. Spatial and socio-behavioral patterns of HIV prevalence in the Democratic Republic of Congo. Soc Sci Med; 2010,71(8): 1428–35.
9. Daw MA, El-Bouzedi A. Prevalence of hepatitis B and hepatitis C infection in Libya: results from a national population based survey. BMC Infect Dis 2014; 14:17. [https://doi.org/10.1186/1471-2334-14-17, PMID: 24405790].
10. Daw MA, Elkaber MA, Drah AM, et al. Prevalence of hepatitis C virus antibodies among different populations of relative and attributable risk. Saudi Med J. 2002;23:1356–60 [PMID: 12506296].
11. Daw MA, El-Bouzedi A, Ahmed MO etal., Epidemiology of hepatitis C virus and genotype distribution in immigrants crossing to Europe from North and Sub-Saharan Africa. Travel Med Infect Dis 2016;15. https://doi.org/10.1016/j.tmaid.2016.05.020. PMID: 2C7502972.
12. Daw MA, El-Bouzedi A, Dau AA. Geographic distribution of HCV genotypes in Libya and analysis of risk factors involved in their transmission. BMC Res Notes. 2015;8:367 [PMID: 26293137. https://doi.org/10.1186/s13104-015-1310-x.
13. Organization WH (2014) Guidelines for the screening, care and treatment of persons with hepatitis C infection.
14. OnyekwereC A, Hameed L. Hepatitis B and C virus prevalence and association with demographics: report of population screening in Nigeria. Trop Dr. 2015;45:231–5.
15. Daw MA, Dau AA. Hepatitis C virus in Arab world: a state of concern. SciWorldJ. 2012;2012. https://doi.org/10.1100/2012/719494 PMID:22629189.
16. Daw MA, El-Bouzedi A. Viral haemorrhagic fever in North Africa; an evolving emergency. J ClinExpPathol. 2015;5:2161–0681.
17. Kauhl B, Heil J, Hoebe CJ, Schweikart J, Krafft T, Dukers-Muijrers NH. The spatial distribution of hepatitis C virus infections andAssociated determinants--an application of a geographically weighted Poisson

regression for evidence-based screening interventions in hotspots. PLoS One. 2015;10:e0135656. https://doi.org/10.1371/journal.pone.0135656. PMID: 26352611.
18. Wang L, Xing J, Chen F, Yan R, Ge L, Qin Q, Wang L, Ding Z, Guo W, Wang N. Spatial analysis on hepatitis C virus infection in mainland China: from 2005 to 2011. PLoS One. 2014;9(10):e110861.
19. Pandey V, Bharaj TS, Hans U. Improving Healthcare Management System using Efficient Geo-Spatial Data Analysis–An Approach using QGIS. 2015
20. Cromley EK, McLafferty SL. GIS and public health. New York: Guilford Press; 2011.
21. Meyers DJ, Hood ME, Stopka TJ. HIV and hepatitis C mortality in Massachusetts, 2002–2011: spatial cluster and trend analysis of HIV and HCV using multiple cause of death. PLoS One. 2014;9(12):e114822.
22. Moran PA. Notes on continuous stochastic phenomena. Biometrika. 1950;37: 17–23. PMID: 15420245.
23. Anselin L. Exploring Spatial Data with GeoDaTM: A Workbook. Urbana: Spatial Analysis Laboratory, Department of Geography, University of Illinois at Urbana-Champaign; 2005.
24. Zehender G, Ebranati E, Gabanelli E, et al. Spatial and temporal dynamics of hepatitis B virus D genotype in Europe and the Mediterranean Basin. PLoS One. 2012;7(5):e37198.
25. Wu SQ, Wu FQ, Hong RT, He J. Incidence analyses and space-timecluster detection of hepatitis C in Fujian province of China from 2006 to 2010. PLoS One. 2012;7:e40872.
26. Kwon GY, Lee H, Gwack J, Lee SW, Ki M, Youn SK. Regional distribution of hepatitis C virus infection in the Republic of Korea, 2007-2011. Gut Liver. 2014;8:428–32.
27. Daw MA, Shabash A, El-Bouzedi A, Aghnya A. Dau in association with the Libyan study group of hepatitis &HIV.Seroprevalence of HBV, HCV & HIV co-infection and risk factors analysis in Tripoli-Libya. PLoS One. 2014;9(6): e98793. https://doi.org/10.1371/journal.pone.009879. PMID: 24936655. https://doi.org/10.1371/journal.pone.0098793.
28. The Guardian- Guardian Africa network, 2015.Why Egyptians are risking their lives to work in Libya. https://www.theguardian.com/world/2015/feb/20/egyptians-risk-lives-work-libya. Accessed on 17 Apr 2017.
29. Zulu LC, Kalipeni E, Johannes E. Analyzing spatial clustering and the spatiotemporal nature and trends of HIV/AIDS prevalence using GIS: the case of Malawi, 1994-2010. BMC Infect Dis 2014; 23:14(1):1.
30. Kharsany A, Karim QA. HIV infection and AIDS in sub-Saharan Africa: current status, challenges and opportunities. Open AIDS J. 2016;10(1).
31. Ismail SM, Eisa AA, Ibrahim F. HIV-infected people in Sudan moving toward chronic poverty: possible interventions. J Assoc Nurses AIDS Care. 2016;27(1):30–43.
32. Oliveira-Filho AB, Sawada L, Pinto LC, Locks D, Bahia SL, Castro JA, Hermes RB, Brasil-Costa I, Amaral CM, Lemos JAR. Epidemiological aspects of HCV infection in non-injecting drug users in the Brazilian state of Pará, eastern Amazon. Virol J. 2014;11(1):38.
33. Cook C, and Kanaef N The Global State of Harm Reduction 2008: Mapping the response to drug-related HIV and hepatitis C epidemics. London: International Harm Reduction Association; 2008.
34. Nelson PK, Mathers BM, Cowie B, et al. Global epidemiology of hepatitis B and hepatitis C in people who inject drugs: results of systematic reviews. Lancet. 2011;378(9791):571–83.
35. Tanser F, Barnighausen T, Cooke GS, Newell ML. Localized spatial clustering of HIV infections in a widely disseminated rural South African epidemic. Int J Epidemiol. 2009;38:1008–16. https://doi.org/10.1093/ije/dyp148. PMID: 19261659.
36. Bush KR, Henderson EA, Dunn J, Read RR, Singh A. Mapping the core: chlamydia and gonorrhea infections in Calgary, Alberta. Sex Transm Dis. 2008;35:291–7. https://doi.org/10.1097/OLQ.0b013e31815c1edb. PMID: 18490871.
37. Kirby RS, Delmelle E, Eberth JM. Advances in spatial epidemiology and geographic information systems. Ann Epidemiol. 2016,27(1):1–9.
38. Daw MA, Shabash A, El-Bouzedi A, Dau AA, Habas M. Modelling the prevalence of hepatitis C virus amongst blood donors in Libya: an investigation of providing a preventive strategy. World J Virol. 2016;5:14–22 [PMID: 26870670. https://doi.org/10.5501/wjv.v5.i1.14.
39. Kauhl B, Heil J, Hoebe CJ, Schweikart J, Krafft T, Dukers-Muijrers NH. The spatial distribution of hepatitis C virus infections and associated determinants—an application of a geographically weighted poisson regression for evidence-based screening interventions in hotspots. PLoS One. 2015;10(9):e0135656.
40. Edwards DJ, Coppens DG, Prasad TL, Rook LA, Iyer JK. Access to hepatitis C medicines. Bull World Health Organ. 2015;93(11):799–805.
41. Sifaki-Pistolla D, Karageorgos SA, Koulentaki M, Samonakis D, Stratakou S, Digenakis E, Kouroumalis E. Geoepidemiology of hepatocellular carcinoma in the island of Crete, Greece. A possible role of pesticides. Liver International. 2015. PMID: 26610175. https://doi.org/10.1111/liv.13034.
42. Gökengin D, Doroudi F, Tohme J, Collins B, Madani N. HIV/AIDS: trends in the Middle East and North Africa region. Int J Infect Dis. 2016;44:66–73.
43. Daw MA, Daw AM, Sifennasr NE, Draha AM, Daw AM, Daw AM, Ahmed MO, Mokhtar ES, El-Bouzedi A, Daw IM. The Epidemiology of Hepatitis D Virus in North Africa: A Systematic Review and Meta-Analysis. ScientificWorldJournal. 2018;2018:1–11.

Early sofosbuvir-ledipasvir treatment for acute HCV infection induced severe immune thrombocytopenia

Vincent Alcazer[1,2*], Patrick Miailhes[3], Christophe Ramière[2,4,5], Caroline Charre[2,4,5] and Laurent Cotte[3]

Abstract

Background: Hepatitis C virus (HCV) infection is a recognised cause of secondary immune thrombocytopenia (ITP). While its incidence has been largely described during chronic HCV infection, only one case of ITP secondary to acute HCV infection has been reported at this time.

Case presentation: We report herein the case of severe ITP secondary to an acute HCV genotype 1a reinfection in a human immunodeficiency virus (HIV)-negative man having sex with men who had been cured several years before of a previous acute genotype 4d HCV infection. After an unsuccessful standard therapy with two courses of intravenous immunoglobulin (at 1 g/kg daily for 2 days) associated with methylprednisolone 1 mg/kg daily, antiviral treatment with sofosbuvir-ledipasvir rapidly achieved virological response and normalised the platelet count.

Conclusions: As a direct effect of HCV on megakaryocytes could be the predominant cause of ITP during acute infection, early antiviral treatment may be beneficial in this case.

Keywords: Hepatitis C virus, Sofosbuvir-ledipasvir, Acute immune thrombocytopenia

Background

Immune thrombocytopenia (ITP) is an acquired thrombocytopenia caused by immune platelet destruction. Most adults (80%) present a primary ITP in which different mechanisms contribute to a reduced platelet lifespan, involving mostly antibody- or T cell-mediated platelet destruction and impaired megakaryocytopoiesis [1]. Secondary ITP pathogenesis is slightly different and relates to underlying disorders among which infections, auto-immune diseases, and lymphoproliferative disorders are the leading causes [2].

Hepatitis C virus (HCV) infection is a recognised cause of secondary ITP [3]. Its occurrence has been well described in the case of chronic infection where the diagnosis can be difficult as different factors can contribute to thrombocytopenia including cross-reactive antibodies directed against platelet antigens, bone-marrow viral infection of progenitor cells, decreased production of thrombopoietin and splenic sequestration secondary to portal hypertension [2]. However, few cases of ITP secondary to acute hepatitis C virus (HCV) infection have been reported to date.

Herein we report the case of a patient with severe secondary ITP during an acute HCV genotype 1a reinfection. Early treatment with sofosbuvir-ledipasvir allowed the prompt recovery of thrombocytopenia.

Case presentation

In July 2017, a 54-year-old male was hospitalised for the recent appearance of multiple purpuric spots on the legs associated with gum bleeding. The patient was an HIV-negative man having sex with men, receiving HIV pre-exposure prophylaxis with tenofovir/emtricitabine for over a year. His medical history was significant for a primary syphilis in 2014 and multiple episodes of urethritis in the recent years. He reported frequent unprotected anal sex, with occasional bleeding, insertive and receiving fisting without gloves, and the use of nasal mephedrone during sexual encounters. He was previously diagnosed with an

* Correspondence: vincent.alcazer@chu-lyon.fr
[1]Département d'hématologie clinique, Hospices Civils de Lyon, Centre Hospitalier Lyon Sud, 69495 Pierre-Bénite, France
[2]Inserm U1052, Centre de Recherche en Cancérologie de Lyon, 69008 Lyon, France
Full list of author information is available at the end of the article

acute genotype 4 HCV infection in 2011 (Versant HCV genotype 2.0 assay (LiPA), Siemens Healthineers, Erlangen, Germany), cured following a 6-month course of pegylated interferon (IFN) and ribavirin. Acute genotype 1a HCV reinfection was diagnosed on 2017, June 26th (NS5A Sanger sequencing), while HCV-RNA was still negative on 2017, April 4th (Abbott RealTime HCV, Abbott, Molecular, Des Plaines, USA). The patient was asymptomatic at that time, platelet count was normal and HCV-RNA surveillance was scheduled, following the recommendations from the European AIDS clinical society [4].

Initial physical examination found no other symptoms apart from a petechial purpura of the lower extremities and oral haemorrhagic blister. Blood pressure was 130/97 mmHg, heart rate 60 bpm with no fever, lymphadenopathy, or splenomegaly. There was no evidence of severe haemorrhage. Laboratory data at the admission are resumed in Table 1. Complete blood count found a severe thrombocytopenia (5 G/L) without any other cytopenia. Thrombocytopenia was confirmed on the peripheral blood smear which exhibited no morphological abnormalities and the absence of schistocytes. No other associated haemostasis abnormality was present (normal fibrinogen and factor V). Serum protein electrophoresis found no clonal gammopathy. Thyroid-stimulating hormone was normal. HIV serology was repeatedly negative and Hepatits B surface antibodies were detectable following a previous vaccination. At that time, mild elevation in aspartate transaminase (AST, 6 times the upper limit of normal (ULN)) and alanine transaminase (ALT, 7 x ULN) was found associated with a detectable HCV viral load of 4.9 log IU/mL (Fig. 1). There was no evidence of other replicating viruses including cytomegalovirus, parvovirus B19, human herpes virus type 6 and type 8 (except a slight Epstein-Barr virus replication which was considered insignificant (348 UI/mL). Cryoglobulin investigation was negative. No circulating anti-platelet IgG antibodies were detected. A bone marrow aspiration was performed; normal cellularity with an increased number of megakaryocytes and normal erythropoiesis and myelopoiesis was found, thus confirming the diagnosis of ITP secondary to acute HCV infection.

An initial administration of intravenous immunoglobulin (IVIG; at the dose of 1 g/kg on day 1 and day 3) had clinical benefit (regression of gum bleeding and purpura), but did not have any effect on the platelet count which remained below 10G/L. A second administration of IVIG (1 g/kg daily for 2 days) combined with methylprednisolone (1 mg/kg daily) improved platelet count which reached 40G/L but a normal value was not attained (Fig. 1). At which point it was decided after collegial discussion to start treating the infectious trigger. Pegylated IFN and ribavirin combination was contra-indicated because of severe thrombocytopenia,

Table 1 Laboratory data at the admission

Parameter	Baseline value	Normal value (range)
Complete blood count		
Leucocytes	5.69 G/L	4.00–10.00
Haemoglobin	149 g/L	130–170
MCV	95.0 fL	80–100
Platelet	< 10 G/L	150–400
Schistocytes	< 1%	< 1%
Neutrophils	3.27 G/L	1.8–7.5
Eosinophils	0.19 G/L	0.02–0.8
Lymphocytes	1.65 G/L	1–4
Monocytes	0.52 G/L	0.2–0.9
Haemostasis	Normal PT and aPTT	
Fibrinogen	2.23 g/L	2.13–4.22
Factor V	> 150%	61–142
Blood chemistry		
Creatinine	86 µmol/L	59–104
eGFR	87.8 mL/min/1.73 m^2	90.0–120.0
AST	202 IU/L	15–37
ALT	483 IU/L	16–61
Alkaline phosphatase	101 IU/L	50–136
GGT	292 IU/L	15–85
Total bilirubin	13 µmol/L	3–17
Conjugated bilirubin	4 µmol/L	0–3
Lacticodehydrogenase	254 IU/L	87–241
Serum protein electrophoresis	Normal	
Cryoglobulin	Negative	
Myelogram	Normal cellularity	
Serology		
Syphilis	Negative	
HIV	Negative	
HBV	Positive for Hbs Ab	
CMV	Positive for IgG	
EBV	Positive for IgG	
Blood / plasma viral load		
HCV RNA	82,004 IU/mL	< 12
CMV DNA	0 IU/mL	150–500
EBV DNA	348 IU/mL	182–500
HIV RNA	< 40 copies/mL	< 40
Parvovirus B19 DNA	0 copies/mL	70–87
HHV6 DNA	0 copies/mL	
HHV8 DNA	0 copies/mL	500–2000

GGT Gamma Glutamine Transferase, *PT Prothrombine time, aPTT Activated Partial Thromboplastin Time*

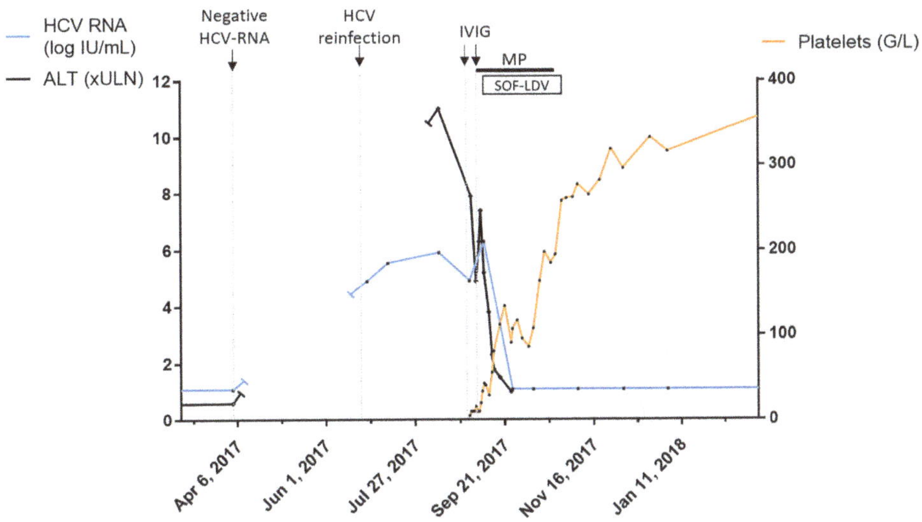

Fig. 1 Platelet and HCV viral load. Acute genotype 1a HCV reinfection was diagnosed on August 2017 on a systematic survey, with 11 xULN ALT and 5.91 log IU/mL HCV RNA. Platelets were found at 5 G/L for the unit admission on August 30, 2017. First course of IVIG was administrated on August 31, at the dose of 1 g/kg on day 1 and day 3, with clinical benefit but no effect on the platelet count. Second IVIG course was administrated on September 05 in association with methylprednisolone 1 mg/kg daily. Sofosbuvir-ledipasvir was started on September 11, allowing a sustained recovery of the platelet count with a quick viral load control (basal blue line represents an undetectable HCV viral load, inferior to 12 IU/mL). IVIG: intravenous immunoglobulin, MP: methylprednisolone, SOF-LDV: sofusbuvir-ledispavir, ALT: Alanine transaminase, HCV: Hepatitis C virus

therefore a 12 weeks course of sofosbuvir-ledipasvir was indicated. At initiation of the treatment, the platelet count was 43 G/L and HCV viral load was 6.3 log IU/mL. At day 15 of antiviral treatment, HCV viral load was undetectable (< 12 IU/ml) and the platelet count had increased to 108 G/L allowing rapid tapering and discontinuation of corticosteroids before the end of antiviral therapy. HCV viral load remained undetectable until week 12 post-treatment, confirming HCV cure (Fig. 1). Platelet count fully normalised 5 weeks following treatment initiation and remained within normal range thereafter. The patient went through his 12 weeks course of sofosbuvir-ledipasvir with a good tolerance, without any specific adverse event reported.

Discussion and conclusions

Chronic HCV infection has been associated with immune thrombocytopenia; the incidence is estimated to be 30.2–53 cases / 100,000 person-years [5, 6]. Conversely, HCV antibodies have been found in 10 to 36% of patients with chronic ITP in cross-sectional studies [5, 6]. However, our case is a rare report of ITP in the context of acute hepatitis C. Only one similar case has already been reported by Narita et al. in 2003 [7]. According to this report, ITP also occurred at the second HCV infection after a first HCV infection cured by 6 months of IFN-α2b. HCV genotype was found to be 2a in this reinfection case, versus 2b for the first one. In contrary to our findings, platelet associated immunoglobulins (PAIgG) were found positive in this report, with no other circulating antibodies (anti-nuclear antibody and rheumatoid factor were negative). Additionally, platelet count increased up to 39,000 /μL spontaneously and the PAIgG returned to the normal ratio without any specific therapy while in our case, platelet count only recovered after specific antiviral therapy. Considering these differences, a distinct physiopathological mechanism may have been the source of ITP in these two cases.

Thrombocytopenia is frequent in viral infection. In such situations, a complex crosstalk between platelet and the virus is engaged and different mechanisms may contribute to two major events [8]: first, a decreased platelet production which can be induced by direct infection of megakaryocytes, infection of haematopoietic stem cells, induction of a type-1 IFN response leading to suppression of platelet formation, or modulation of liver thrombopoietin production; second, an increased platelet destruction, either by a direct contact during viraemia, interaction with immune complexes, cross-reactive antibodies directed against the virus, or proinflammatory events induced by the infection [8].

The exact mechanism of HCV-induced ITP is still not clear. Extra-hepatic manifestations are common in HCV-infected patients, most of which are immune-related manifestations including mixed cryoglobulinaemia, arthralgia/myalgia, and auto-antibody production [9]. Importantly, the presence of only anti-platelet antibodies is not associated with thrombocytopenia [10]. This leads to consider the potential role of immune complexes promoted by the presence of cross-reactive antibodies or a compensating mechanism following a decrease in thrombopoietin production [10]. A direct effect of the virus on megacaryocytes may also be suspected as HCV can bind to CD81 on the platelet membrane, and HCV-RNA has also been detected in washed platelets of infected patients [11]. Platelets could thus either favour the spread of the virus or contribute to its immune recognition by providing targetable antigens [10]. Moreover, detection of HCV-RNA with a higher frequency in platelets of thrombocytopenic patients suggest that HCV is directly involved in this process [12]. At this time, there is no evidence for a particular association between specific HCV genotypes and incidence of ITP [12].

The treatment of HCV-related ITP, particularly in the case of acute infection, is not standardized. Dufour et al. reported the outcome of 8 patients with HCV-related ITP [13]. Patients had a poor response to initial corticosteroids therapy, with only one complete response and three partial response. IVIG led to transient efficacy in three other patients. Of eight patients treated by antiviral therapy associating IFN-α with ribavirin, five responded. Normalisation of platelet count occurred in three responders, and normalisation of viral load was usually slow. Other authors have reported the increase of platelet count associated with complete HCV eradication after IFN therapy [14, 15]. However, kinetic of platelet recovery was usually low in these cases.

Herein, we describe the case of a severe ITP associated with acute HCV reinfection. IVIG was chosen as the first-line therapy, owing to their efficacy in primary ITP and secondary ITP related to chronic HCV infection [6]. The absence of effect on the platelet count led to a second course of IVIG and administration of methylprednisolone, which improved only slightly the thombocytopenia. Sofosbuvir-ledipasvir treatment was then initiated which rapidly decreased viral load to under the limit of detection and normalised the platelet count. Interestingly, no drop back of platelet following corticosteroid discontinuation was observed. The acute installation of the thrombocytopenia, its refractoriness to the first-line immunomodulatory and immunosuppressive therapy, the rapid improvement following antiviral treatment and the absence of circulating anti-platelet antibodies suggest a predominant effect of direct viral-mediated platelet destruction in this context where the other adaptive mechanisms might not had the time to develop. Notably, the first HCV infection in the patient presented herein did not trigger any thrombocytopenia. There is currently no data on the risk on ITP following HCV reinfection and we can only speculate on the relation between the first infection and the ITP case.

In summary, we report herein the case of a secondary ITP associated with an acute genotype 1a HCV reinfection in a 54-year-old patient. Early treatment with sofosbuvir-ledispavir was followed by a rapid virological response and a sustained platelet count recovery, suggesting a viral-mediated platelet destruction corrected by the antiviral therapy.

Abbreviations

HCV: Hepatitis C Virus; ITP: Immune thrombocytopenia; IVIG: Intravenous Immunoglobulin

Acknowledgements

Not applicable

Funding

This manuscript did not benefit from any funding.

Authors' contributions

VA, PM, CR, CC, and LC analysed and interpreted the patient data. VA wrote the final manuscript. PM and LC reviewed and gave correction on the final version. All authors read and approved the final manuscript.

Consent for publication

Written consent for publication was obtained from the patient.

Competing interests

The authors declare that they have no competing interests.

Author details

[1]Département d'hématologie clinique, Hospices Civils de Lyon, Centre Hospitalier Lyon Sud, 69495 Pierre-Bénite, France. [2]Inserm U1052, Centre de Recherche en Cancérologie de Lyon, 69008 Lyon, France. [3]Service des maladies infectieuses et tropicales, Hospices Civils de Lyon, Hôpital de la Croix Rousse, 69004 Lyon, France. [4]Laboratoire de virologie, Hospices civils de Lyon, Hôpital de la Croix Rousse, 69004 Lyon, France. [5]INSERM U1111, Centre International de Recherche en Infectiologie, Lyon, France.

References

1. Lambert MP, Gernsheimer TB. Clinical updates in adult immune thrombocytopenia. Blood. 2017;129(21):2829–35.
2. Cines DB, Liebman H, Stasi R. Pathobiology of secondary immune thrombocytopenia. Semin Hematol. 2009;46(1 Suppl 2):S2–14.
3. Chiao EY, Engels EA, Kramer JR, Pietz K, Henderson L, Giordano TP, et al. Risk of immune thrombocytopenic purpura and autoimmune hemolytic anemia among 120 908 US veterans with hepatitis C virus infection. Arch Intern Med. 2009;169(4):357–63.
4. Ryom L, Boesecke C, Gisler V, Manzardo C, Rockstroh JK, Puoti M, et al. Essentials from the 2015 European AIDS clinical society (EACS) guidelines for the treatment of adult HIV-positive persons. HIV Med. 2016;17(2):83–8.
5. Pawlotsky JM, Bouvier M, Fromont P, Deforges L, Duval J, Dhumeaux D, et al. Hepatitis C virus infection and autoimmune thrombocytopenic purpura. J Hepatol. 1995;23(6):635–9.
6. Dimitroulis D, Valsami S, Stamopoulos P, Kouraklis G. Immunological HCV-Associated Thrombocytopenia: Short Review. Clin Dev Immunol. 2012;2012 Available from: https://www.ncbi.nlm.nih.gov/pmc/articles/PMC3400398/. [cited 2018 Apr 24].
7. Narita R, Asaumi H, Abe S, Nakamura H, Tabaru A, Yoshikawa I, et al. Idiopathic thrombocytopenic purpura with acute hepatitis c viral infection. J Gastroenterol Hepatol. 2003;18(4):462–3.

8. Assinger A. Platelets and Infection – An Emerging Role of Platelets in Viral Infection. Front Immunol. 2014;5 Available from: https://www.frontiersin.org/articles/10.3389/fimmu.2014.00649/full. [cited 2018 Jan 24].
9. Cacoub P, Comarmond C, Domont F, Savey L, Desbois AC, Saadoun D. Extrahepatic manifestations of chronic hepatitis C virus infection. Ther Adv Infect Dis. 2016;3(1):3–14.
10. Panzer S, Seel E, Brunner M, Körmöczi GF, Schmid M, Ferenci P, et al. Platelet autoantibodies are common in hepatitis C infection, irrespective of the presence of thrombocytopenia. Eur J Haematol. 2006;77(6):513–7.
11. Hamaia S, Li C, Allain JP. The dynamics of hepatitis C virus binding to platelets and 2 mononuclear cell lines. Blood. 2001;98(8):2293–300.
12. de Almeida AJ, Campos-de-Magalhães M, de Melo Marçal OP, Brandão-Mello CE, Okawa MY, de Oliveira RV, et al. Hepatitis C virus-associated thrombocytopenia: a controlled prospective, virological study. Ann Hematol. 2004;83(7):434–40.
13. Dufour J-F, Pradat P, Ruivard M, Hot A, Dumontet C, Broussolle C, et al. Severe autoimmune cytopenias in treatment-naive hepatitis C virus infection: clinical description of 16 cases. Eur J Gastroenterol Hepatol. 2009; 21(3):245.
14. Karasawa T, Togashi H, Tajima K, Suzuki A, Onodera S, Haga H, et al. Case of chronic type C hepatitis complicated with idiopathic thrombocytopenic purpura that was successfully treated by interferon therapy. Nihon Shokakibyo Gakkai Zasshi Jpn J Gastro-Enterol. 2009;106(3):405–10.
15. d'Alteroche L, Assor P, Lefrou L, Senecal D, Gaudy C, Bacq Y. Severe autoimmune neutropenia and thrombopenia associated with chronic C hepatitis: effect of antiviral therapy. Gastroenterol Clin Biol. 2005;29(3):297–9.

17

Confirmation of HCV viremia using HCV RNA and core antigen testing on dried blood spot in HIV infected peoples who inject drugs in Vietnam

Truong Tam Nguyen[1,2*], Véronique Lemee[3], Karine Bollore[2], Hai Vinh Vu[4], Karine Lacombe[5], Xuan Lien Truong Thi[6], Que Anh Luong[6], Charline Dubos[3], Jean-Christophe Plantier[3], Huong Duong Thi[7], Didier Laureillard[8], Maud Lemoine[9] and Edouard Tuaillon[2]

Abstract

Background: Nucleic acid tests performed on blood samples collected on Dried Blood Spot (DBS) and detection of HCV core antigen (HCVcAg) are two approaches that may facilitate access to HCV diagnosis in low and middle incomes countries. In this study we evaluate HCV RNA and HCV antigen testing on DBS in HIV/HCV co-infected peoples who inject drugs in Vietnam.

Method: One hundred and four HIV/HCV seropositive patients managed in outpatient care at the Haiphong Viet Tiep hospital were included in this study from February to March, 2014 (ANRS 12262 study).

Results: Eighty-six subjects were tested positive for HCV RNA in serum, median (IQR): 6.9 $\log_{10}$ IU/ml (5.6–7.4 $\log_{10}$ IU/ml). Genotypes consisted of 57 G1 (69%), 3 G3 (4%), and 22 G6 (27%). HCV RNA was detected on DBS specimens in 79 out 86 subjects with chronic hepatitis C (sensitivity 92.5%; 95% CI: 85.1–96.9%). HCV RNA level on DBS and serum was moderately correlated ($r = 0.24$; $p = 0.05$) suggesting a degradation of HCV RNA due to transportation and storage conditions. HCVcAg was detected in 75/86 dB specimens (sensitivity: 87.2%; 95% CI: 78.3–93.4%), with a strong positive relationship between DBS HCVcAg and serum HCV RNA levels ($r = 0.80$; $P < 0.0001$).

Conclusions: Quantification of HCVcAg on DBS appears to benefit from substantial stability under prolonged storage conditions but with a lower analytical sensitivity compared to DBS HCV RNA testing. Detection of HCV RNA on DBS is an interesting approach for confirming viral replication in HCV seropositive persons but the impact of pre-analytical conditions on the integrity of HCV RNA needs to be controlled.

Keywords: Hepatitis C virus (HCV), Human immunodeficiency virus (HIV), HCV core antigen, HCV RNA, Vietnam

Background

Decisive breakthrough was recently achieved in hepatitis C virus (HCV) antiviral therapy but the limited access to reliable and low-cost HCV diagnosis tools is a key barrier in the global fight against HCV epidemic [1]. The World health organization (WHO) has recently incorporated HCV elimination in its 2030 agenda and has called for a 90% decrease in HCV incidence and 65% of HCV-related mortality [2]. In order to achieve these objectives, it is critical to simplify HCV testing in particular in high risk populations. However, HCV infection is frequently undiagnosed because the course of the disease is generally asymptomatic until end stage of liver disease. In low- and middle-income settings, where the burden of HCV is high, it is estimated that more than 95% of people are unaware of their HCV status [3, 4]. Screening for HCV infection is currently based on the detection of anti-HCV antibodies (HCVAb) followed by HCV RNA detection to confirm active infection. Rapid diagnosis

* Correspondence: ntruongtam@yahoo.fr
[1]University of Medicine Pham Ngoc Thach, Ho Chi Minh City, Vietnam
[2]Pathogenesis and Control of Chronic Infections, INSERM, Université de Montpellier, CHU Montpellier, Montpellier, France
Full list of author information is available at the end of the article

test format provides a valuable alternative to laboratory tests for the scaling-up of HCV testing [4]. Over the last years whilst simple rapid diagnosis tests for HCVAb detection have been developed with two manufacturers fulfilling requirements for the WHO prequalification [5, 6], access to molecular assays is still limited in resource-limited countries. Poor laboratory capacities and logistical difficulties represent key barriers for the scaling testing and the treatment, particularly in rural areas and difficult to reach populations.

Serological methods assessing HCV core antigen (HCVcAg) can be surrogate assays to nucleic acid tests for detection of HCV viremia. HCVcAg detection can be less costly than PCR and may have a clinical utility in low and middle income countries [7]. Conditional recommendation has recently been published by WHO to consider the use of HCVcAg assays as a possible method to confirm HCV infection [4]. In this first global guidelines directed at low- and middle-incomes countries, the capillary sampling on blotting paper (DBS) is also considered as an easily transportable and simple alternative to peripheral venous sampling for confirmation of HCV infection based on RNA detection [1, 4]. In rural and resource-limited areas, DBS offer a simple transportable alternative to peripheral venous sampling and represents an appealing method for scaling up testing.

In Vietnam, the presence of anti-HCV antibodies has been reported between 1 to 6% of the general population and is dramatically higher (up to 90%) in people who inject drugs [8, 9]. The Vietnamese Ministry of Health has recently developed a national HCV guidance upon the release of the first WHO Guidelines on HCV care and treatment [10]. We previously reported a high proportion of advanced liver fibrosis among HIV-HCV co-infected peoples who inject drugs in Haiphong, Northern Vietnam [11]. In this study we evaluate the performance of HCV RNA and HCV antigen detection on DBS collected in Haiphong Viet Tiep Hospital and compared to serum PCR using open polyvalent PCR platform.

Patients and methods

Study population

The source population was HIV-infected outpatients reporting past injection or ongoing drug use who also participated in a cross-sectional study conducted at the Viet Tiep hospital in Haiphong between February and March 2014 (ANRS 12262). Eligibility criteria were: age over 18 years, positivity for anti-HCV antibodies and HCV RNA, HCV treatment-naïve status, ART initiated for more than 6 months, CD4+ T cells count over 200/mm^3. Patients tested positive for HCV antibodies using both a rapid test (SD Bioline anti-HCV rapid test, Standard Diagnostics Inc., Korea) and laboratory test (Phamatech anti HCV EIA kit, USA) were prospectively enrolled after providing written consents. Sample size calculation was performed based on an expected sensitivity of 0.85 (95% acceptable lower CI: 0.70) using HCVcAg on DBS for identification of HCV chronic hepatitis, to control the design accuracy [12]. HCV RNA quantification and HCV genotyping were assessed as previously described [10]. Briefly, HCV RNA in serum was extracted using the MagNa Pure 96 system and quantified using a CE marked HCV kit (HCV Real-time Quant, Sacace Biotechnologies, Italy) on LightCycler 480 instrument (Roche, USA). HCV genotyping was performed for samples with HCV RNA level above 1000 copies/mL as previously described. HCV subtypes were identified using the Los Alamos Hepatitis C sequence (www.hcv.lanl.gov). Blood samples from HCV infected outpatients followed in the Montpellier University hospital and having provided informed consent were used for the validation of PCR and HCVcAg methods on DBS specimens (DC-2008-417). HCV RNA levels of HCV samples collected in France were quantified using the COBAS® AmpliPrep/COBAS® TaqMan® V2.0 assay (Roche), and genotypes were determined using the HCV Versant Genotype 2.0 assay (LiPA) (Siemens Healthcare Diagnostics, Tarrytown, NY). HCV genotypes consists of G1 ($n = 18$), G2 ($n = 2$), G3 ($n = 9$), G4 ($n = 8$), G5 ($n = 1$). The study protocol and written informed consent form were approved by the Ethic Committee of the Viet Tiep Hospital and the Institutional Review Board (IRB) of the Haiphong Medical Services (n° 01BVVT/HDKH). Then, the written informed consent was obtained from all participants before blood sampling.

DBS specimen preparation

Fifty microliters of venous whole-blood collected in ethylene diamine tetraacetic acid tube was spotted onto the filter paper card (Whatman 903; GE Healthcare Europe, Freiburg, Germany). The filter paper was dried at ambient temperature, stored in an individual sealed plastic bag with a desiccant package at − 20 °C. DBS samples collected from the Montpellier University Hospitals were stored at − 20 °C until used. Samples from the Viet Tiep hospital in Haiphong were defrosted and transported at ambient temperature during 72 h, and stored again at − 20 °C for a mean duration of 18 months until HCV RNA and HCVcAg testing.

HCV RNA testing on DBS specimens

HCV RNA were quantified in DBS using the HCV Generic assay (Generic HIV Viral Load, Biocentric, France) with a detection limit of 80 IU/mL using 0.2 mL of serum. For DBS elution, 2 punched disks with a 6 mm diameter was eluted into 200 µl of elution buffer (PBS, BSA 10%, Tween 0,05%) at 4 °C with gentle agitation for 1 h. The nucleic acid extraction was done using 140 µL of DBS eluate on the Qiacube apparatus, and the amplification - using the LigthCycler 480 thermocycler (Roche). An estimated input plasma volume of 2–3 µL per PCR were used instead of 40 µL per PCR on serum. Then, DBS samples collected in the Haiphong Viet Tiep hospital were tested for HCV RNA in the Montpellier University Hospital using the same procedure.

HCVcAg testing on DBS specimens

HCVcAg testing was performed using an automated chemiluminescent microparticle immunoassay (Architect HCV antigen assay; Abbott Diagnostics, Chicago, Illinois) as previously described [13]. Briefly, a punched disk of 6 mm diameter was eluted into 1 mL of 0.05% Tween 20 PBS at 4 °C with gentle agitation for 60 min. A total of 20 µL of DBS supernatant was used for the assay.

Statistical analysis

Continuous variables were described as median and inter-quartile range (IQR). HCV RNA concentrations were converted to Log_{10} values before performing statistical analysis. Relationships between quantitative variables were studied by means of Pearson correlation. Bland-Altman bias plots were used to assess the differences between the different assays and clinical samples. For each plot, mean bias and 95% confidence interval (95% CI) of the bias were calculated and the mean biases were compared using Student's t-test. The agreement between the detection of DBS HCV RNA and DBS HCVcAg was analyzed using Cohen's kappa test. All statistical analyses were done with MS Excel and Graphpad Prism 6.0 (GraphPad Software, Inc., San Diego, CA).

Results

Comparison of HCV RNA quantification on serum and DBS specimens

HCV RNA values on DBS specimens were compared to serum HCV RNA values quantified in matched serum samples collected in 37 HCV-infected patients followed in the Montpellier University Hospital, France. HCV RNA were detected in all DBS samples. The median IQR HCV RNA were 5.5 log IU/mL on serum and 3.8 log IU/mL on DBS elution buffer. We observed a good correlation between DBS using the Biocentric assay and serum HCV RNA using the Roche assay (Fig. 1a) ($r = 0.9488$; $P < 0.0001$). The mean difference (bias ± SD) between the results on DBS and the reference HCV RNA level was 1.391 ± 0.32 log IU/mL. Bland–Altman analysis shown that 36 (97%) results were seated within the 95% confidence interval (Fig. 1b). The limit of detection (LOD) for HCV RNA on DBS was estimated at 3000 IU/mL (data not shown).

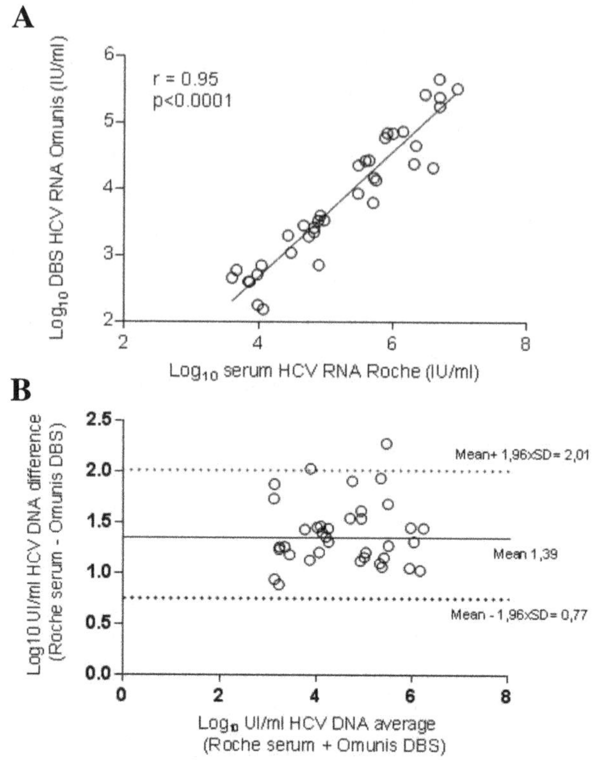

Fig. 1 Regression analysis of HCV RNA levels and Bland-Altman plot of titer differences in paired DBS and serum samples collected in Montpellier University Hospital, France. **a** Linear regression analysis HCV RNA levels for 37 matched DBS–serum pairs. **b** Agreement between the HCV RNA quantification by plotting the differences between serum and DBS specimen averages of the two techniques using the Bland-Altman analysis

HCV RNA detection and quantification on DBS specimens collected from HIV/HCV co-infected patients from Viet Tiep hospital, Hai Phong, Vietnam

One hundred and four patients were tested positive for HCV antibodies. DBS samples were available for 101 of them. Patients' characteristics were summarized in Table 1. Eighty-six subjects (85%) were tested positive for HCV RNA in serum, median (IQR): 6.9 log10 IU/mL (5.6–7.4 log_{10} IU/mL). Genotypes were determined in 82/86 samples (95%) samples: G1 ($n = 57$), G3 ($n = 3$), G6 ($n = 22$). HCV RNA was detected in 79/86 dB samples (sensitivity 92.5%; 95% CI: 85.1–96.9%; negative predictive value 68.2%; 95% CI: 51.2–81.4%). Fifteen patients (15%) were tested positive for anti-HCV antibodies using rapid diagnosis test and laboratory method but were found negative for HCV RNA. None of above mentioned samples were found positive for HCV RNA on DBS (specificity: 100%; 95% CI: 78.2–100%; positive predictive value: 100%). Among seven specimens collected from viremic patients but tested negative for HCV RNA on DBS, the viral load in the matching serum ranged from 711 to 339,000 IU/mL (median 121,000 IU/mL; IQR: 10,600 to 261,000). Four DBS were

Table 1 Clinical characteristics of study participants

Characteristics	
Patients (total)	101
Sex Male/Female	97/4
Age years (IQR)	34.3 (31.2–40.3)
IV drug use (n)	72 (69.2%)
HCV and HIV diseases characteristics	
Fibrosis > F2 (n)	24 (23%)
CD4 T cell count (µl, IQR)	504 (357–624)
Nadir of CD4 T cells (µl, IQR)	82 (35–173)
2NRTI and NNRTI	97 (96%)
2NRTI and IP	5 (4%)
HIV RNA < 50 copies/ml (n)	97 (96%)

Median and interquartile range (IQR) were used for continuous variables
SD Standard deviation, *NRTI* Nucleosidique Reverse Transcriptase Inhibitors, *NNRTI* Non Nucleosidique Reverse Transcriptase Inhibitors

positive for HCV RNA but with concentration seated below the lower limit of detection of the PCR assay (80 IU/mL), whereas in the matching serum the HCV RNA ranged from 35,500 to 32,600,000 IU/mL (median 16,360,000 IU/mL; interquartile range: 856,625 to 31,800,000). HCV RNA was successfully quantified in 75/86 samples (87%), (median HCV RNA: 1840 IU/mL of DBS elution buffer, IQR 957 to 4060). We observed a low correlation between DBS and serum HCV RNA measurements (Fig. 2a) ($r = 0.24$; $p = 0.0135$). Mean difference between HCV RNA values obtained with DBS vs. serum on Bland-Altman plot was 2.9 log IU/mL, with limits of agreement (mean difference ± 2 standard deviation) ± 3.28.log IU/mL (Fig. 2b). All the values were within the 95% confidence interval.

HCVcAg detection and quantification on DBS specimens collected from HIV/HCV co-infected patients from Viet Tiep hospital, Hai Phong, Vietnam

DBS were tested for the presence of HCVcAg using the Architect HCV antigen assay. HCVcAg was detected on DBS in 75/86 (sensitivity: 87.2%; 95% CI: 78.3–93.4%; negative predictive value: 57.7%; 95% CI: 43.9–70.3%). All serum samples tested negative for HCV RNA were undetectable for HCVcAg in matched DBS samples (specificity 100%; 95% CI: 78.2–100%; positive predictive value: 100%). As shown in Fig. 2c, we observed a strong positive relationship between HCVcAg levels measured in DBS specimens and serum HCV RNA level ($r = 0.80$; $P < 0.0001$), regardless of the HCV genotype. Among the 11 dB samples collected from patient with chronic HCV infection but tested negative for HCVcAg on DBS, serum HCV-RNA viral load ranged from 711 to 88,600 IU/mL (median: 29300 IU/mL; IQR: 23,800 to 36,900 IU/mL). Of these samples tested negative for HCVcAg on DBS specimen but positive for serum HCV RNA, seven were positive for HCV RNA on DBS. By

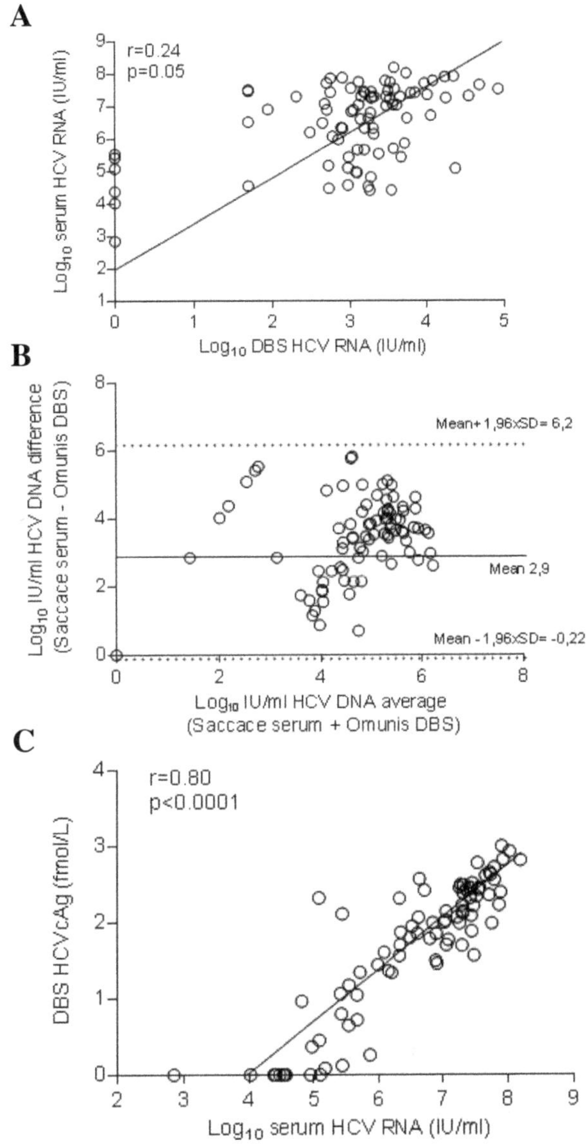

Fig. 2 Assessment of HCV RNA and HCVcAg on DBS specimens collected from HIV/HCV co-infected patients care in Haiphong Viet Tiep Hospital, Vietnam. **a** Linear regression analysis HCV RNA levels for 86 matched DBS–serum pairs collected from subjects with chronic HCV infection. **b** Agreement between the HCV RNA quantification by plotting the differences between serum and DBS specimen averages of the two techniques using the Bland-Altman analysis. **c** Correlation between DBS HCVcAg and serum HCV RNA

comparison, four DBS samples not tested negative for HCV RNA were found reactive for HCVcAg. A good agreement was observed between the HCV RNA and the HCVcAg Ag tests performed on DBS (Kappa coefficient: 0.65) in Table 2.

Discussion

Research evaluations are needed regarding novel laboratory techniques that would allow confirmation of HCV

Table 2 Clinical performance and agreement of HCV RNA and HCVcAg detection on DBS

	Specificity % (n)	Sensitivity % (n; 95% CI)	Cohen coefficient
DBS HCV RNA	100% (15/15)	92.0% (79/86; 86.3–97.7)	
DBS HCVcAg	100% (15/15)	87.2% (75/86; 79.9–94.1)	
HCV RNA/HCVcAg agreement			0.65

replication without the need for expensive laboratory equipment or trained personnel at the site of blood collection. Testing the feasibility, diagnostic accuracy, cost-effectiveness and clinical impact of HCVcAg or HCV RNA assays on DBS in field conditions remain some of the research gaps. In this study, the detection of HCV RNA using an open polyvalent PCR platform, and the detection of HCV core antigen on DBS confirmed the HCV replication in almost 9 out of 10 patients with chronic HCV infection. The nucleic acid tests on DBS provided a better sensitivity than the detection of HCVcAg, however, the HCVcAg antigen test on DBS appears to benefit from substantial stability under prolonged storage conditions.

HCVcAg detection may contribute to improve an access to HCV diagnosis in low- and middle-income countries. Blood collection on DBS, make possible to combine decentralized capillary blood collection with simple transportation from remote areas to regional laboratories [15]. Based on a systematic reviews and evidence summaries of the of the primary literature, recommendation was made by WHO to consider the use of DBS specimens as an option to facilitate an access to HCV antibodies and nucleic acid testing [16]. Good performance of nucleic acid tests on DBS have been reported for HCV RNA detection, with an overall sensitivity and specificity estimated to 96.0% (95% CI: 93.4–97.6%) and 97.7% (95% CI: 94.7–99.0%), respectively [17]. In this study we have concomitantly evaluated HCV RNA and HCVcAg on DBS in HIV/HCV co-infected people living in Vietnam. The sensitivity for HCV RNA detection on DBS collected in Vietnam were seated around the lower limit of the lower bounds values reported in previous studies [17]. Some samples with high serum HCV viremia were found undetectable for HCV RNA on DBS collected in Vietnam and we observed a low correlation for HCV RNA values between DBS and serum specimens. These DBS samples collected from the Hanoi Hospital were transported to France at ambient temperature, undertaken frozen-thawed cycles and were stored during a prolonged period. Thus, a partial degradation of HCV RNA can be suspected. DBS specimens are considered as generally stable over time, maintaining good accuracy in tropical conditions. However, degradation of RNA on DBS has been reported suggesting that HCV RNA levels can decrease over the prolonged transportation, long term storage at ambient temperature and freeze-thaw cycles [15, 19–21]. Our results confirm that assessment and control of the pre-analytical conditions remains critical for the accurate quantification of HCV RNA on DBS. In line with previous studies, we observed a high positive predictive value using HCVcAg detection on DBS [13, 18] showing that the assay is highly performing to confirm HCV replication. Laboratory performances of HCVcAg testing on DBS have been evaluated by Soulier et al. [13] but evaluation should be done in the field, in low-resource countries. High rate of HCVcAg detection on DBS was recently reported in HCV infected peoples who inject drugs in Tanzania, suggesting that HCVcAg on DBS may be an alternative to serum HCV PCR [18]. HCVcAg quantitation performed after 18 months of DBS collection was remarkably well correlated to serum HCV RNA level. This good correlation is in line with previous reports using serum specimens [20, 22], or DBS [13, 18] for HCVcAg quantitation. This observation suggests that HCVcAg is less susceptible to degradation than HCV RNA under the undesirable storage and transportation conditions that the DBS collected in our study underwent. HCVcAg detection on DBS can be a simple and useful alternative method to confirm HCV replication but the limit of serum HCVcAg detection estimated to about 3000 UI/mL HCV RNA [14, 22] is lower than serum HCV RNA assays. Furthermore, it is substantially reduced compared to the LOD of DBS HCV RNA,. Hence, the LOD of HCVcAg can be estimated equivalent around 10^5 IU/mL HCV RNA [13, 18]. In our study all serum samples tested negative for HCVcAg on paired DBS have HCV RNA level below 10^5 IU/mL. Even with such suboptimal sensitivity, the detection HCVcAg on DBS is able to confirm HCV replication in the majority of seropositive patients since the HCV RNA level is generally higher than 10^5 IU/mL during the chronic HCV infection [23, 24]. Diagnostic algorithm based on HCVcAg detection has been proposed to directly identify chronic HCV infection [7, 18]. Predictive negative values over 90% [14] in blood but below 60% on DBS [13, 18] have been reported suggesting that the performances of HCVcAg testing may be insufficient as a one-step HCV screening and confirmation test when DBS are used. Furthermore, the HCVcAg test performed on the Abbott Architect platform is the only assay extensively studied and widely available [14]. The characteristics of this automated laboratory apparatus limit the access to this marker to well-equipped laboratories. No HCVcAg point of care tests are currently available to confirm HCV replication in subjects tested positive for HCV antibodies.

In conclusion, the quantification of HCVcAg on DBS appears to benefit from substantial stability under prolonged storage conditions but with a higher LOD than for HCV RNA on DBS. Detection of HCV RNA on DBS is an efficient approach for confirming viral replication in HCV seropositive individuals but should be accompanied by an assessment of the pre-analytical conditions observed during the transportation and HCV RNA preservation before the tests. Although the lack of qualification of the HCV tests on DBS specimens, and the absence of technological solutions adapted to resource-limited countries for HCVcAg testing are important limitations, one of the most feasible and cost-effective strategy to confirm HCV replication in many countries may be the collection of DBS for testing HCV RNA or HCVcAg in central locations.

Conclusions

Quantification of HCVcAg on DBS appears to benefit from substantial stability under prolonged storage conditions but with a lower analytical sensitivity compared to DBS HCV RNA testing. Detection of HCV RNA on DBS is an interesting approach for confirming viral replication in HCV seropositive persons but the impact of pre-analytical conditions on the integrity of HCV RNA needs to be controlled.

Abbreviations

ANRS: France REcherche Nord&Sud Sida-hiv Hépatites; DBS: Dried Blood Spot; HCV RNA: hepatitis C virus ribonucleic acid; HCVcAg: Hepatitis C virus core antigen; HIV: Human immunodeficiency virus; PCR: Polymerase chain reaction; RNA: Ribonucleic acid; WHO: World Health Organization

Acknowledgements

This work was supported by a doctoral scholarships awarded to TTN by the Ambassy of France in Vietnam. The authors thank the participants and the team of the HIV outpatient clinic working at the Viet Tiep Hospital in Haiphong.

Funding

This study formed part of a grant from the French National Agency for Research on AIDS and Viral Hepatitis [ANRS 12336].

Authors' contributions

TTN and ET designed the study; KL, TTN, ML and ET performed statistical analysis and drafted the first version of this manuscript; VL, KB, JCP, CD and ET carried out the virological studies; TTN, DL, HVV, QAL, XLTT and HDT collected sample and the demographic data. All other authors read and approved the final manuscript.

Ethics approval and consent to participate

The study protocol and written informed consent form were approved by the Ethic Committee of the Viet Tiep Hospital and the Institutional Review Board (IRB) of the Haiphong Medical Services (n° 01BVVT/HDKH). Then, the written informed consent was obtained from all participants before blood sampling. Privacy and confidentiality as well as the anonymity of the participants were ensured at all stages of data collection.

Consent for publication

Not applicable.

Competing interests

The authors declare that they have no competing interests.

Author details

[1]University of Medicine Pham Ngoc Thach, Ho Chi Minh City, Vietnam. [2]Pathogenesis and Control of Chronic Infections, INSERM, Université de Montpellier, CHU Montpellier, Montpellier, France. [3]Normandie Univ., CHU Rouen, Laboratoire de Virologie, Rouen, France. [4]Department of Infectious and Tropical Diseases, Viet Tiep Hospital, Hai Phong, Vietnam. [5]Department of Infectious and Tropical Diseases, Saint-Antoine Hospital, AP-HP, Sorbonne Universités, Université Paris 06, INSERM S 1136, iPLESP, Paris, France. [6]Pasteur Institute, Ho Chi Minh City, Vietnam. [7]Department of Public Health, University of Medicine and Pharmacy, Hai Phong, Vietnam. [8]Pathogenesis and Control of Chronic Infections, INSERM, Université de Montpellier, CHU Nîmes, Montpellier, France. [9]Department of Hepatology, St Mary's Hospital, Imperial College, London, UK.

References

1. Easterbrook PJ, WHO guidelines development group. WHO to test and how to test for chronic hepatitis C infection - 2016 WHO testing guidance for low- and middle-income countries. J Hepatol. 2016;65(1 Suppl):S46–66.
2. WHO. Combating hepatitis B and C to reach elimination by 2030. 2016. Available at http://www.who.int/hepatitis/publications/hep-elimination-by-2030-brief/en/
3. Polaris Observatory HCV Collaborators. The global burden of viral hepatitis from 1990 to 2013: findings from the Global Burden of Disease Study 2013. Lancet. 2016; 388(10049):1081–88.
4. WHO. Global health sector strategy on viral hepatitis, 2016–2021. Available from: http://www.who.int/hepatitis/strategy2016-2021..
5. WHO. Guidelines on Heaptitis B and C Testing 2017. Available from: http://apps.who.int/iris/bitstream/10665/254621/1/9789241549981-eng. Accessed 6 Feb 2017.
6. WHO Prequalification of In Vitro Diagnostics PUBLIC REPORT Product: OraQuick HCV Rapid Antibody Test Kit WHO reference number: PQDx 0244–055-00. Available from: http://www.who.int/diagnostics_laboratory/evaluations/pq-list/hcv/170301_final_pq_report_PQDx_0244_055_00.pdf. Accessed 1 Mar 2017.
7. Duchesne L, Njouom R, Lissock F, Tamko-Mella GF, Rallier S, Poiteau L, Soulier A, Chevaliez S, Vernet G, Rouveau N, Pawlotsky JM, Girard PM, Lacombe K. HCV Ag quantification as a one-step procedure in diagnosing chronic hepatitis C infection in Cameroon: the ANRS 12336 study. J Int AIDS Soc. 2017;20(1):21446.
8. Berto A, Day J, Van Vinh Chau N, Thwaites GE, My NN, Baker S, Darton TC. Current challenges and possible solutions to improve access to care and treatment for hepatitis C infection in Vietnam: a systematic review. BMC Infect Dis. 2017;17(1):260. https://doi.org/10.1186/s12879-017-2360-6.
9. Duong HT, Jarlais DD, Khuat OHT, Arasteh K, Feelemyer J, Khue PM, Giang HT, Laureillard D, Hai VV, Vallo R, Michel L, Moles JP, Nagot N. Drive study group. Risk behaviors for HIV and HCV infection among people who inject drugs in Hai Phong, Viet Nam, 2014. AIDS Behav. 2017. https://doi.org/10.1007/s10461-017-1814-6.
10. Ministry of Health. Plan of preventing viral Hepatits Deseases in Vietnam 2015–2019. 2015. Information on: http://www.wpro.who.int/vietnam/mediacentre/releases/2015/worldhepatitisday2015/en/
11. Nguyen Truong T, Laureillard D, Lacombe K, Duong Thi H, Pham Thi Hanh P, Truong Thi Xuan L, Chu Thi N, Luong Que A, Vu Hai V, Nagot N, Tuaillon E, Dominguez S, Lemoine M. High proportion of HIV-HCV Coinfected patients with advanced liver fibrosis requiring hepatitis C treatment in Haiphong, northern Vietnam (ANRS 12262). PLoS One. 2016;11(5):e0153744.
12. Flahault A, Cadilhac M, Thomas G. Sample size calculation should be performed for design accuracy in diagnostic test studies. J Clin Epidemiol. 2005;58(8):859–62.
13. Soulier A, Poiteau L, Rosa I, Hézode C, Roudot-Thoraval F, Pawlotsky JM, Chevaliez S. Dried blood spots: a tool to ensure broad access to hepatitis C screening, diagnosis, and treatment monitoring. J Infect Dis. 2016;213(7):1087–95.
14. Freiman JM, Tran TM, Schumacher SG, White LF, Ongarello S, Cohn J, Easterbrook PJ, Linas BP, Denkinger CM. Hepatitis C Core antigen testing for diagnosis of hepatitis C virus infection: a systematic review and meta-analysis. Ann Intern Med. 2016;165(5):345–55.

15. Tuaillon E, Montain A, Meroueh F, Ottomani L, Picot MC, Nagot N, et al. Dried blood spot for hepatitis C virus serology and molecular testing. Hepatology. 2010;51(3):752–8.
16. Lange B, Cohn J, Roberts T, Camp J, Chauffour J, Gummadi N, Ishizaki A, Nagarathnam A, Tuaillon E, van de Perre P, Pichler C, Easterbrook P, Denkinger CM. Diagnostic accuracy of serological diagnosis of hepatitis C and B using dried blood spot samples (DBS): two systematic reviews and meta-analyses. BMC Infect Dis. 2017;17(Suppl 1):700.
17. Lange B, Roberts T, Cohn J, Greenman J, Camp J, Ishizaki A, Messac L, Tuaillon E, van de Perre P, Pichler C, Denkinger CM, Easterbrook P. Diagnostic accuracy of detection and quantification of HBV-DNA and HCV-RNA using dried blood spot (DBS) samples - a systematic review and meta-analysis. BMC Infect Dis. 2017;17(Suppl 1):693.
18. Mohamed Z, Mbwambo J, Shimakawa Y, Poiteau L, Chevaliez S, Pawlotsky JM, Rwegasha J, Bhagani S, Taylor-Robinson SD, Makani J, Thursz MR, Lemoine M. Clinical utility of HCV core antigen detection and quantification using serum samples and dried blood spots in people who inject drugs in Dar-es-salaam, Tanzania. J Int AIDS Soc. 2017;20(1):21856.
19. Abe K, Konomi N. Hepatitis C virus RNA in dried serum spotted onto filter paper is stable at room temperature. J Clin Microbiol. 1998;36(10):3070–2.
20. J G, Roberts T, Cohn J, Messac L. Dried blood spot in the genotyping, quantification and storage of HCV RNA: a systematic literature review. J Viral Hepat. 2015;22(4):353–61.
21. Mederacke I, Wedemeyer H, Ciesek S, Steinmann E, Raupach R, Wursthorn K, Manns MP, Tillmann HL. Performance and clinical utility of a novel fully automated quantitative HCV-core antigen assay. J Clin Virol. 2009;46(3):210–5.
22. Descamps V, Op de Beeck A, Plassart C, Brochot E, François C, Helle F, Adler M, Bourgeois N, Degré D, Duverlie G, Castelain S. Strong correlation between liver and serum levels of hepatitis C virus core antigen and RNA in chronically infected patients. J Clin Microbiol. 2012;50(2):465–8.
23. Ottiger C, Gygli N, Huber AR. Detection limit of architect hepatitis C core antigen assay in correlation with HCV RNA, and renewed confirmation algorithm for reactive anti-HCV samples. J Clin Virol. 2013;58(3):535–40.
24. Ticehurst JR, Hamzeh FM, Thomas DL. Factors affecting serum concentrations of hepatitis C virus (HCV) RNA in HCV genotype 1-infected patients with chronic hepatitis. J Clin Microbiol. 2007;45(8):2426–33.

18

Increased hepatitis C virus co-infection and injection drug use in HIV-infected fishermen in Myanmar

Janet Ousley[1,3*†], Robin Nesbitt[1†], Nang Thu Thu Kyaw[1], Elkin Bermudez[1], Kyi Pyar Soe[1], Rey Anicete[1], Phyu Ei Mon[1], Win Le Shwe Sin Ei[1], Susannah Christofani[1], Marcelo Fernandez[1] and Iza Ciglenecki[2]

Abstract

Background: In Southeast Asia, though fishermen are known to be a key population at high risk of HIV, little is known about their co-infection rates with Hepatitis C virus (HCV), or how illness and risk behaviors vary by occupation or type of fishermen. In Myanmar, this lack of knowledge is particularly acute, despite the fact that much of the country's border is coastline.

Methods: We conducted a retrospective analysis to assess clinical, demographic, and risk characteristics of HIV-infected, ≥15-year-old males under HIV care from 2004 to 2014. Subgroups of fishermen were categorized according to the location of fishing activities, boat ownership, and length of time at sea. Generalized linear models assessed odds of high risk behaviors, including MSM (men who have sex with men), transactional sex, injection drug use (IDU), and HCV co-infection among international, local subsistence, and national migrant fishermen.

Results: Of 2798 adult males who enrolled in HIV care between 2004 and 2014, 41.9% ($n = 1172$) were fishermen. Among these, migrants had the highest odds of engaging in risk behaviors such as sex work (Myanmar national migrants: OR 3.26 95% CI: 2.20 to 4.83), and injecting drugs (international migrants: OR 2.93, 95% CI: 1.22 to 3.87) when compared to the general male HIV clinic population. 15.9% of all fishermen reported past or current IDU (23.0% of international migrants). 22.8% of all fishermen were also co-infected with HCV, and though predictably injectors had the highest odds (OR 20.1, 95% CI: 13.7 to 29.5), even after controlling for other risk factors, fishermen retained higher odds (OR 2.37 95% CI: 1.70 to 3.32).

Conclusions: HIV positive fishermen in Myanmar had higher odds of HCV co-infection. They also disproportionally injected drugs and engaged in transactional sex more than other patients. This is especially pronounced among international migrant fishermen. HIV-infected fishermen should be counseled on high risk activities, screened for HCV, and targeted by harm reduction programs.

Keywords: Migration, Risk behaviors, Southeast Asia, Epidemiology-HIV/AIDS

Background

Due to the mobile nature of seafaring, fishing industry communities' close sexual networks, and their relative access to cash and income (and often, thus, the frequency with which they engage in transactional sex), fishermen have long been recognized as vulnerable to HIV infection [1–4]. In Southeast Asia, where fisheries employ an estimated 30 million people and supply a quarter of global fish production annually, a prior review found HIV seroprevalence rates among fishing communities to be between 4.6 and 14 times higher than in the general population, ranging from 15.5% in Thailand ($n = 818$), 16.2% in Cambodia ($n = 465$), and 12.4% in Malaysia ($n = 398$) [5–8]. In Myanmar, despite an abundance of coastline and fishing related economic activity, fishermen remain mostly unmonitored by HIV surveillance

* Correspondence: janetousley1@gmail.com
†Janet Ousley and Robin Nesbitt contributed equally to this work.
[1]MSF-Switzerland, Myanmar Project, #101 Dhama Zedi Road, Kamayut Tsp, Yangon, Myanmar
[3]Medecins Sans Frontiers, 333 7th Avenue, 2nd Floor, New York, NY 10001, USA

systems, international organizations, and national AIDS programming [9]. What's more, the very behaviors that leave fishermen susceptible to HIV infection may also expose them to other infections such as hepatitis C virus (HCV), particularly among injection drug users [10]. This study describes the clinical, demographic, and treatment characteristics of HIV-infected fishermen attending an MSF HIV clinic, and compares their risk characteristics with non-fishermen HIV-infected males at the same clinical site. It is the first to look at this patient population in Myanmar.

Methods

Study design

A retrospective cohort analysis was conducted using a convenience sample of anonymized medical data for all patients presenting between 2004 and 2014.

Study context

Medecins Sans Frontiers (MSF) has been operating an HIV clinic in Dawei District, Tanintharyi Division, in southern Myanmar, since 2004. One of the two largest fish producing areas in the country, Tanintharyi generated 650,000 tons of fish during the 2009–2010 seasons, over twice the yield of the next most productive state, according to recent data [11]. The entire Western border of the region is coastline bordering the Andaman sea, and much of the population lives along this coast or along multiple rivers and tributaries, providing ample opportunities for fishing both within Myanmar waters and in the international waters off of Thailand and beyond [12]. MSF is providing HIV testing, treatment and care for high risk groups, including those working in fishing related industries.

All data used in this analysis were gathered as part of routine clinical assessments at the MSF facility and research procedures were in accordance with the Declaration of Helsinki. Analysis fulfilled the exemption criteria set by the Médecins Sans Frontières Ethics Review Board for a posteriori analyses of routinely collected, de-identified clinical data and thus did not require ERB review, nor did it require Myanmar National ERB approval as a review of anonymized programmatic information [13].

Study population

All adult male (≥15 years) HIV positive patients who accessed HIV care at the MSF Dawei clinic from 2004 to 2014 were included. For the purposes of our study, a fisherman was defined as a person who, upon presentation to care, self-reported catching fish as their primary income generating activity (though were not necessarily involved in the resale, transfer, or processing of fish). Occupation was established during an interview at the initial clinic visit, and data were de-identified using an anonymous patient number. Three subgroups of fishermen existed and were categorized according to the location of fishing activities, boat ownership, and length of time at sea: 1) local subsistence fishermen worked on smaller boats, owned by themselves or another Myanmar citizen, and spent shorter lengths of time at sea, sometimes even returning home the same day; 2) Myanmar migrant fishermen were those whose fishing occurred further away from Dawei along Myanmar's coastline and may have spent somewhat longer lengths of time at sea, a few days to a few weeks, also in a vessel owned by a Myanmar citizen; and 3) international migrant fishermen worked on boats owned by a foreigner, often deep-sea vessels traveling in international waters, and often spending months away from home.

Statistical analyses

Baseline demographic and treatment characteristics were compared between fishermen and non-fishermen patients using means with their standard deviations (SD), or medians with corresponding interquartile ranges (IQR) for continuous variables, and frequencies and proportions for categorical data. Tests for differences between fishermen and the general male cohort were performed using Mann-Whitney U tests or t-tests for continuous variables and chi squared tests for categorical variables.

Three behavioural risk factors for HIV were investigated in the total male cohort enrolled in HIV care (i.e. those who initiated antiretroviral therapy as well as those who do not): transactional sex with a commercial sex worker (CSW); men who have sex with men (MSM); and intravenous drug use (IDU). Odds ratios for these factors were analyzed using generalized linear models with binomial distribution and robust standard errors. Risk factors for HCV co-infection (expressed as positive HCV seroprevalence using Oraquick Rapid Antibody Test) were investigated amongst patients who had been tested whilst on ART, using the same statistical procedures; these included clinical and demographic characteristics (age, BMI, CD4 count, marital status, WHO stage) as well as behavioural risk factors for HIV.

Results

Demographic characteristics

There were a total of 2798 HIV positive adult males who accessed HIV care at the MSF clinic from July 2004 until December 2014 (Fig. 1). Amongst those enrolled in HIV care, fishing was reported as the most common occupation ($n = 1172$, 41.9%). Other migrant work (non-fishing; 31.0%) and manual workers (14.8%) were also common. Of the fishermen who enrolled in HIV care, 453 (38.6%) were local subsistence fishermen, 239 (20.4%) were Myanmar migrants and 480 (41.0%) were international migrant fishermen. There was no difference in mean age

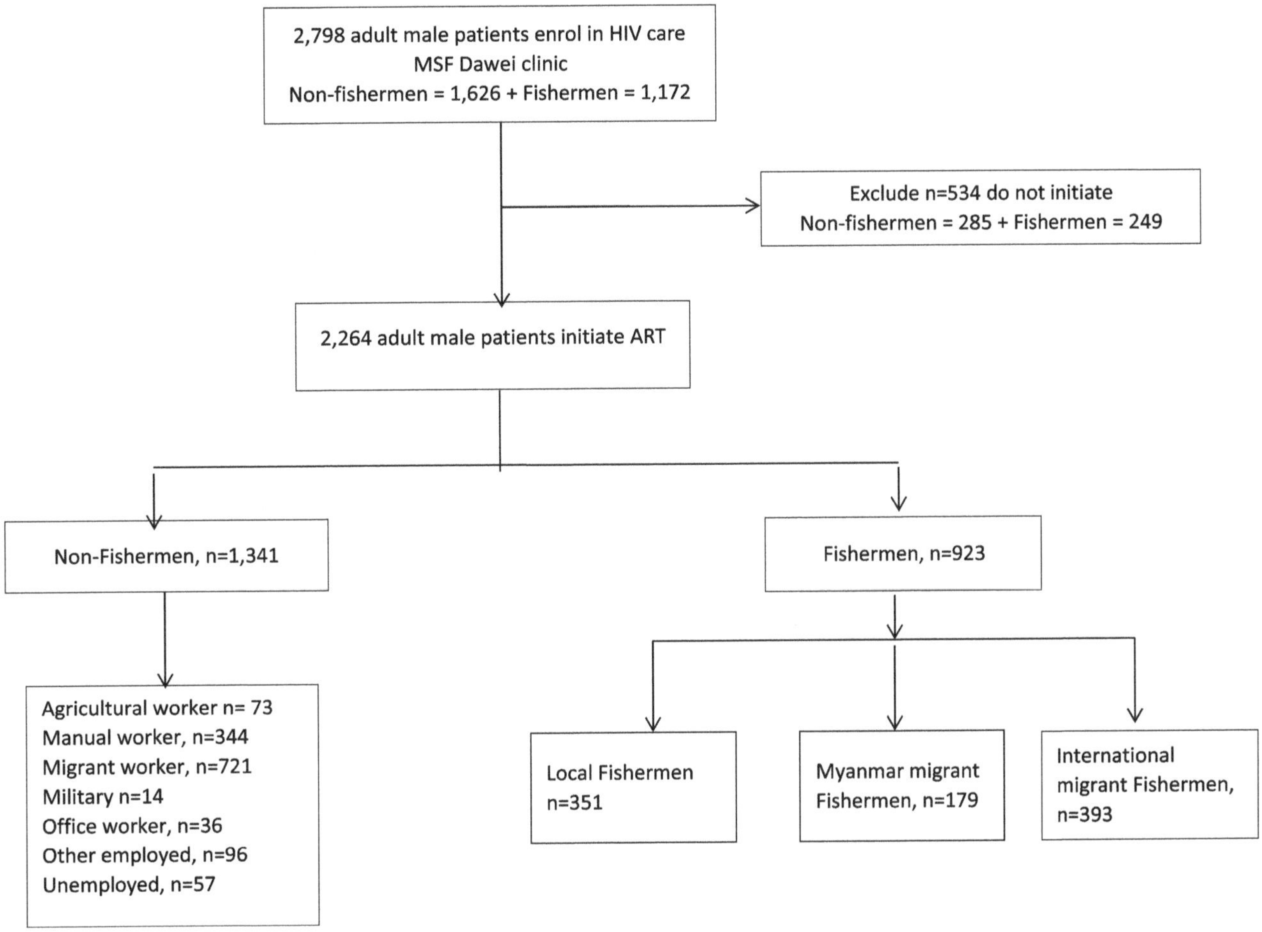

Fig. 1 Patients included in analysis

at enrolment in HIV care between fishermen and non-fishermen (36.9 and 37.1 years respectively, $p = 0.6$), although a higher proportion of fishermen were 30–49 years (Table 1). Fishermen and non-fishermen differed in their marital status, with fewer fisherman married (51.6% vs 58.6%, $p = 0.003$).

High risk behaviour

Male fishermen in care engaged in high-risk activities more than non-fishermen enrolled in HIV care. Fishermen had 2.5 times higher odds of buying sex from a CSW than the general cohort (OR 2.53 95% CI: 2.09 to 3.06), the highest odds among Myanmar migrant fishermen (OR 3.26 95% CI: 2.20 to 4.83), of whom 87% reported buying sex from a CSW (Table 2). In addition, fishermen had almost 90% higher odds of current or past IV drug use than non-fishermen (OR 1.89 95% CI: 1.49 to 2.39). This was driven by the higher prevalence of drug use in international fishermen, who had almost three times the odds of IDU in adjusted models (OR 2.93, 95% CI: 2.22 to 3.87) and among whom 23% reported past or current drug use, compared to 13% of local fishermen and 8% of both non-fishermen and Myanmar migrant groups. There were lower odds of MSM among fishermen compared to non-fishermen (OR 0.34, 95% CI: 0.23 to 0.48), also in all fishermen subgroups.

Clinical, immunological, and treatment characteristics

At presentation, fishermen had a slightly higher median BMI (19.0 IQR 17.4–20.6) than non-fishermen (18.7 IQR 17–20.5, $p = 0.01$), though no statistical difference in CD4 count between the two groups (90 IQR 30–233 vs 84 IQR 39–198, $p = 0.18$ Table 1). Slightly more fishermen enrolled later in HIV care than non-fishermen (78.8% WHO stage 3/4, vs 75.4%, $p = 0.038$), failed to initiate ART (78.8 vs 82.5%, $p = 0.014$), and had a longer median time to ART initiation (42 days vs 32 days, $p = < 0.01$).

Hepatitis C virus (HCV) CO-INFECTION

Of the HIV patients on ART, 1648 (72.8%) were screened for HCV, with equal proportions screened from both occupational groups (72.1% fishermen vs 73.3% non-fishermen, $p = 0.51$). Significantly more fishermen were HCV seropositive than non-fishermen (23.2% vs

Table 1 Baseline characteristics of male HIV+ adults at enrolment in HIV care at Dawei clinic- n=2798[1]

Characteristics		General ($n = 1626$)		Fishermen ($n = 1172$)		p-value
		n	%	n	%	
Age (years)	15–29	355	21.7	191	16.3	< 0.001
	30–49	1141	70.3	906	77.3	
	50+	130	8.0	75	6.4	
	Mean (sd)	37.1	(8.8)	36.9	(7.5)	0.6
Marital status	Married	952	58.6	605	51.6	0.003
	Single	427	26.3	350	29.9	
	Divorced	140	8.6	127	10.8	
	Widow	107	6.6	90	7.68	
BMI	> 18.5[2]	791	48.7	598	51.0	0.001
	< 18.5	699	43.0	435	37.1	
	Missing	136	8.4	139	11.9	
	Median (IQR)	18.7	(17–20.5)	19.0	(17.4–20.6)	0.01
CD4 count	< 50	415	25.5	292	24.9	0.025
	50	421	25.9	305	26.0	
	200	173	10.6	105	9.0	
	350	89	5.5	52	4.4	
	500	83	5.1	41	3.5	
	Missing	445	27.4	377	32.2	
	Median (IQR)	90	(30–233)	84	(39–198)	0.18
WHO Stage	1	165	10.2	73	6.2	0.004
	2	235	14.5	176	15.0	
	3	833	51.2	633	54.0	
	4	393	24.2	290	24.7	
Risk factors for HIV acquisition	IDU	138	8.49	186	15.9	< 0.001
	CSW	1086	66.9	980	83.7	< 0.001
	MSM	157	9.7	47	4.02	< 0.001
Initiate ART		1341	82.5	923	78.8	0.014
HCV positive [3]		93	9.5	154	23.2	< 0.001

[1]Total includes $n = 2$ non-fishermen who are < 15 at enrolment but > 15 at ART initiation, p-values from chi square or Mann-Whitney U test for BMI and CD4 count and t-test for age; [2] this category includes 37 patients with BMI > 24.9 and 3 patients with BMI > 30; [3] amongst 1648 screened for HCV. *ART = antiretroviral therapy*

Table 2 Crude and adjusted odds ratios for MSM, CSW, IDU in male HIV+ adults at enrolment in HIV care at Dawei clinic (include those who initiate and do not initiate ART)- comparing fishermen and fishermen subtypes to the general non-fishermen cohort

	MSM ($n = 2781$)					CSW ($n = 2793$)					IDU ($n = 2974$)				
		Crude		Adjusted			Crude		Adjusted			Crude		Adjusted	
	%	OR	95% CI	OR	95% CI	%	OR	95% CI	OR	95% CI	%	OR	95% CI	OR	95% CI
Non-fishermen	9.7	1		1		66.9	1		1		8.5	1		1	
Fisherman	4.0	0.39	0.28–0.54	0.34	0.23–0.48	83.7	2.53	2.10–3.05	2.53	2.09–3.06	15.9	2.03	1.61–2.57	1.89	1.49–2.39
Non-fishermen	9.7	1		1		66.9	1		1		8.5	1		1	
Local	3.5	0.34	0.20–0.57	0.29	0.17–0.50	79.3	1.88	1.47–2.42	1.91	1.48–2.46	12.6	1.55	1.12–2.15	1.49	1.07–2.06
International	3.8	0.36	0.22–0.60	0.31	0.18–0.52	86.2	3.09	2.33–4.09	3.07	2.31–4.08	23.0	3.21	2.44–4.22	2.93	2.22–3.87
Myanmar	5.5	0.54	0.30–0.96	0.49	0.26–0.91	87.0	3.31	2.24–4.90	3.26	2.20–4.83	8.0	0.93	0.56–1.53	0.85	0.52–1.41

% with outcome (MSM, CSW, IDU) Reference group is always general non-fishermen cohort; adjusted models include age at enrolment and marital status

9.5%, $p < 0.001$), with 28.5% of international fishermen and 21.5% of local fishermen screening positive for the disease, respectively, corresponding to 2.4 times higher odds of HCV co-infection compared to the general cohort in adjusted models (Table 3). When disaggregated by fisherman subtype, local and international fishermen had 2.6 times higher odds of HCV co-infection. The biggest risk factor for HCV infection was past or current IV drug use, and 67% of adult males on ART who reported IDU also screening HCV seropositive. IDU was associated with a 20-fold increased odds of infection (OR 20.1, 95% CI: 13.7 to 29.5), though even after accounting for IDU in an adjusted model, fishermen retained higher odds of HCV infection (OR 2.37, 95% CI: 1.70–3.32, Table 3, adjusted model 1).

Discussion

This analysis establishes the clinical, demographic, and risk characteristics of a cohort of adult HIV patients about which, to date, no information has been published in Myanmar or in Southeast Asia. Occupations that demand mobility or migration are, by definition, less stable. In this case, they may also hold more health risks: Fishermen often have little access to health facilities and sources of health information while at sea, and they may be socially marginalized and endure real physical risks as part of their work. Weekly, seasonal, or long term migration is an expected part of the occupation, and close knit peer networks replacing family and community while far from home can increase the frequency of unsafe activities fishermen engage in [8].

Table 3 HCV co-infection in HIV + males initiated on ART at MSF clinic in Dawei- 2004-2014, $n = 1648$

Characteristics		HCV+	Crude $n = 1648$		Adjusted model 1 $n = 1639$		Adjusted model 2 $n = 1639$	
		%	OR	95% CI	OR	95% CI	OR	95% CI
Occupation	Non-fisherman	9.5			1			
	Fisherman	23.2	2.88	2.18–3.81	2.37	1.70–3.32		
Fisherman sub-groups	Non-fisherman	9.5						
	Local	21.5	2.62	1.80–3.81			2.66	1.75–4.04
	International	28.5	3.82	2.73–5.34			2.59	1.70–3.96
	Myanmar	15.1	1.7	1.02–2.84			1.50	0.77–2.91
Age at initiation	15–29 yrs	7.2			1			
	30–49 yrs	17.2	2.68	1.65–4.38	2.26	1.40–3.65	2.25	1.39–3.63
	50+	8.4	1.18	0.53–2.63	1.59	0.70–3.64	1.59	0.69–3.65
Marital status	Married	13.2						
	Single	19.1	1.56	1.15–2.10	1.23	0.84–1.79	1.23	0.84–1.79
	Divorced	16.1	1.26	0.78–2.05	0.9	0.50–1.64	0.92	0.50–1.67
	Widow	11.8	0.88	0.48–1.62	0.9	0.41–1.93	0.9	0.42–1.93
BMI at initiation	< 18.5	12.4						
	> 18.5	16.2	1.37	0.90–2.08	1.21	0.71–2.06	1.22	0.72–2.09
	Missing	15.1	1.26	0.84–1.88	1.25	0.73–2.14	1.23	0.72–2.12
CD4 count at initiation	< 50	14.7						
	50	17.9	1.27	0.85–1.89	1.49	0.88–2.53	1.55	0.91–2.64
	200	7.7	1.03	0.71–1.49	0.86	0.41–1.83	1.26	0.74–2.16
	350	16.9	0.49	0.26–0.91	2.01	0.92–4.37	0.86	0.40–1.83
	500	18.9	1.18	0.61–2.31	1.29	0.40–4.20	2.02	0.92–4.44
	Missing	15.0	1.36	0.56–3.26	1.29	0.76–2.18	1.35	0.42–4.42
WHO Stage	1/2	8.9	1		1			
	3/4	16.1	1.98	1.26–3.11	1.45	0.84–2.50	1.46	0.85–2.52
Risk factors for HIV acquisition[a]	IDU	67.0	22.81	15.99–32.54	20.1	13.69–29.52	19.73	13.45–28.94
	MSM	5.7	0.32	0.16–0.66	0.45	0.20–1.01	0.46	0.21–1.03
	CSW	16.2	1.45	1.05–2.02	1.00	0.67–1.50	1.02	0.68–1.53

Population includes only n = 1648 screened for HCV during follow up and excludes 534 who did not initiate ART. Model 1 compares fishermen to general non-fishermen cohort. Model 2 compares fishermen subgroups to general cohort. [a]For each risk factor, baseline for odds ratio is those without risk factor

Our results confirm that Myanmar fishermen also lead lifestyles suffused with risk, yet remain largely untargeted as a subgroup by social services and health and risk education providers in the country. Over 80% of fishermen under MSF's care reported engaging in commercial sex (especially common in migrants away from their homes and families), which was particularly troubling since past meta-analyses have found that up to 90% of fishermen use condoms infrequently with their primary partners [14]. High risk IDU, especially among international fishermen, is also troubling in the world's second largest opium producer (Myanmar is home to the notorious "Golden Triangle," a major drug producing region that spans Myanmar, Laos, and Thailand) [15]. For certain occupations in Myanmar, such as miners in the north of the country, drug use is understood to be a problematic driver of morbidity, and programs target these groups with harm reduction and HIV interventions accordingly [9]. Yet fishermen in the south of the country fall almost entirely outside of these efforts, and national HIV surveillance data largely overlooks them and the Tanintharyi region in strategic documents [9]. Because of the retrospective, clinical nature of the data available for this analysis, an in-depth investigation of these factors was unavailable for this cohort and are worthy of future research. However our results make clear that HIV and harm reduction actors in Myanmar would do better to coordinate their activities to target fishermen with these programs.

Furthermore, risk factors such as IDU may be leading to increased proportions of HCV seroprevalence among fishermen. Rates seen in this analysis were higher than those found in other parts of Myanmar [16]. This is a serious issue. HCV therapies are not yet widely available in Myanmar, especially to vulnerable or indigent populations, and official guidance has only recently recommended using Direct Acting Anti-retrovirals (DAAs) rather than older, less expensive interferon based therapies that can interact with ART. Recent evidence has also suggested that people co-infected with HIV and HCV have a higher incidence of other illnesses, such as an almost two-fold risk of developing cancer [17]. The HIV/HCV co-infection rates seen in these fishermen, as well as the inter-related patterns of fishing, injecting drugs, and transactional sex, warrant further in depth study to better target HIV and HCV prevention and screening efforts, as well as better treatment of both diseases.

Limitations

Some risk behavior related information may have been underestimated as 1) self-reported information about high risk sex and drug use is sensitive in the Myanmar cultural context, 2) in some cases, patients engaging in multiple high risk behaviors may not have had all their risk factors captured in clinic databases 3) risk information was asked about during initial clinic visits and may not account for changes in behavior during follow up. As with all operational research, some subtle inconsistencies in reporting due to staff transition may have occurred over a decade of data collection, particularly distinctions between types of fishermen.

Conclusion

In Southeast Asia, the HIV epidemic is not generalized, but resides within specific higher risk groups. This analysis shows that in Myanmar, outside of the traditional CSW, MSM, and IDU risk group categories, fishermen disproportionally inject drugs, are HCV co-infected, and engage in transactional sex. Since many of these men are migrating internationally, they are of note to HIV actors across the region. A better understanding how lengths of time at sea and destinations may affect their risk for disease transmission could better target this group. Introducing systematic HCV screening and harm reduction services for fishermen in Myanmar could be important to curbing both the HIV and HCV epidemics there.

Abbreviations

AIDS: Acquired Immunodeficiency Syndrome; ART: Anti-Retroviral Therapy; CD4: A glycoprotein in t-cells which are counted as an indicator of immune health; CI: Confidence Interval; HCV: Hepatitus C Virus; HIV: Human Immunideficiency Virus; IQR: Inter-Quartile Range; MSF: Medecins Sans Frontieres; OR: Odds Ratio; TB: Tuberculosis

Acknowledgements

We thank the many MSF staff in Dawei, Yangon, and Geneva who provided support and input at various points during the study.

Funding

The study was funded entirely with MSF project funds without external financing.

Author's contributions

All authors contributed to this study as part of regular duties as staff with Medecins Sans Frontieres-Switzerland in Myanmar and have read and approved the final manuscript. JO conceived of the study and participated in its design, coordination, statistical analysis, and drafted the manuscript. RN conducted the statistical analysis, drafted parts of the manuscript, and provided technical review, NTTK and EB participated in the design, and provided technical review of it. KPS participated in the design and data collection of the study and technical review of the manuscript, including drafting some manuscript content. RA provided input into the study design, data cleaning, and technical review of the manuscript. PEM, KPS coordinated the data collection and cleaning and provided technical insight during analysis and manuscript drafting. SC, MF, and WLS provided technical review of the manuscript throughout the study process (from conception through analysis and reporting). WLS also presented preliminary results at MSF's international research congress. IC oversaw the study, participated in its design and conception, and IC and SC provided final technical and editorial review of the manuscript as well as its final authorization. All authors read and approved the final manuscript.

Ethics approval and consent to participate

This research fulfilled the exemption criteria set by the Médecins Sans Frontières Ethics Review Board for a posteriori analyses of routinely collected clinical data and thus did not require MSF ERB review. It was conducted with permission from Micaela Serafini, Medical Director, Operational Centre Geneva Médecins Sans Frontières. Additionally, formal Myanmar ERB approval was not sought for this retrospective analysis of routinely collected anonymized clinical and program data since national regulations currently do not require a formal ERB submission for reviews of program implementation, of which this research constitutes (more information can be found at http://www.ercdmrlm.org/welcome/index).

These data and findings have been shared formally at MoH public meetings and informally with counterparts from the Myanmar national AIDS and TB programs. All clinical care received by participants during the course of their treatment and reviewed in this analysis followed established medical ethical practice, and all research procedures conducted were in accordance with the Declaration of Helsinki.

Consent for publication

Not applicable.

Competing interests

All authors are staff with Medecins Sans Frontiers and declare no competing financial or non-financial relationships that could influence the outcome of this analysis.

Author details

[1]MSF-Switzerland, Myanmar Project, #101 Dhama Zedi Road, Kamayut Tsp, Yangon, Myanmar. [2]MSF, Geneva, Switzerland. [3]Medecins Sans Frontiers, 333 7th Avenue, 2nd Floor, New York, NY 10001, USA.

References

1. Kissling E, Allison E, Russell S, Bachmann M, Musgrave S, Heck S. Fisherfolk are among the groups most at-risk of HIV: cross-country analysis of prevalence and numbers infected. AIDS. 2005;19:1939–46.
2. Camlin C, Kwena Z, Dworkin S. *Jaboya* vs. *Jakambi*: status, negotiation, and HIV risks among female migrants in the "sex for fish" economy in Nyanza province, Kenya. AIDS Educ Prev. 2013;25(3).
3. Serwadda D, Sewankambo N, Carswell JW, Kirwa GB, Bayley A, Downing R, et al. Slim Disease: a new disease in Uganda and its association with HTLV-III Infection. Lancet. 1985:849–52.
4. Seeley J, Allison E. HIV/AIDS in fishing communities: challenges to delivering antiretroviral therapy to vulnerable groups. AIDS Care. 2005;17(6):688–97.
5. MKK C, El-Bassel N, PCG A, Gilbert L, Wu E, West BS, et al. Prevalence and correlates of HIV and hepatitis C virus infections and risk behaviors among Malaysian fishermen. PLoS One. 2015. https://doi.org/10.1371/journal.pone.0118422.
6. Samnang P, Leng H, Kim A, Canchola A, Moss A, Mandel J, et al. HIV prevalence and risk factors among fishermen in Sihanouk Ville, Cambodia. Intl J STD AIDS. 2004;15:479–83.
7. West B, Choo M, El-Bassel N, Gilbert L, Wu E, Kamarulzaman A. Safe havens and rough waters: networks, place, and the navigation of risk among injection drug using Malaysian fishermen. Intl J Drug Policy. 2014;25(3).
8. Thawatwiboonpol EA, Ruffolo VP, Chinveschakitvanich V, Soskolne V, van Griensven GJ. HIV-1 prevalence, HIV-1 subtypes and risk factors among fishermen in the Gulf of Thailand and the Andaman Sea. AIDS. 2000;14(8):1027–34.
9. HIV Sentinel Sero-Surveillance Survey Report, National AIDS Programme, Department of Health, Ministry of Health, Myanmar. 2013.
10. Backmund M., Reimer J., Meyer K., Gerlach JT., Zachoval R. Hepatitis C virus infection and injection drug users: prevention, risk factors, and treatment. Clin Inf Disease 2005; 40(5) https://doi.org/10.1086/427475
11. UNHCR South-east Myanmar Information Management Unit. Tanintharyi Region Profile. (2014). http://data.unhcr.org/thailand/download.php?id=221. Accessed 11 May 2014.
12. Entz, A; Prachuabmoh, V, Van Griensven, F., Soskine V. STD history, self-treatment, and healthcare behaviours among fishermen in the Gulf of Thailand and the Andaman Sea. Sex Trans Infections 2001; 76:436–440.
13. Ethics Review Committee. Department of Medical Research, Ministry of Health and Sports, Republic of the Union of Myanmar. http://www.ercdmrlm.org/. Accessed 11 May 2014.
14. Smolak A. A meta-analysis and systematic review of HIV risk behaviour among fishermen. AIDS Care. 2014;26(3):282–91.
15. United Nations Office on Drugs and Crime. Southeast Asia Opium Survey 2015: Lao PDR, Myanmar.http://www.unodc.org/documents/southeastasiaandpacific/Publications/2015/Southeast_Asia_Opium_Survey_2015_web.pdf. Accessed online May 2014.
16. Zaw SK, Tun ST, Thida A, Aung TK, Maung W, Shwe M, et al. Prevalence of hepatitis C and B virus among patients infected with HIV: a cross-sectional analysis of a large HIV care programme in Myanmar. Trop Dr. 2014;43(3):113–5.
17. Meijide H, Pertega S, Rodriguez-Osorio I, Castro-Iglesias A, Balinas J, Rodriguez-Martinez G. Increased incidence of cancer observed in HIV/hepatitis C coinfected patients versus HIV-monoinfected. AIDS. 2017;31(8):1099–107. https://doi.org/10.1097/QAD.0000000000001448.

19

Changing the odds: motives for and barriers to reducing HCV-related sexual risk behaviour among HIV-infected MSM previously infected with HCV

Femke Lambers[1*], Wendy van der Veldt[1], Maria Prins[1,2], Udi Davidovich[1] and on behalf of the MOSAIC study

Abstract

Background: Among HIV-infected MSM who have been treated for HCV infection, the HCV reinfection rate is high. It is therefore essential to understand their perceptions of HCV risk behaviour and risk-reducing strategies.

Methods: This qualitative study among 20 HCV-infected MSM, the majority treated in the era before direct acting antivirals, provides insight into their ideas, motives, and barriers concerning HCV risk reduction, and aims to strengthen prevention strategies for both primary HCV infection and HCV reinfection.

Results: The strongest motive to implement risk reduction strategies was the reward of avoiding HCV retreatment and its side effects, but this may change with the current implementation of less burdensome HCV treatment. Also, the sexual risk norms in the MSM scene, including social pressure towards risk-taking, HCV stigma, and non-disclosure of HCV status, all form barriers to safe sex. Drug use, strongly present in the context of clubs and group sex, directly impedes the self-efficacy of men to take risk reduction measures.

Conclusions: Tailored prevention messages, empowerment of self-efficacy for risk reduction, and more insight into risk behaviour over time are ingredients for effective HCV prevention among these men.

Keywords: HCV, HIV, Men who have sex with men, Sexual health, Protection motivation theory, Qualitative

Background

The emergence of an epidemic of hepatitis C virus (HCV) infections among HIV-infected men who have sex with men (MSM) has become a new public health problem in high-income countries [1, 2]. Previously, the transmission of HCV, a bloodborne virus, was exclusively related to injecting drug use, surgical procedures, or usage of contaminated blood products. Studies among heterosexuals found the risk for sexual transmission of HCV to be extremely low [3]. Prevention of HCV infection was therefore focused on harm reduction strategies such as needle exchange programs, methadone provision, and screening of blood products [4]. However, the main risk factors for HCV transmission in HIV-infected MSM appear to be sexual [2]. Several studies have demonstrated that sexual practices such as fisting and sharing of toys, but also unprotected anal intercourse, specifically in a group-sex setting and under influence of drug use, are associated with acute HCV infection among HIV-infected MSM [5–7]. Unlike HIV infection, HCV infection can be cleared spontaneously or, in the last three decades, by increasingly successful treatment [8–10]. Until 2011, treatment of HCV consisted of weekly peg-interferon in combination with daily ribavirin, with modest success rates and side effects such as depression and anemia. Since the introduction of direct acting antivirals (DAA), it is highly successful with fewer side effects [11]. Accessibility to DAA differs according to disease stage (grade of fibrosis) and differs per country. Also, DAA is not yet approved for acute HCV infection in every country.

Most important, HCV clearance does not preclude reinfection if risk exposure continues. The incidence of

* Correspondence: femke.lambers@gmail.com
[1]Department of Infectious Diseases, Research and Prevention, Public Health Service of Amsterdam, Amsterdam, the Netherlands
Full list of author information is available at the end of the article

HCV reinfection in the HIV-infected MSM population is high, at 5–15 per 100 person-years [12–15]. This suggests that some MSM are not able to implement HCV risk reduction measures after HCV clearance. To diminish the HCV epidemic among MSM, it is necessary to understand the bottlenecks for the implementation of risk reduction strategies. It is important to understand the motives regarding the practice of HCV-related sexual risk behaviour and the motives and barriers as to application of risk-reducing strategies. Such information will help strengthen strategies to prevent both primary HCV infection and HCV reinfection. The purpose of this qualitative study among 20 MSM with previous HCV infection was to provide this much-needed information.

Methods

Recruitment and sample

The study is based on in-depth interviews held from January 2011 to December 2012. In total, 19 HIV-infected MSM who were HCV-co infected, plus 1 HCV mono-infected MSM were interviewed to gain insight into their motives and barriers as to implementation of HCV risk reduction strategies. Men were recruited from the 'MSM Observational Study of Acute Infection with hepatitis C' (MOSAIC) at several HIV outpatient clinics or through the HCV facebook page of 'Poz and Proud,' a subcommittee of the HIV Organization Netherlands, a non-governmental organization which works in the interests of persons infected with HIV. Written information on the study was provided by the HIV nurse or study coordinator at recruitment. If men chose to enroll, they were invited by phone or email for an interview at their regular HIV-treatment location or at the offices of the Public Health Service of Amsterdam, depending on their preference. Recruitment continued until data saturation was reached, i.e. until no new motives or barriers to reducing sexual risk behavior and using risk reduction strategies emerged during the interviews.

Procedure

In total, 20 face-to-face in-depth interviews, one per participant, were conducted (average duration: 60–75 min) by a medical anthropologist trained in qualitative research methods. At the beginning of each interview, the participants were provided with information on the aim of the study and the established conditions for anonymity and confidentiality, followed by an oral informed consent. The interviews were semi-structured and allowed the interviewer to deeply explore the participant's feelings and perspectives on the relevant subjects.

The main focus concerned the impact of sexually-acquired HCV infection on sexual risk-taking and the motives and barriers to reducing risk behaviour. A topic list (Table 1) was used to initiate rapport between interviewer and participant, and themes were developed according to participant disclosures. The interviewer was free to pursue areas of interest or to probe responses further for clarification. All interviews were audio-taped and transcribed verbatim. Participants received a gift certificate (€20) for their participation.

Theoretical background

The Protection Motivation Theory was used as a theoretical base for the interpretation of the data. Protection motivation refers to the motivation to protect oneself against a health threat like an HCV infection. The theory proposes that the intention to protect oneself depends upon two concepts. One consists of the *threat appraisal* of a disease, in this case HCV infection: its perceived *severity*, one's perceived *vulnerability* (probability of becoming infected), and the perceived *rewards* of implementing preventative measures. The other concept consists of the *coping mechanisms* for implementing protective measures: the perceived *response efficacy* of the measures (the belief that they are truly preventative), the perceived *self-efficacy* (the belief that one is able and likely to perform the preventative measures), and the *costs* of their implementation [16]. The probability of implementing HCV risk reduction strategies increases with higher perceptions of HCV severity, one's vulnerability to HCV reinfection, response efficacy, self-efficacy for implementing the strategies, and rewards of preventative behaviour. When one or more of these perceptions/factors is low, behavioural change to protect against HCV reinfection is less likely to occur.

Analysis

The transcribed interviews were entered into a database for coding, using qualitative data analysis software

Table 1 Main themes from topic list used during interviews with 20 (previously) HCV-infected MSM in the Amsterdam area from January 2011 to December 2012

Theme	Topics
Circumstances of HCV diagnosis	- Knowledge about HCV prior to diagnosis - Sexual behaviour prior to diagnosis - Feelings about HCV diagnosis
HCV infection	- Current HCV status - Perception of HCV since diagnosis - Experiences with treatment of HCV - Knowledge about reinfection
Sexual behaviour	- Current sexual behaviour - Sexual behaviour between diagnosis and treatment - Sexual behaviour during HCV treatment - Sexual behaviour after HCV treatment
Risk reduction strategies	- Risk reduction strategies prior to HCV infection - Risk reduction strategies after HCV infection - Influences of HCV infection on risk reduction - Perception of HCV risk in future - Perception of self-efficacy of risk reduction

(MAXQDA 10) which allowed for coding of data segments using a flexible set of categories. In the first phase of data analyses, open coding by two researchers (a medical doctor and a medical anthropologist) was performed to explore the subjective experiences of the participants regarding HCV diagnosis, treatment, sexual behaviour, risk reduction, etc. Transcripts were repeatedly examined to discover emerging themes which were discussed and, if found relevant, added to the initial topic list of the interviews. This iterative method allowed us to adjust data collection according to what was learned [17] and ultimately to establish saturation. The two researchers coded the same data from all transcripts to ensure that codes being used were the best fit for the segments. Where disagreements were noted, they discussed their difficulties, clarified their opinions, and agreed to a final classification after discussion with the study supervisor, a social and clinical psychologist. Upon reaching consensus, the researchers continued to perform coding to excerpt and sort segments of data into subcodes. In the second phase of analyses, focussing on the research aim, the researchers grouped relevant codes into categories based on the theoretical background of the Protection Motivation theory. They produced a list of categories covering motives and barriers to changes in sexual behaviour for use in analyzing the remaining transcripts. This procedure was followed until a definite database was created containing a definite list of categories. The final results, interpretations, and conclusions were based on that database and supported by quotes from the interviews.

Ethical framework

This study is part of the MOSAIC study which is approved for by the Medical Ethics committee of the Academid Medical Center in Amsterdam, the Netherlands.

Information on the aims, procedures, and use of findings was provided to each participant. Participants were informed that answering the interview questions was voluntary and they could withdraw from participation at any time. During the consent process, participants were informed about the confidentiality of transcripts and publications and assured that all identifying markers would be removed. The consent was recorded on audiotape and documented by transcription together with the interview.

Results

Characteristics

Participants' average age was 39 years (range 27–59), most were born in the Netherlands (95%), and approximately half of the men were in a steady relationship. Of the 20 participants, 5 were still undergoing HCV treatment during the time of the interview; 11 had been successfully treated in the (recent) past; 2 had been unsuccessfully treated and were chronically infected; 1 was chronically infected and had never received treatment, and 1 had spontaneously cleared the HCV virus. Of the 5 in treatment, 4 men had contracted HCV more than one time: 2 had been reinfected once, and 2 had been reinfected for the second time.

Interview results

First, we will describe the risk reduction strategies that were implemented by the participants, followed by the motives and barriers to changing sexual risk behaviour and applying HCV risk reduction strategies.

Implemented HCV risk reduction strategies

Participants described a wide range of strategies used to prevent HCV reinfection.

Preventing direct transmission

Several strategies concern reducing direct transmission of HCV during sex, e.g. using condoms; not sharing gloves, toys or lubricant; and limiting mucosal damage:

> "No sharing of gloves, condoms, toys, et cetera (....), surely these kind of essential things, which may give blood-to-blood contact (.....). Well, using a toy or something like that, while being with more persons at the same time, it could happen that we exchanged it. But now [after HCV diagnosis] I'm very cautious that this won't happen to me again." (MSM 5).

> "Sometimes Crisco [lubricant] is being used. So then you should be using your own jar. If you go through it [Crisco] and then someone else goes through it, you could just as well have unsafe sex." (MSM 4).

> "Using drugs anally is something I definitely don't do anymore (...). I suspect it is unhealthy for the mucosa, by which you increase the risk of being more susceptible to not only HCV but also other STI." (MSM 8).

HCV serosorting

Some strategies to diminish risk of reinfection depend on choosing sex partners based on their assumed HCV status:

> "When someone is HCV-infected, I don't want sex with him. Just because of the risk of infection." (MSM11).

> "Well, we still have unsafe sex with each other, but not at the moment, because he is HCV-infected and I

absolutely don't want to become infected again." (MSM5).

Avoiding risk-related contexts

Some risk reduction strategies involve simply trying to avoid specific sexual contexts that are perceived by participants as encouraging risk. Group sex, sex in clubs, or sex under influence of drugs are perceived as contexts associated with risk-taking:

"During group sex at a club, you are more likely to meet somebody with HCV, because you have sex with more men. Also it is more likely to skip the use of a condom, especially near the end of the evening after four glasses of vodka. So I am eliminating that kind of group sex at those clubs. I am going one-on-one. That lowers the risk of contracting HCV." (MSM19).

"I think drugs are a risk factor anyway, and that is why I would like to eliminate them." (MSM11).

"I'm totally done with drugs. You know, I can say that drugs were partly the cause, and that's true, but in the end I myself am responsible for my actions. So I did it myself. So I don't want to blame it all on drugs, but drugs have certainly been a catalyst. If I hadn't used it, I would have certainly used a condom during sex." (MSM17).

Being cautious on the internet

Negotiating safe sex with partners met through internet dating is perceived to be challenging, as disclosure of HIV and HCV status and safe-sex intention are sometimes not apparent or transparent over the internet. Some men are therefore more cautious when dating through the internet or using the information put online to screen their choices:

"I will never date somebody who fills in 'needs discussion' [answer to question about safe-sex intention on internet profile], because that means that they do not always have safe sex. And I can't trust them, especially when drugs are involved." (MSM18).

"Do you make new contacts through the internet?" (interviewer).

"We really don't feel like that anymore. We think that world can't be trusted. They never say what's going on, what they have. That risk is too big for us. You never know what you get into your home. No, we don't do that anymore." (MSM2).

Motives for implementing risk reduction strategies

Effect of diagnosis and treatment on sexual desire and self-perceived attractiveness

Men reported changing behaviour shortly after start of HCV treatment due to its impact on sexual desire. Many men suffered from side effects such as extreme fatigue, flulike symptoms, and depression which lowered sexual desire and the ability to take sexual initiatives. Reducing sexual behaviour during treatment could therefore be not so much driven by deliberate rational or emotional motives but rather by physical circumstances:

"The medication is heavy, I agree; because of that you don't have sex anymore, you don't feel like going out, you don't do any drugs. So, the medication is heavy, but the choices you have to make are actually made for you, which is very easy. But what happens when you have finished the treatment?" (MSM 5).

"You get a lot of side effects, you feel really sick, every weekend again, so you won't be able to do a thing." (MSM15).

Moreover, men feel too unattractive to have sex, partly due to the stigma of HCV infection:

"Did the HCV diagnosis influence your sexual life? You mentioned that at the beginning you did not feel like it [having sex]." (interviewer).

"Well, I felt dirty. You know, dirty not in a sense that nobody was allowed to touch me but, well, there is quite a taboo against HCV. It is also being called the new HIV, comparable to some years ago. HIV is sort of seen as something normal, but HCV is not." (MSM 6).

Fear of HCV treatment side effects

Almost all participants perceive HCV to be a severe infection, like or even more severe than HIV infection or other STI. This is mainly due to the negative perception of HCV treatment. As stated above, HCV treatment side effects have a strong impact on physical and mental health and day-to-day life, including work, social life, and relationships, and are therefore mentioned as an important motive for behavioural change:

"Well, you see, I always say I would a hundred times rather have an HIV infection than an HCV- infection, and I really mean it. Because HIV really means nothing compared to it [HCV]." (MSM9).

"That's what [HCV] changed my behaviour. You see, an infection with gonorrhea or chlamydia sometimes means taking a pill, not a treatment you want very often, but it's not a disaster when it sometimes happens. But this [HCV] is really something that has great impact and simply takes six or, when unlucky, twelve months of your life. It's not worth it." (MSM5).

"It is such a demanding treatment, if I were to go through it again, I fear things might go wrong. I simply don't want that to happen. So from now on I do it safe or not at all." (MSM3).

Fear of infecting others

In addition, an often mentioned motive for changing behaviour is the fear of infecting somebody else:

"both times that I was HCV-infected I did not have sex during the treatment period...[tells reasons]. I also wanted to be sure that I did not infect anybody with HCV." (MSM19).

Knowledge and high perceived susceptibility

The fear of becoming infected yourself is related to the perceived personal susceptibility for HCV infection. For some, experiencing previous infection and subsequently gaining knowledge about transmission has increased the perceived susceptibility for a new infection and contributed to changing behaviour in the future:

"Well, on the other side, I wasn't totally aware how easy you can become infected with HCV. I always assumed you really had to do a lot: so really have rough sex or long-lasting sex, you know, that there really should be blood. That's what I thought, about the way you get HCV through sex, and that's not what I did. Now that I know that the HCV virus can stay alive outside your body for a long time, it becomes a whole different story [...] If I had known that back then, I would not have done that." (MSM11).

Barriers to implementing HCV risk reduction strategies

Although most participants were motivated to implement one or more of the above-mentioned risk reduction strategies, a wide range of barriers to do so was mentioned.

Lack of HCV knowledge and low response efficacy

The intention of implementing risk reduction strategies may be absent or hampered when the participant does not know how HCV transmission can be prevented or does not believe in the efficacy of preventative strategies:

"Well of course you have this idea, you can contract anything, when you don't know how you contract it, you can't prevent it anyway. I might better live in a bubble then. I mean, you can't protect yourself if you don't know what to protect yourself against. It's no use." (MSM7).

"I should stop having any sex at all, because it really doesn't matter what I do to prevent HCV. Whether I am having safe sex or not, I will contract it either way." (MSM19).

Heat of the moment

Sex has been described as a non-rational act that does not always line up with considering and actively introducing protective measures in the heat of the moment:

"It's like, postponing thinking about the possible consequences at the moment you have sex; the heat of the moment, but also thinking that you won't catch it again. Afterwards, you naturally think 'how stupid of me'." (MSM19).

Negative impact on sex quality

The use of condoms can negatively influence an erection, and is therefore an obstacle to performing sex:

"With a condom, it's always difficult and because it's a hassle, you lose your erection. It makes me nervous because I'm not used to it." (MSM 11).

Challenging settings

Certain sexual contexts, such as club settings or group sex are described as having an impact on the capability to use condoms or implement other risk reduction strategies:

"Sometimes I go to certain clubs. It's much easier there to let go of certain things and to be less careful than you normally are [....] It's the group process and also exhibitionism, to a certain extent." (MSM19).

"[...] sometimes such a party goes on for two days and at a certain point people just go on, and things get a bit, well, messy: a hand goes in or a dildo, I don't know. Thinking becomes less sharp." (MSM17).

"No, you're not with the same partner the whole evening. It happens, but mostly not. No, four, five, six....At a certain point, hands don' t get washed that well anymore." (MSM12).

Drug use

Drug use was reported to lead to impulsivity and to impede the ability to consistently implement risk reduction strategies.

"During which situations did it [safe sex] go by the board?" (interviewer).

"When you're under influence of drugs, I would say. You become less careful, you're not really aware anymore." (MSM2).

Sexual risk habits and peer pressure

A commonly mentioned barrier is the habit of not using condoms when those around you are not using them either. Many men became part of the "bare-scene" after having been diagnosed with HIV. They became used to not needing a condom anymore to prevent HIV infection. Breaking that norm by re-starting condom use to prevent HCV-infection proves to be difficult:

"In a very short period, the behaviour of many people changed [to bare sex], including mine."

Do you have an explanation for that?

"Yes, I do. Firstly I think that at a certain moment it's almost strange to use a condom if everybody does it [bare sex]. That's because the risks and the quality of [HIV] treatment have improved. It's kind of backwards: just because you know that your life is not (or less) at stake, you start taking more risks." (MSM5).

"Every person that's [HIV] positive, in my surrounding, does it unsafe."

"So, unsafe sex is actually the norm?"

"Yes, for positive persons it is." (MSM6).

"It's not like just using a condom again, it's a total switch in your behaviour." (MSM14).

Disclosure-related barriers

Being part of a sex environment that does not use condoms also leads to the fear of losing sexual partners when making HCV infection and condom-use part of sexual negotiation, as this necessitates the disclosure of the HCV status. Participants confirmed that disclosure of HCV status is therefore complicated and often not done:

"It's not desirable to contract HCV, certainly not since most are already HIV-positive. They feel like, 'That's something I can't handle [on top of HIV] as well, and I won't tell it once I have it.' It's like that for me, because I don't tell it either. I feel like, no one is talking about it, why should I? If I would, I know for sure that I won't receive any invitations [for sexual contact] anymore." (MSM17).

In addition, for men who have not disclosed their HIV status, the disclosure of HCV status can mean two disclosures at once:

"When someone hears hepatitis C and starts googling it, then it becomes evident that the person in question is also HIV-positive [...] That feels like a nasty blow. I thought, I'm doing it the wrong way, I should not disclose it this easily." (MSM18).

Open disclosure of HIV or HCV status online occurs often. The internet is a low-threshold way to meet sexual partners and is often used by MSM. Statements about wanting to have safe sex only or about one's negative HIV/HCV status are sometimes visible on online user profiles. However, study participants have experienced that these statements are not always trustworthy:

"It's not like, when somebody says safe sex [preferred type of sex expressed on the internet profile], it will automatically be like that." (MSM5).

"Well, then [when posting you want condomless sex] you actually show you are HIV- seropositive. Consequently you also sort of admit you are HCV-positive. So, you actually contradict your own status. Many rather not do that. So, you post 'safe'." (MSM17).

"On the other side, I have also had a chat session with somebody literally asking me 'you don't have an STI?' My thoughts at that moment were: I'm not going to tell you I have HCV, I don't even know you. I mean, you will pull out, but what will you do with that information? You've got my chat name, perhaps we have contacts in common, so it's easy to blab to others about it."

"So what did you do?" (interviewer).

"I told him I did not have anything." (MSM18).

"And you met up with him?" (interviewer).

"Yes." (MSM18).

"And the subject was not brought up again?" (interviewer).

"No." (MSM18).

"(.....) *So, it's difficult to make it open to discussion?" (interviewer).*

"Yes, it's really very complicated." (MSM18).

Mental health

Some men reported their ability to implement risk reduction was influenced by their mental condition. Symptoms of depression are described as posing another barrier for implementing risk reduction strategies:

"(...) when you care less about yourself, (...), a sort of neglect [takes place]. That's in fact what in a way also happened to having safe sex." (MSM 16).

Declining perceived severity due to decline of side effects

When treatment has been successful, the motivation to prevent HCV reinfection may decline due to the fact that the experienced discomfort declines:

"I mean, the first months [after HCV treatment] you start feeling better and you have good intentions; it's not going to happen to me again. But I know what I'm like. At a certain moment, when it's a year later, you start crossing your boundaries again, doing this and that." (MSM5).

Discussion

The main focus of this study concerns the impact of sexually acquired HCV infection on sexual risk behaviour among HCV-infected MSM, exploring which risk reduction strategies are being implemented and what are the motives for and barriers to their implementation.

We will discuss our results within the theoretical framework of the Protection Motivation Theory and existing literature. Accordingly, we will suggest strategies to improve interventions for MSM with and at risk of HCV (re-)infection.

Threat appraisal of HCV infection

Severity

In contrast to another qualitative study [18], possible complications of HCV infection such as chronic liver disease and its maligne interaction with HIV infection did not profoundly contribute to the perceived threat of HCV among our participants. It could be that the fear of complications was not specifically mentioned during the interviews because other topics, such as the severity of HCV treatment, were more salient. It could be that expectations of favourable treatment outcome are predominantly high. For treatment with peg-interferon and ribavirin, starting treatment shortly after diagnosis of acute HCV, the success rate of HCV treatment is indeed high, even in HIV-coinfected patients [19]. As a result, men perhaps do not perceive the severe consequences of untreated HCV infection as a likely scenario for their future, considering their high intention to get treated. Still, when treatment fails, complications such as liver cirrhosis can become severe and may occur more quickly as suggested by Fierer et al. [20]. Finally, our participants may simply be unaware of HCV complications, as was found among MSM participating in the Amsterdam Cohort Studies [21].

Addressing complications of HCV infection in the at-risk population through HCV-specific information campaigns can contribute to more accurate threat appraisal. Particularly when information is provided by HCV-infected peers, the consequences of infection may become more explicit and recognizable.

As the success rates of treatment are increasing with the introduction of new anti-HCV agents, physicians should clearly discuss with their patient the still possible side effects, the risk of reinfection and how to address it and, if relevant, the effort and financial cost that are involved.

Vulnerability

Besides the perceived severity of a disease, the perceived vulnerability to that disease determines the threat appraisal and accordingly the behavioural response.

Some of our participants did not perceive themselves as belonging to a high-risk group since they did not engage behaviour that they considered risky, such as group sex or techniques such as fisting. The emphasis of study results and prevention messages on the extremes of risky sexual behaviour as a main cause of infection seems to have anchored the feeling that *only* such behaviours can lead to HCV-infection. For some men, the fact that their infection occurred despite the avoidance of such extremes caused them to doubt the efficacy of certain risk reduction strategies. Consequently, while some men became more careful and started implementing more rigorous risk reduction strategies, some felt there are no realistic behavioural steps they can take to make themselves any less vulnerable. Ambivalent perceptions of risk make it challenging to develop effective prevention messages. Focussing on the most risky subpopulations and highest-risk techniques may help those most at risk, but it might also create the illusion that lower-risk techniques are completely safe from HCV infection. Tailored prevention messages need to be constantly updated as the transmission dynamics within a risk population change, e.g. when HCV spreads to HIV-negative MSM, presumably because of the protective effect PrEP (pre-exposure prophylaxis) has on the acquisition of HIV [22, 23]. Furthermore, addressing only high-risk subgroups may increase the stigma around HCV and indirectly raise a barrier to risk reduction strategies, as it increases avoidance behaviour and prevents free communication and HCV status disclosure [24]. Regular consultation on preventative interventions should offer realistic messages regarding high-risk techniques and should focus on the full range of techniques that can lead to HCV infection. Discussing such techniques should be paired directly with realistic suggestions of risk reduction strategies even for techniques that are considered more low-risk.

Rewards of applying risk reduction strategies

Classic HCV treatment (peg-interferon and ribavirin) often had a temporary but severely negative effect on patients' well-being through serious physical and psychological side effects, and it consequently negatively influenced work participation, daily activities, sexual experiences and partnerships. Not wanting to go through these negative treatment-related experiences was an important motivator for behavioural change among our participants and was seen by some as an important reward for applying risk reduction strategies. Eventually though, treatment-related complaints will decline due to new less burdensome treatment options, with possibly a decline in motivation to prevent reinfection and an increase in risk-taking. Interestingly, this concern was expressed by participants themselves [data not shown]. Some expected that with new HCV treatment regimens, HCV infection will be 'just another' STI that is 'easily' treatable. Future studies should examine whether avoiding HCV retreatment is still a motive for risk reduction in the DAA-era, and close attention needs to be paid in future HCV prevention programs to the effect of new HCV treatments on declining motivation to change behaviour to avoid HCV reinfection. Counter measures could include communication of treatment costs and the low but existing possibility of treatment failure.

An additional motive to implement risk reduction strategies was the reward of not infecting somebody else. The issue of responsibility for one's own or one's partner's health seems affected on the one side by social commitment and, on the other side, by fear of stigmatization after status disclosure. How these conflicting forces are resolved seem to determine whether a person will or will not engage in risk reduction behaviour or status disclosure with a partner. The balance between these motives should be addressed in prevention messages for both sides of the spectrum, both to increase responsibility towards sex partners and also to decrease HCV-related stigma.

Coping appraisal of HCV risk reduction strategies

For many MSM, the barriers to risk reduction implementation are related to limited coping mechanisms for behavioural change. They question or feel challenged by both the response-efficacy of risk reduction strategies and the self-efficacy of applying these strategies.

Response efficacy

To start with the response efficacy, the ongoing discussion about risk factors for HCV infection in this population apparently leaves men in doubt about what risk reduction strategies are actually effective. Some men choose to be very careful and apply all recommended strategies; others find that they still might become (re) infected even when applying these strategies. The indistinctness of risk factors leads to lack of faith in the suggested strategies and results in a perception of low response efficacy. Providing a constant, clear, and uncomplicated prevention message linked to an accessible and tailored HCV testing policy may reduce doubts about response efficacy. Using an HCV risk score to determine the need for testing, as developed by Newsum et al. [25], may be such a method.

Self-efficacy

Although low response efficacy is a major issue for some men, the majority of our participants experience barriers related to low self-efficacy. Implementing risk reduction strategies such as condom use, proper glove usage, sterilization of toys, and separate and hygienic lubricant containers is challenging in certain sexual contexts such as group sex or public venues. Helping men to improve their skills for implementing these strategies and facilitating these strategies under these conditions can improve uptake.

External factors that influence self-efficacy are difficult to tackle. In the interviews it became apparent that interpersonal interaction and situational circumstances during sex have a high impact on the self-efficacy of implementing risk reduction strategies. Since the HCV epidemic has specifically affected HIV-infected MSM, a number of our participants confirmed being part of a social network of HIV-infected MSM who practice condomless sex. They stressed that being part of this scene creates peer-based and contextual barriers to HCV risk reduction strategies that are hard to overcome. The norms and social pressure during, for example, sex parties or group sex make it more difficult to disclose HCV-status and to request safe sex. The significance of condomless sex is multifold, ranging from pleasure-seeking to identity-forming [26, 27]. To change the norms within this social-sexual structure is challenging, but reducing HCV stigma and increasing awareness for HCV prevention within such networks is imperative. Innovative social-network approaches, e.g. using online social media and mobile phone technologies, can facilitate the dissemination of information and support within social and sexual circles and help make HCV a more overt topic of consideration.

In addition, lowering HCV testing thresholds and increasing test frequency could support men in high-risk sexual networks. For example, the development and dissemination of client-initiated HCV home-collection tests would facilitate frequent testing and distribution of tests among the high-risk networks.

Another important factor influencing self-efficacy among our participants was drug use. The percentage of HCV-infected MSM using recreational drugs before and/or during sex ("chemsex") is high [7, 28]: 84% of MSM with acute HCV who participated in the MOSAIC study compared to 53% of MSM without acute HCV. The association of HCV infection with drug use may reflect a direct transmission route of HCV through sharing needles or snorting equipment [6, 7]. However, the negative effect of drugs on self-efficacy and thereby its association with other high-risk sexual behaviour is most probable. The specific drugs used, particularly ketamine and methamphetamine, increase sexual desire and endurance, but at the same time they lessen the capability for risk assessment and behavioral adaptation. This effect was strongly emphasized by our participants. It is one of the risk behaviours that men intend to change after HCV diagnosis, but being the norm in some sexual networks, drug use is difficult to reduce. For many, it has become the only way to perform and sustain their desired sexual activity, despite the danger of slipping into generalized addictive behaviour. Changing sexually-related drug use is challenging, and emphasizing its negative consequences is not sufficient to bring long-lasting change. HCV prevention measures could perhaps integrate components of drug use interventions, such as cognitive behavioural therapy or related interventions [29, 30], into their approach. Such interventions should be tailored to the personal context and possible comorbid mental illness of the user, while also building on existing interventions [31].

The challenges that come with condom use were mentioned by our participants as a behavioural barrier to risk reduction strategies. Condom use can negatively influence their erection and impede the intimacy experienced between partners [32]. This makes them less able to use condoms, even when they intend to. However, strategies effective for increasing condom use to prevent HIV and other STI may also be effective in preventing HCV. Motivational interviewing and skills training, combined with tailored cognitive behavioral interventions, are several of these evidence-based strategies [33].

Last but not least, as described by our participants, mental health problems may also reduce self-efficacy and can be exacerbated by HCV treatment with interferon. While depressive symptoms can reduce sexual desire, they can also make one indifferent to the threat of sexually transmitted diseases. The fact that syndemic factors such as mental disorders and drug use often coincide with high-risk behavior among MSM [34, 35] is an issue that public health workers and physicians should bear in mind when discussing safe sex and related topics. Even though patient with depressive symptoms receive professional attention during HCV treatment, more post-treatment attention is perhaps needed and would help to prevent HCV reinfection.

Costs of applying risk reduction strategies

Some men consider the costs of changing their sexual way of life (using condoms, reducing number of sex acts, giving up group sex) as too high. For them the pleasure of sex outweighs the risk of reinfection.

Furthermore, our participants indicated that reducing risk behaviour to protect others might directly or indirectly signal their HCV and HIV positivity to old or new sexual partners, leading to rejection. This is considered one of the highest costs of implementing risk reduction strategies within the existing sexual context of our study participants. A study among MSM by Owen et al., one of two other qualitative studies on HCV stigmatization, describes its negative consequences on status disclosure and its effect on implementation of risk reduction strategies [36]. Clearly, addressing issues of HCV stigma, generating more open discourse regarding HCV transmission, and improving HCV testing and cure in high-risk MSM are more imperative than ever. Empowerment of men through interactive online training modules that allow them to practice management of disclosure issues may be one method to facilitate this.

Conclusions

With this qualitative study, we are among the first to describe the implementation of risk reduction strategies after HCV diagnosis among MSM previously infected with HCV, with emphasis on the motives and barriers to engage in such strategies. An important motive to implement risk reduction strategies was the reward of not having to go through peg-interferon/ribavirin treatment and its side effects again. This motive may lose strength in the future, as less burdensome treatments with DAA are becoming common practice. Future HCV prevention strategies should take such treatment-related changes in motivation into account. Instead of a focus on avoiding treatment, perhaps a more useful focus would be self-efficacy, since the lack of it was found to be a prominent barrier to behavioural change. Particularly sexual norms prevalent within the sexual network of HCV- positive MSM are described as difficult to manage and result in social pressure, HCV stigma, and non-disclosure of status. Drug use, strongly present in the sexual contexts of many HCV-infected MSM, also directly influences self--efficacy. Specific training modules targeting drug use in sexual contexts should be developed, evaluated, and integrated into HCV prevention initiatives. Prevention messages should be provided on a tailored basis, considering the dynamic nature of risk behaviour and sexual networks and therefore developed and disseminated with peer cooperation, possibly using online technologies and social networking. Each HCV-positive MSM's thoughts and feelings about sexual activity, risk reduction, and HCV reinfection should be periodically explored after both HCV diagnosis and treatment to raise physician and patient awareness of possible changes in threat appraisal.

Abbreviations

DAA: Direct Acting Antivirals; HCV: Hepatitis C Virus; HIV: Human Immunodeficiency Virus; MOSAIC: MSM Observational Study of Acute Infection with hepatitis C; MSM: Men who have Sex with Men; PrEP: Pre-Exposure Prophylaxis; STI: Sexually Transmitted Infection

Acknowledgements

The authors would like to thank all participants for providing their time and sharing their personal experiences, as well as research nurses at the HIV outpatient clinics for recruiting participants and L. Philips for editing the manuscript.

Funding

This qualitative study was funded by the "AIDS Fonds" Netherlands (grant number 2012017). F. Lambers was supported by a grant from "AIDS Fonds" Netherlands (grant number 2008026) and funding for the MOSAIC study from the Public Health Service Amsterdam Research & Development.
The funding bodies did not play any role in the design of the study and collection, analysis, and interpretation of data, neither in writing the manuscript.

Authors contributions

MP, FL, and UD are responsible for conception of the study and first design; FL, UD and WV are responsible for the final design and methods. WV interviewed participants. FL and WV analyzed the patient data and interpreted it in close collaboration with UD, and subsequently MP. FL and WV are responsible for writing the first draft of the manuscript. UD and MP contributed to critically rewriting the manuscript. All authors read and approved the final manuscript.

Ethics approval and consent to participate

This study is part of the MOSAIC study which was approved for by the Medical ethics committee of the Academic Medical Center Amsterdam (Medisch Ethische Toetsings Commissie AMC). The participants gave written consent for participating in the MOSAIC study and verbal consent for participating in the interview (substudy) and using the collected data for the study; the consent was documented by audio recording and and transcription together with the interview.

Consent for publication

Not applicable.

Competing interests

The authors declare that they have no competing interests.

Author details

[1]Department of Infectious Diseases, Research and Prevention, Public Health Service of Amsterdam, Amsterdam, the Netherlands. [2]Department of Infectious Diseases (Centre for Infection and Immunology Amsterdam (CINIMA), Academic Medical Centre (University of Amsterdam), Amsterdam, the Netherlands.

References

1. van de Laar TJ, et al. Acute hepatitis C in HIV-infected men who have sex with men: an emerging sexually transmitted infection. AIDS. 2010;24(12):1799–812.
2. van de Laar TJ, Richel O. Emerging viral STIs among HIV-positive men who have sex with men: the era of hepatitis C virus and human papillomavirus. Sex Transm Infect. 2017;93(5):368–73.
3. Terrault NA, et al. Sexual transmission of hepatitis C virus among monogamous heterosexual couples: the HCV partners study. Hepatology. 2013;57(3):881–9.
4. van den Berg CH, et al. Major decline of hepatitis C virus incidence rate over two decades in a cohort of drug users. Eur J Epidemiol. 2007; 22(3):183–93.
5. Danta M, Rodger AJ. Transmission of HCV in HIV-positive populations. Curr Opin HIV AIDS. 2011;6(6):451–8.
6. Schmidt AJ, et al. Trouble with bleeding: risk factors for acute hepatitis C among HIV-positive gay men from Germany--a case-control study. PLoS One. 2011;6(3):e17781.
7. Vanhommerig JW, et al. Risk Factors for Sexual Transmission of Hepatitis C Virus Among Human Immunodeficiency Virus-Infected Men Who Have Sex With Men: A Case-Control Study. Open. Forum Infect. Dis. 2015;2(3):ofv115.
8. Micallef JM, Kaldor JM, Dore GJ. Spontaneous viral clearance following acute hepatitis C infection: a systematic review of longitudinal studies. J Viral Hepat. 2006;13(1):34–41.
9. Brillanti S, et al. A pilot study of combination therapy with ribavirin plus interferon alfa for interferon alfa-resistant chronic hepatitis C. Gastroenterology. 1994;107(3):812–7.
10. Doyle JS, et al. Response to treatment following recently acquired hepatitis C virus infection in a multicentre collaborative cohort. J Viral Hepat. 2015; 22(12):1020–32.
11. Guidelines for the Screening Care and Treatment of Persons with Chronic Hepatitis C Infection: Updated Version. Geneva; 2016.
12. Lambers FA, et al. Alarming incidence of hepatitis C virus re-infection after treatment of sexually acquired acute hepatitis C virus infection in HIV-infected MSM. AIDS. 2011;25(17):F21–7.

13. Martin TC, et al. Hepatitis C virus reinfection incidence and treatment outcome among HIV-positive MSM. AIDS. 2013;27(16):2551–7.
14. Thomas XV, et al. Genetic characterization of multiple hepatitis C virus infections following acute infection in HIV-infected men who have sex with men. AIDS. 2015;29(17):2287–95.
15. Ingiliz P, et al. HCV reinfection incidence and spontaneous clearance rates in HIV-positive men who have sex with men in Western Europe. J Hepatol. 2017;66(2):282–7.
16. Rogers RW. Cognitive and physiological processes in fear appeals and attitude change: A Revised theory of protection motivation. In: Cacioppo JT, Petty R, editors. Social psychophysiology. New York: Guilford Press; 1983.
17. Prachi Srivastava NH. A Practical Iterative Framework for Qualitative Data Analysis. International Journal of Qualitative Methods, 2009. 8(Issue 1).
18. Le Talec JY. When 'raw sex' turns to a 'raw deal'. taking the opportunity to think about sex? Interviews with HIV-positive gay men diagnosed with acute hepatitis C. Cult. Health Sex. 2013;15(10):1133–47.
19. Vogel M, Boesecke C, Rockstroh JK. Acute hepatitis C infection in HIV-positive patients. Curr Opin Infect Dis. 2011;24(1):1–6.
20. Fierer DS, et al. Rapid progression to decompensated cirrhosis, liver transplant, and death in HIV-infected men after primary hepatitis C virus infection. Clin Infect Dis. 2013;56(7):1038–43.
21. Lambers FA, et al. High awareness of hepatitis C virus (HCV) but limited knowledge of HCV complications among HIV-positive and HIV-negative men who have sex with men. AIDS Care. 2014;26(4):416–24.
22. Urbanus AT, et al. Hepatitis C virus infections among HIV-infected men who have sex with men: an expanding epidemic. AIDS. 2009;23(12):F1–7.
23. Hoornenborg E, et al. Men who have sex with men starting pre-exposure prophylaxis (PrEP) are at risk of HCV infection. AIDS. 2017;31(11):1603–10.
24. Dowson L, et al. Why some MSM present late for HIV testing: a qualitative analysis. AIDS Care. 2012;24(2):204–9.
25. Newsum, A.M., et al., Development and validation of the HCV-MOSAIC risk score to assist testing for acute hepatitis C virus (HCV) infection in HIV-infected men who have sex with men (MSM). Euro Surveill, 2017. 22(21): pii 30540.
26. Berg RC. High rates of unprotected sex and serosorting among men who have sex with men: a national online study in Norway. Scand J Public Health. 2012;40(8):738–45.
27. van den Boom W, et al. Is anyone around me using condoms? Site-specific condom-use norms and their potential impact on condomless sex across various gay venues and websites in the Netherlands. Health Psychol. 2015; 34(8):857–64.
28. Heiligenberg M, et al. Recreational drug use during sex and sexually transmitted infections among clients of a city sexually transmitted infections clinic in Amsterdam, the Netherlands. Sex Transm Dis. 2012;39(7):518–27.
29. Mimiaga MJ, et al. A pilot trial of integrated behavioral activation and sexual risk reduction counseling for HIV-uninfected men who have sex with men abusing crystal methamphetamine. AIDS Patient Care STDs. 2012;26(11):681–93.
30. Semple SJ, et al. Drug assertiveness and sexual risk-taking behavior in a sample of HIV-positive, methamphetamine-using men who have sex with men. J Subst Abus Treat. 2011;41(3):265–72.
31. Bourne A, Weatherburn P. Substance use among men who have sex with men: patterns, motivations, impacts and intervention development need. Sex Transm Infect. 2017;93(5):342–6.
32. Lammers M, Davidovich U, Prins M, Stolte I. Condom induced erectile dysfunction (COINED): a unique predictor of deliberate sexual risk. In: 17th International AIDS Conference; August 5–8, 2008. Mexico City: Abstract THPDC205. http://www.aids2008.org/Pag/PSession.aspx?s=320; 2008.
33. Hart TA, et al. A pilot trial of a sexual health counseling intervention for HIV-positive gay and bisexual men who report anal sex without condoms. PLoS One. 2016;11(4):e0152762.
34. Herrick A, et al. Pathways towards risk: syndemic conditions mediate the effect of adversity on HIV risk behaviors among young men who have sex with men (YMSM). J Urban Health. 2014;91(5):969–82.
35. Mimiaga MJ, et al. High prevalence of multiple syndemic conditions associated with sexual risk behavior and HIV infection among a large sample of Spanish- and Portuguese-speaking men who have sex with men in Latin America. Arch Sex Behav. 2015;44(7):1869–78.
36. Owen G. An 'elephant in the room'? Stigma and hepatitis C transmission among HIV-positive 'serosorting' gay men. Cult Health Sex. 2008;10(6):601–10.

Comorbidities and co-medications in populations with and without chronic hepatitis C virus infection in Japan between 2015 and 2016

Daniel J. Ruzicka[1*], Jumpei Tetsuka[1], Go Fujimoto[2] and Tatsuya Kanto[3]

Abstract

Background: Direct-acting anti-viral agents have improved the treatment of chronic hepatitis C virus (HCV) infection, but this treatment is challenging for patients using co-medications because of potential drug–drug interactions. This study aimed to examine the comorbidities and co-medications of Japanese chronic HCV patients by age group, compared with a non-HCV patient population.

Methods: This was a retrospective observational study using a hospital-based medical claims database. We extracted data of patients with chronic HCV aged ≥18 years, and age-, sex-, and hospital-matched patients without HCV, for the period from January 2015 to November 2016, and then examined chronic comorbidities, long-term co-medications, and medications prescribed at least once during the study period.

Results: We analysed data from 128,967 chronic HCV patients and 515,868 non-HCV patients. The median age was 70 years, and 51.0% of patients were male. More chronic HCV patients than non-HCV patients (70.5% vs. 47.1%) had at least one comorbidity, and older patients had more comorbidities than younger patients. The most common comorbidities in chronic HCV patients were diseases of oesophagus, stomach and duodenum (41.7%), followed by hypertensive diseases (31.4%). Chronic HCV patients used co-medications more commonly than non-HCV patients, and older patients used more co-medications. The most common long-term co-medications in chronic HCV patients were proton pump inhibitors (14.0%), which were prescribed to 31.9% of chronic HCV patients at least once during the study period.

Conclusions: Patients with chronic HCV in Japan had more comorbidities than patients without chronic HCV regardless of age. Particularly older patients, who constitute the majority of the HCV patient population in Japan, commonly had multiple comorbidities and used co-medications. To optimise HCV treatment, physicians need to know the exact medication profiles of patients and take appropriate action to manage drug–drug interactions.

Keywords: Chronic hepatitis C, Comorbidity, Drug interactions, Japan, Polypharmacy

* Correspondence: daniel.ruzicka@merck.com
[1]Medical Affairs, MSD K.K, Kitanomaru Square, 1-13-12 Kudan-kita, Chiyoda-ku, Tokyo 102-8667, Japan
Full list of author information is available at the end of the article

Background

The advent of direct-acting anti-viral agents (DAAs) has dramatically improved the treatment of hepatitis C virus (HCV) infection. Treatment with these agents can achieve high sustained virologic response rates with a favourable tolerability and shortened treatment duration [1, 2]. However, DAA treatment is challenging for patients who use co-medications, especially drugs metabolised by cytochrome P450 CYP3A4, because of potential drug–drug interactions (DDIs) [3].

Chronic HCV infection causes persistent inflammation, which can result in the development of both liver diseases (e.g. cirrhosis, hepatocellular carcinoma) and extrahepatic diseases [4, 5]. Chronic HCV patients therefore tend to have various comorbidities. Some comorbidities such as HIV or hepatitis B virus (HBV) co-infection, obesity, and insulin resistance can contribute to the progression of liver fibrosis, which can lead to advanced liver diseases [6, 7]. Moreover, it has been reported that chronic HCV patients also have an increased risk of death from extrahepatic diseases such as circulatory diseases, renal diseases, and non-liver cancers compared with non-HCV patients [8]. Thus, management of these comorbidities is important to prevent disease progression and reduce mortality from both liver diseases and extrahepatic diseases. However, the use of co-medication to treat comorbidities, regardless of whether it is long- or short-term, can complicate HCV treatment because of the risk of DDIs with DAAs [3, 9]. The situation is even more challenging when treating older patients because they tend to have more comorbidities and use more co-medications [10].

Physicians therefore need to understand the comorbidities and co-medication profiles of chronic HCV patients to appropriately manage chronic HCV infection along with their comorbidities. In the US, studies have examined the comorbidities and co-medications of chronic HCV patients [9, 11]. However, to our knowledge, no such studies have been conducted in Japan, although the profile of chronic HCV patients there may differ from elsewhere. In Japan, the prevalence of HCV infection is higher in older people [12, 13]. HCV started to spread in the 1930s through intravenous drug abuse or medical procedures such as blood transfusion and the use of contaminated needles. However, transmission through blood transfusion has dramatically decreased over the past 50 years thanks to the discovery of HCV and the introduction of HCV antibody screening of donor blood [14], resulting in a low prevalence of HCV infection among younger people [15]. Because of the age distribution of the patient population and potential international differences in treatment patterns, it is important to obtain real-world data about comorbidities and co-medications in chronic HCV patients in Japan.

The aim of this study was therefore to describe the prevalence of comorbidities and the use of co-medications in chronic HCV patients in Japan by age group, compared with an age-, sex-, and hospital-matched non-HCV patient population, using a large-scale medical claims database. This study will create new data that are not yet available in Japan, which will provide physicians with the better understanding of chronic HCV patients in Japan.

Methods

Study design and data source

This was a retrospective, observational database study to examine the number and types of comorbidities and co-medications by age group in patients with and those without chronic HCV. Data were extracted from a hospital-based medical claims database in Japan, which was constructed by Medical Data Vision Co., Ltd. As of January 2017, the database contained data on over 17 million patients in 288 hospitals in Japan, all of which are hospitals with advanced medical care capabilities (e.g., acute care hospitals, general hospitals) and use the diagnosis procedure combination/per-diem payment system. Of these hospitals, 176 (61.1%) had 200–499 beds, 59 (20.5%) had fewer than 200 beds, and 53 (18.4%) had 500 beds or more. The database contained both inpatient and outpatient claims data from any department of the hospitals, including age, sex, diagnoses, medical procedures, prescriptions (inpatient/outpatient prescription, claim name and code, dose, prescription days), and hospitalisation details (if any). Because this hospital-based claims database was not linked to patients' medical records, any medical and treatment histories recorded at different hospitals could not be traced.

Study population

We extracted data on patients aged ≥18 years with at least one record of chronic HCV (the International Statistical Classification of Diseases and Related Health Problems 10th Revision [ICD-10] code: B18.2) between January 2015 and November 2016 (the study period). As non-HCV controls, we extracted data of patients who had no record of chronic HCV (B18.2) during the study period, who were matched to chronic HCV patients according to age (age group), sex, and hospital. The matching ratio of chronic HCV patients to non-HCV controls was 1:10. Patient age was calculated in the month of the first record during the study period, and patients were grouped into the following age ranges: 18–24, 25–29, 30–34, 35–39, 40–44, 45–49, 50–54, 55–59, 60–64, 65–69, 70–74, 75–79, 80–84, 85–89, and ≥ 90 years.

Chronic HCV patients who had prescription records of either DAAs or peginterferon plus ribavirin were defined as treated. The type of HCV treatment was defined as either DAAs or peginterferon plus ribavirin depending on the patients' latest record of HCV treatment. Patients who had no record of DAAs or peginterferon plus ribavirin combination therapy during the study period were considered to be untreated.

Definitions of comorbidities and co-medications

Comorbidities

A comorbidity was identified using ICD-10 codes and defined as another disease (i.e. excluding chronic HCV [B18.2] and chronic hepatitis [K73]) recorded over a time frame of 6 months or more during the study period. If the time from the first to the last record of a particular disease was 6 months or more, the disease was treated as a comorbidity. The minimum time frame of 6 months was set to target chronic diseases from a clinical viewpoint. Comorbidities were classified using the ICD-10 three-character code block categories (e.g. A00–A09 for intestinal infectious diseases) [16].

Among comorbidities, the ten relevant systemic diseases of interest were defined as follows: metabolic disorders (E70–E90); diabetes mellitus (E10–E14); cardiovascular diseases (ischaemic heart diseases [I20–I25], heart failure [I50], and cerebrovascular diseases [I60–I69]); hypertensive diseases (I10–I15); renal failure (N17–N19); dermatitis and eczema (L20–L30); diseases of oesophagus, stomach and duodenum (K20–K31); liver cancers (C22); neoplasms other than liver cancers (C00–D49 except for C22); and psychiatric disorders (mental and behavioural disorders [F00–F99] and sleep disorders [G47]).

Co-medications

Medications were classified using the fourth level of the EphMRA Anatomical classification system codes (ATC codes) [17]. A non-HCV-related medication was considered to be a co-medication if 1) it was supplied for a total of ≥180 days or 2) the ATC code was recorded in 6 or more consecutive months during the study period. DAAs, ribavirin, peginterferon, ursodeoxycholic acid, and monoammonium glycyrrhizinate/glycine/L-Cysteine hydrochloride hydrate were considered to be HCV-related medications, and not co-medications.

We targeted co-medications used for a long period. The total of 180 prescription days was a strict requirement because the study period was about 2 years. However, because patients need to visit the same hospital at least twice to receive medications to cover 180 days, we considered that the co-medications identified could probably be those used for the treatment of each patient's chronic comorbid conditions.

Although we focused on long-term co-medications, we also examined the use of non-HCV-related medications prescribed at least once during the study period because even one-off or short-term use of a medication can influence the patient's treatment regimen. As with co-medications, non-HCV-related medications prescribed at least once during the study period were classified using the fourth level of ATC codes. Examining medications used for a short period will shed light on the types of medications commonly used in Japanese chronic HCV patients, which might otherwise be underestimated using our strict definition of co-medications.

Statistical analysis

The patients' demographic and clinical characteristics were summarised descriptively for chronic HCV patients and non-HCV patients; these included age; sex; hospitalisation (the number of patients with hospital admission, the total length and number of hospital admissions); mental behavioural disorders due to use of alcohol (ICD-10 code F10), tobacco (F17), psychoactive substances (F12–16, F18–19), or opioids (F11); HIV co-infection (B20–24); and HBV co-infection (B18.0, B18.1). Disease names coded as chronic HCV (B18.2) and types of HCV treatment were summarised descriptively for chronic HCV patients.

Different types of comorbidities were summarised descriptively for each group. To compare the prevalence of different types of comorbidities in chronic HCV and non-HCV patients, the chi-square test was performed. The number of comorbidities by patient was summarised by age group for each patient group. Co-medications and non-HCV-related medications prescribed at least once during the study period were summarised descriptively by age group for each patient group, as was the number of co-medications by patient.

All statistical analyses were performed using SAS release 9.4 (SAS Institute Inc., Cary, NC, USA).

Results

Patient characteristics

We analysed data from 128,967 chronic HCV patients and 515,868 non-HCV patients (Table 1). The median age was 70 years and 70% of patients were aged between 60 and 84 years; 51.0% of patients were male. Patients with a record of hospital admission during the study period accounted for 43.0% of chronic HCV patients and 27.5% of non-HCV patients. In the chronic HCV group, 11,533 (8.9%) patients had HCV-related cirrhosis, and 17,244 (13.4%) patients were treated. Of these, 16,338 (94.7%) patients received DAAs and 906 (5.3%) received peginterferon plus ribavirin.

Comorbidities

Overall, 70.5% of chronic HCV patients and 47.1% of non-HCV patients had at least one comorbidity. Proportions of patients with 1–3, 4–6, and ≥ 7 comorbidities

Table 1 Demographic characteristics of chronic HCV patients and non-HCV patients

	Chronic HCV patients (n = 128,967)		Non-HCV patients (n = 515,868)	
	n	(%)	n	(%)
Male	65,781	(51.0)	263,124	(51.0)
Age (years), median (range)	70	(18–107)	70	(18–109)
Age category (years)				
18–24	556	(0.4)	2224	(0.4)
25–29	779	(0.6)	3116	(0.6)
30–34	1388	(1.1)	5552	(1.1)
35–39	2095	(1.6)	8380	(1.6)
40–44	3252	(2.5)	13,008	(2.5)
45–49	4639	(3.6)	18,556	(3.6)
50–54	7008	(5.4)	28,032	(5.4)
55–59	9221	(7.1)	36,884	(7.1)
60–64	13,581	(10.5)	54,324	(10.5)
65–69	19,222	(14.9)	76,888	(14.9)
70–74	20,376	(15.8)	81,504	(15.8)
75–79	20,279	(15.7)	81,116	(15.7)
80–84	16,881	(13.1)	67,524	(13.1)
85–89	7525	(5.8)	30,100	(5.8)
≥ 90	2165	(1.7)	8660	(1.7)
Chronic HCV disease[a]				
Chronic hepatitis C	85,282	(66.1)		–
Hepatitis C	42,802	(33.2)		–
HCV-related cirrhosis	11,533	(8.9)		–
Hepatitis C virus infection	2560	(2.0)		–
Decompensated HCV-related cirrhosis	645	(0.5)		–
Compensated HCV-related cirrhosis	434	(0.3)		–
With treatment of HCV	17,244	(13.4)		–
DAA	16,338	(94.7)		–
Peginterferon + ribavirin	906	(5.3)		–
Mental and behavioural disorders due to[b]				
Alcohol	515	(0.4)	1114	(0.2)
Tobacco	345	(0.3)	607	(0.1)
Psychoactive substance use	137	(0.1)	135	(0.0)
Opioid use	0	(0.0)	0	(0.0)
Co-infection[b]				
HIV	336	(0.3)	167	(0.0)
HBV	5368	(4.2)	4823	(0.9)
Hospital admission[c]	55,423	(43.0)	141,817	(27.5)

Table 1 Demographic characteristics of chronic HCV patients and non-HCV patients *(Continued)*

	Chronic HCV patients (n = 128,967)		Non-HCV patients (n = 515,868)	
	n	(%)	n	(%)
Total length of hospital admissions (days), median (range)	18	(1–678)	13	(1–684)
Total number of hospital admissions				
Once	32,492	(25.2)	100,483	(19.5)
Twice or more	22,931	(17.8)	41,334	(8.0)

Notes: HCV, hepatitis C virus; DAA, direct-acting antiviral agent; HBV, hepatitis B virus

[a]For diseases coded as chronic HCV (B18.2), the number and proportion of patients with that specific disease were shown

[b]For the following diseases, the number and proportion of patients with at least one disease record during the study period were shown: mental and behavioural disorders due to use of alcohol (F10); tobacco (F17); psychoactive substances (F12–16, F18–19); opioids (F11), HIV (B20–24), and HBV (B18.0, B18.1)

[c]All-cause hospital admissions during the study period were counted

were 17.9, 15.9, and 36.7% in chronic HCV patients, and 17.6, 12.2, and 17.3% in non-HCV patients. Figure 1 shows the number of comorbidities by age group. In all age groups, the proportion of patients with at least one comorbidity was larger in chronic HCV patients than that in non-HCV patients. Patients in the older age groups tended to have more comorbidities than patients in the younger age groups, and 44.9% of chronic HCV patients aged 75–79 years had ≥7 comorbidities. In those aged 80 years or older, however, the proportions of patients with at least one comorbidity decreased.

The 20 most common comorbidities in chronic HCV patients are listed in Table 2. Diseases of oesophagus, stomach and duodenum were the most common (41.7%), followed by hypertensive diseases (31.4%) and metabolic disorders (28.2%). Aside from liver diseases, malignant neoplasms of digestive organs and gallbladder/biliary tract/pancreas disorders were much more prevalent in chronic HCV patients than in non-HCV patients (15.0% vs 4.6 and 11.2% vs 2.9%).

The prevalence of each type of relevant systemic diseases was higher in chronic HCV patients than that in non-HCV patients (Table 2). Neoplasms other than liver cancers were common in both groups, and present in 20.4% of chronic HCV patients and 15.3% of non-HCV patients. Only 4.0% of chronic HCV patients had renal failure.

The prevalence of each systemic disease by age group is shown in Fig. 2. Diseases of oesophagus, stomach and duodenum were present in over 10% of chronic HCV patients, even in the youngest age group. Diabetes was more prevalent in chronic HCV patients aged between 60 and 79 years: about 30% vs. under 15% in non-HCV

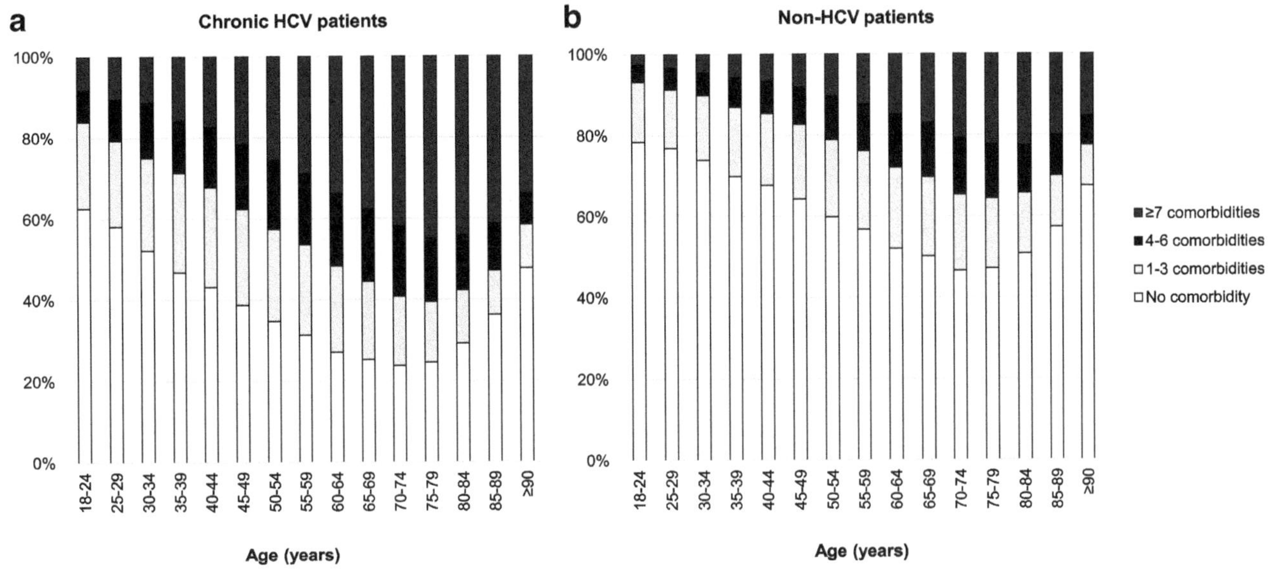

Fig. 1 Proportions of patients with different numbers of comorbidities by age group. **a** chronic HCV patients and **b** non-HCV patients. Comorbidities were counted based on the ICD-10 three-character code block classification categories

patients. Psychiatric disorders were common in chronic HCV patients aged 45 years or older, with a prevalence of approximately 20–25%. The prevalence of cardiovascular diseases was low in the younger age groups in both groups, but increased in older chronic HCV patients with a peak of 29.2% in the 85–89 year group. Although the prevalence of neoplasms other than liver cancers was similar in both groups in patients aged < 60 years, its prevalence exceeded 20% in chronic HCV patients aged 65–69 years and reached 25.2% in the 75–79 year group, in comparison to a peak prevalence of 18.4% in non-HCV patients aged 70–74 years.

Co-medications

Overall, 41.9% of chronic HCV patients and 26.0% of non-HCV patients used at least one co-medication supplied for ≥180 days or recorded in at least 6 consecutive months. Of chronic HCV patients, 19.0% used 1–3 co-medications, 11.0% used 4–6, and 11.9% used ≥7 co-medications, compared with 13.8, 6.5, and 5.8% of non-HCV patients. Figure 3 shows the number of co-medications by age group. In all age groups, the proportion of patients with at least one co-medication was larger among chronic HCV patients. Patients in the older age groups tended to use more co-medications than patients in the younger age groups, and 16.2% of chronic HCV patients aged 80–84 years used ≥7 co-medications.

The most common co-medications in chronic HCV patients were proton pump inhibitors (14.0%), calcium antagonists (12.5%), and angiotensin-II antagonists (9.0%) (Table 3). Additional separate analysis of treated and non-treated chronic HCV patients revealed no major difference between these groups (Additional file 1: Table S1). Almost twice as many chronic HCV patients as non-HCV patients used these co-medications. In both groups, 5.8% of patients used statins as co-medications. Most common co-medications were used more by older patients. For example, proton pump inhibitors or calcium antagonists were used by over 15% of chronic HCV patients aged 75 years or over but by fewer than 5% of patients aged 18–44 years.

In addition to co-medications, we also examined the non-HCV-related medications prescribed at least once during the study period to identify which medications are commonly used by chronic HCV patients. Table 3 shows the medications prescribed in ≥20% of chronic HCV patients (excluding medications classified as hospital solutions or diagnostic agents). Over 30% of chronic HCV patients aged ≥65 years used proton pump inhibitors or antacids, both of which were also common co-medications. These medications were used more commonly by chronic HCV patients compared with non-HCV patients (proton pump inhibitors, 31.9 and 17.4%; antacids, 28.8 and 15.8%, respectively). Anti-rheumatics were prescribed to approximately 28% of chronic HCV patients across all age groups.

Discussion

To our knowledge, this is the first study to examine comorbidities and co-medications in chronic HCV patients in Japan. We found that chronic HCV patients had more comorbidities and used more co-medications than non-HCV patients. Older chronic HCV patients, who

Table 2 The 20 most common comorbidities in chronic HCV patients and prevalence of relevant systemic diseases

Type of comorbidities/relevant systemic diseases	ICD-10 code blocks	Chronic HCV patients (*n* = 128,967)		Non-HCV patients (*n* = 515,868)	
		n	%	*n*	%
The 20 most common comorbidities					
Diseases of oesophagus, stomach and duodenum[#]	K20-K31	53,817	41.7	94,325	18.3
Hypertensive diseases[#]	I10-I15	40,466	31.4	79,602	15.4
Metabolic disorders[#]	E70-E90	36,403	28.2	71,959	13.9
Diabetes mellitus[#]	E10-E14	33,632	26.1	60,428	11.7
Other diseases of intestines	K55-K64	31,581	24.5	61,083	11.8
Episodic and paroxysmal disorders	G40-G47	25,077	19.4	44,756	8.7
Other dorsopathies	M50-M54	22,629	17.5	39,653	7.7
Diseases of liver	K70-K77	22,080	17.1	20,432	4.0
Malignant neoplasms of digestive organs	C15-C26	19,405	15.0	23,518	4.6
Other forms of heart disease	I30-I52	18,715	14.5	44,546	8.6
Dermatitis and eczema[#]	L20-L30	16,294	12.6	24,107	4.7
Nutritional anaemias	D50-D53	15,433	12.0	20,678	4.0
Disorders of gallbladder, biliary tract and pancreas	K80-K87	14,471	11.2	14,977	2.9
General symptoms and signs	R50-R69	13,548	10.5	22,990	4.5
Ischaemic heart diseases	I20-I25	12,355	9.6	31,462	6.1
Chronic lower respiratory diseases	J40-J47	11,400	8.8	23,630	4.6
Disorders of bone density and structure	M80-M85	10,203	7.9	23,124	4.5
Other diseases of upper respiratory tract	J30-J39	10,168	7.9	20,404	4.0
Disorders of ocular muscles, binocular movement, accommodation and refraction	H49-H52	9941	7.7	30,291	5.9
Cerebrovascular diseases	I60-I69	9914	7.7	28,193	5.5
Relevant systemic diseases[a]					
Psychiatric disorders	–[b]	28,253	21.9	51,813	10.0
Neoplasms other than liver cancers	–[b]	26,286	20.4	79,126	15.3
Cardiovascular diseases	–[b]	24,000	18.6	62,901	12.2
Liver cancers	–[b]	11,878	9.2	1578	0.3
Renal failure	–[b]	5180	4.0	9293	1.8

P-values for the comparisons of the percentages in chronic HCV patients and non-HCV patients using the chi-square test were all < 0.0001

[a]Among the ten relevant systemic diseases of interest, five diseases that were not defined using ICD-10 three-character code block categories are listed under this heading. The other five diseases are listed in the ranking of the 20 most common comorbidities and indicated by a sharp (#)

[b]These five relevant systemic diseases were defined as follows: psychiatric disorders included mental and behavioural disorders (F00–F99) and sleep disorders (G47). Neoplasms other than liver cancers were defined as C00–D49 except for C22. Cardiovascular diseases included ischaemic heart diseases (I20–I25), heart failure (I50), and cerebrovascular diseases (I60–I69). Liver cancers were defined as C22. Renal failure were defined as N17–N19

constitute the majority of the HCV patient population in Japan, commonly had multiple comorbidities and used more co-medications, suggesting the difficulty of appropriate management of this patient population.

In this study, older chronic HCV patients were more likely than younger patients to have comorbidities. Interestingly, however, the proportion of patients with comorbidities decreased in patients aged ≥75 years. This may be because those with fewer comorbidities tended to survive longer. It is also noteworthy that 16.0% of chronic HCV patients aged 18–24 years had four or more comorbidities, showing the relatively common presence of multiple comorbidities in young patients. Given that intravenous drug abuse is an important route of HCV transmission among young people [15], some of these young patients may be injecting drug users and are therefore more vulnerable to developing other diseases. However, these details could not be investigated in this study because of an absence of relevant data within the database.

The patterns of comorbidity distribution among chronic HCV patients were comparable to those of non-HCV patients who were 30 years older. The percentage of patients with no comorbidities decreased

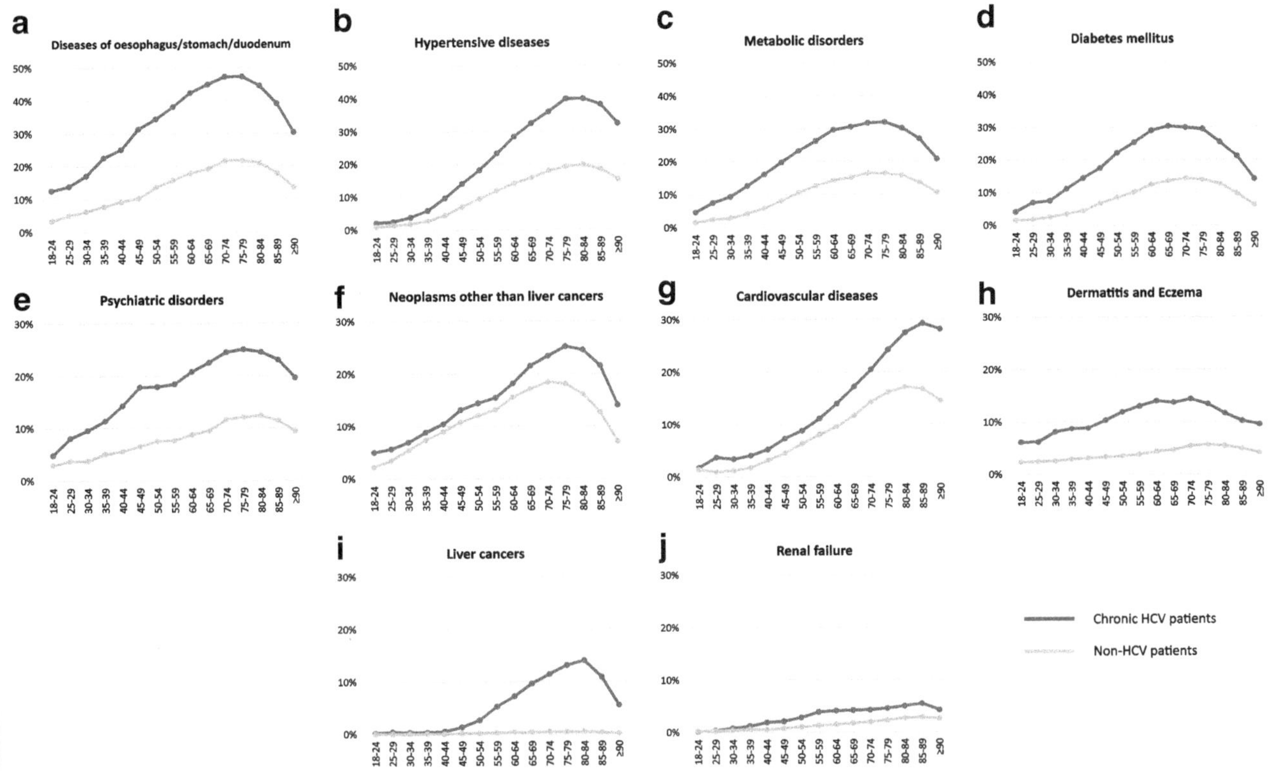

Number of patients in each age group

Age group	18–24	25–29	30–34	35–39	40–44	45–49	50–54	55–59	60–64	65–69	70–74	75–79	80–84	85–89	≥90
Chronic HCV patients	556	779	1388	2095	3252	4639	7008	9221	13581	19222	20376	20279	16881	7525	2165
Non-HCV patients	2224	3116	5552	8380	13008	18556	28032	36884	54324	76888	81504	81116	67524	30100	8660

Fig. 2 Prevalence of systemic diseases by age group in chronic HCV patients and non-HCV patients. **a** diseases of oesophagus, stomach and duodenum; **b** hypertensive diseases; **c** metabolic disorders; **d** diabetes mellitus; **e** psychiatric disorders; **f** neoplasms other than liver cancers; **g** cardiovascular diseases; **h** dermatitis and eczema; **i** liver cancers; and **j** renal failure

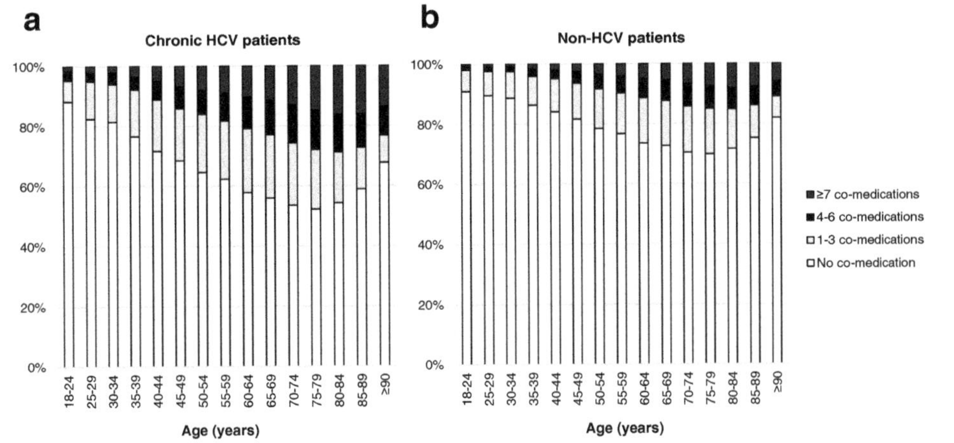

Fig. 3 Proportions of patients with different numbers of co-medications by age group. **a** chronic HCV patients and **b** non-HCV patients

Table 3 Common co-medications and short-term non-HCV-related medications by age group

		Chronic HCV patients					Non-HCV patients				
Drug class	ATC Code	18–44 years	45–64 years	65–74 years	≥75 years	Total	18–44 years	45–64 years	65–74 years	≥75 years	Total
Number of patients		8070	34,449	39,598	46,850	128,967	32,280	137,796	158,392	187,400	515,868
Co-medications[a]											
Proton pump inhibitors	A02B2	4.8	11.8	15.1	16.1	14.0	1.7	4.6	6.6	7.1	6.0
Calcium antagonists, plain	C08A0	1.7	9.1	13.7	15.9	12.5	1.0	4.6	6.7	7.5	6.1
Angiotensin-II antagonists, plain	C09C0	2.0	7.7	9.9	10.4	9.0	1.2	4.2	5.5	5.4	4.8
Non-barbiturates, plain	N05B1	2.9	5.9	7.0	7.2	6.5	1.1	1.8	2.7	3.2	2.5
Plain antacids	A02A1	1.4	3.4	5.7	8.7	5.9	0.6	1.7	3.1	4.3	3.0
Statins (HMG-CoA reductase inhibitors)	C10A1	2.2	5.6	7.0	5.5	5.8	1.3	5.4	6.9	5.8	5.8
All other antiulcerants	A02B9	2.1	4.5	5.8	6.8	5.6	0.8	1.9	2.5	3.2	2.5
Loop diuretics plain	C03A2	1.0	3.8	5.1	7.8	5.5	0.2	1.1	1.6	2.9	1.9
DPP-4 inhibitor antidiabetics, plain	A10N1	1.5	5.2	6.0	4.8	5.1	0.6	2.8	3.4	2.7	2.8
Non-HCV-related medications prescribed at least once[b]											
Anaesthetics local, topical	N01B3	19.1	32.4	41.1	43.2	38.2	11.2	20.4	26.0	26.1	23.6
Non-narcotics and anti-pyretics	N02B0	24.9	26.5	31.2	38.6	32.2	20.8	16.5	18.2	22.2	19.4
Proton pump inhibitors	A02B2	15.8	27.1	32.5	37.7	31.9	8.0	14.5	17.7	20.9	17.4
Stimulant laxatives	A06A2	12.7	21.4	30.3	37.5	29.5	7.6	13.9	19.2	22.7	18.3
Anaesthetics local, medical injectables	N01B1	18.9	23.3	30.1	34.4	29.1	12.5	16.0	19.7	20.7	18.7
Plain antacids	A02A1	13.2	22.3	30.2	35.2	28.8	8.2	11.8	16.8	19.2	15.8
Anti-rheumatics, non-steroidal plain	M01A1	28.0	27.0	28.0	29.8	28.4	24.0	19.9	18.5	18.6	19.3
Plain antiflatulents and carminatives	A02A2	11.2	23.3	29.9	27.6	26.2	5.0	11.5	14.9	13.3	12.8
Injectable cephalosporins	J01D2	13.5	18.1	24.5	32.1	24.8	10.3	11.9	14.9	18.0	14.9
Calcium antagonists, plain	C08A0	4.6	16.3	25.0	33.7	24.6	2.7	9.2	13.7	18.5	13.5
Topical anti-rheumatics and analgesics	M02A0	9.8	16.9	22.7	29.2	22.7	6.2	10.5	14.1	18.2	14.1
Non-barbiturates, plain	N05B1	11.7	18.6	22.6	26.6	22.3	4.8	8.0	11.1	14.0	10.9
All other antiulcerants	A02B9	17.5	19.0	21.6	24.8	21.8	14.3	14.0	14.5	15.4	14.7

Data are percentages of patients in each age categories unless otherwise specified. For readability, patients were categorised into four age groups: 18–44, 45–64, 65–74, and ≥ 75 year groups

[a]Co-medications meet the requirements of either 1) supplied for a total of ≥180 days during the study period, or 2) the ATC codes were identified in 6 or more consecutive months during the study period. Co-medications prescribed in ≥5% of chronic HCV patients are listed

[b]Non-HCV-related medications prescribed at least once during the study period were examined. Medications prescribed in ≥20% of chronic HCV patients are listed. Classes of EphMRA ATC codes starting with K (hospital solutions) or T (diagnostic agents) were excluded from the list because these classes do not exist in WHO ATC classification and are difficult to interpret as "medications": sodium chloride solutions (K01B1), low osmolar angio-urography (T01A0), 1/3 Electrolyte solutions (K01A4), and other electrolyte solutions (K01A9) are not shown in the table

across the age groups in a very similar way in the two groups, although the proportion with no comorbidities was lower from a younger age in the chronic HCV group (see Fig. 1). A similar trend has been described for patients with ongoing HIV infection and it has been hypothesised that this might imply premature aging in those patients, possibly caused by persistent inflammatory and immune changes [18, 19]. Unfortunately, however, we did not examine whether similar changes occurred in chronic HCV patients.

The most common comorbidities in chronic HCV patients were diseases of oesophagus, stomach and duodenum (41.7%), hypertensive diseases (31.4%), and metabolic disorders (28.2%). A US study reported similar findings among chronic HCV patients: gastrointestinal disorders (24.4%), oesophageal disorders (20.5%), essential hypertension (32.6%), and disorders of lipid metabolism (25.9%) [11]. We also found that all ten systemic diseases were more common in chronic HCV patients than non-HCV patients, and that the prevalence of most systemic diseases tended to become higher in older chronic HCV patients. Our findings underscore the importance of age-related comorbidities such as hypertensive diseases, metabolic disorders, cardiovascular diseases and malignancies in older chronic HCV patients.

Chronic HCV patients used more co-medications than non-HCV patients, and more than one in five chronic HCV patients (22.9%) used at least four co-medications. Although direct comparisons of our results with previous findings are not appropriate because of different study methods, German studies have previously reported that 31–34% of HCV patients took at least four regular out-patient medications [3, 20]. An Italian study showed that 31.0% of chronic HCV patients with liver diseases used at least four co-medications, and estimated that 30–44% of chronic HCV patients receiving DAAs and using co-medications were at risk of DDIs [21]. The proportion in our study was slightly smaller than reported in these countries, but this may be because of our strict definition of co-medications. The common use of multiple co-medications in our study implies that chronic HCV patients in Japan may be at similarly high risk of potential DDIs.

The five most common co-medications used by chronic HCV patients were proton pump inhibitors, calcium antagonists, angiotensin-II antagonists, non-barbiturates, and antacids. This is similar to a German study reporting that the five most common co-medications included beta-blockers, proton pump inhibitors, thyroid hormones, angiotensin-II antagonists, and dihydropyridine calcium channel blockers [3]. The common use of gastric acid suppressants and hypertensive agents in our study might be attributed to our finding of a high prevalence of gastric diseases and hypertension in chronic HCV patients in Japan.

Gastric acid suppressants (e.g. proton pump inhibitors, antacids) have potential DDIs with DAAs [20–23]. These medications alter the acid environment, which can result in reduced absorption of certain drugs such as ledipasvir [22, 23]. Calcium antagonists also have potential DDIs with DAAs; plasma concentration of these medications can be increased by the concomitant use of CYP3A inhibitors such as telaprevir and simeprevir [22–24]. In this study, both these co-medications were common, especially in older chronic HCV patients. Although our chronic HCV population included a large proportion of untreated patients, examination of co-medication profiles in treated patients revealed that proton pump inhibitors and calcium antagonist were commonly prescribed to patients treated with DAAs (13.5 and 13.3%, respectively), roughly corresponding to the results of the overall chronic HCV population [see Table 3 & Additional file 1: Table S1]. Because of our strict definition of co-medications, our results probably reflect the medications used for chronic conditions, meaning that these medications may be difficult to stop or substitute. To select the optimal DAA treatment for chronic HCV patients, physicians should pay careful attention to the long-term use of these medications in their patients.

Even short-term use of other medications can influence DAA treatment. However, patients may not always inform their physicians about short-term use of medications, probably because they are not aware of the risks for DDIs. This study also examined short-term use of medications, and found that proton pump inhibitors, antacids, and calcium antagonists were used by about 25–30% of chronic HCV patients. Other classes of medications with potential DDIs with DAAs, such as analgesics, diuretics, and sedatives were also used by many chronic HCV patients [see Additional file 2: Table S2] [24, 25]. These results reinforce the need for physicians to have an exact knowledge of medication profiles of chronic HCV patients to avoid or manage DDIs. When initiating a DAA treatment, physicians may need to consider appropriate action for the management of DDIs, such as discontinuation, dose change, use of alternative medications, and increased monitoring of patients [23].

This study has several limitations. First, the generalisability of its results may be limited because the hospitals included in the database are only those with advanced medical care capabilities (e.g., acute care hospitals, general hospitals). The chronic HCV patients studied may therefore be "sicker" than other patients such as those treated at clinics. Likewise, the non-HCV patients may have severe medical conditions, which would influence the results. Second, the study has limitations inherent in the use of a pre-existing hospital claims database, such as misclassification owing to incorrectly recorded or missing data. For example, the diagnosis of chronic

HCV infection was based on the diagnosis record and its accuracy might vary from hospital to hospital. Patients may have received other medications for other comorbidities at different hospitals, but this could not be traced. The lack of data on the time of HCV clearance in patients may have resulted in under- or overestimation of comorbidities. The low prevalence of HCV-related cirrhosis among chronic HCV patients may also be attributed in part to underestimation stemming from limitations of the database (i.e., miscoding, lack of data). However, this may also be explained by the difficulty of correct diagnosis of cirrhosis, which requires biopsy. Whereas patients usually undergo biopsy when they start HCV treatment, most of our chronic HCV patients were untreated, implying that not many patients who were likely to receive a correct diagnosis of HCV-related cirrhosis were included. Third, we set strict definitions to identify the chronic comorbidities and co-medications most likely to have been used to treat chronic conditions, which may have resulted in underestimation of both comorbidities and co-medications because patients may not constantly visit the hospital. Fourth, we examined ten relevant systemic diseases, but these are not comprehensive. Investigation of other extrahepatic manifestations is needed for a more comprehensive understanding of systemic manifestations in chronic HCV patients in Japan [see Additional file 3: Table S3 for additional data of additional extrahepatic manifestations of chronic HCV infection]. Finally, this study was unable to investigate any causal relationships between the results and chronic HCV infection or DAA treatment because the comorbidities and co-medications were not examined against the timing of diagnosis or treatment. Further studies may shed light on these relationships.

Conclusions

In the present study in Japan, patients with chronic HCV had more comorbidities than those without HCV regardless of age. In particular, older chronic HCV patients commonly had multiple comorbidities and used more co-medications. The results suggest the difficulty of managing chronic HCV patients in Japan, especially older patients constituting the majority of the HCV patient population in Japan, because of the potential for DDIs. To provide optimal DAA treatment for this older patient population, it is important for physicians to closely monitor their medication profiles and take appropriate action to manage DDIs.

Additional files

Additional file 1: Table S1. Common co-medications in treated and non-treated chronic HCV patients. Description of data: The proportions of patients who received common co-medications in treated chronic HCV patients (including patients treated with DAAs and patients treated with peginterferon plus ribavirin) and non-treated chronic HCV patients are summarised. (DOCX 17 kb)

Additional file 2: Table S2. Non-HCV-related medications prescribed at least once during the study period by age group. Description of data: The proportions of patients who received non-HCV-related medications at least once during the study period are summarised by age for both chronic HCV patients and non-HCV patients. (XLSX 184 kb)

Additional file 3: Table S3. Prevalence of other extrahepatic manifestations of chronic HCV infection. Description of data: Prevalence of additional extrahepatic manifestations that were not included in the analysis of 10 relevant systemic diseases in patients with or without chronic HCV. (DOCX 17 kb)

Abbreviations

ATC codes: The EphMRA Anatomical classification system codes; DAA: Direct-acting anti-viral agent; DDI: Drug–drug interaction; HBV: Hepatitis B virus; HCV: Hepatitis C virus; ICD-10: The International Statistical Classification of Diseases and Related Health Problems 10th Revision

Acknowledgements

Medical writing and statistical supports were provided by Clinical Study Support, Inc. The contents of this study were presented at the 27th Annual Conference of APASL in New Delhi, India, on March 14–18, 2018.

Funding

The study was funded by MSD K.K. MSD K.K. had no role in the data collection, but was involved in the study design, data analysis, and preparation of the manuscript.

Authors' contributions

DJR, JT, GF, and TK contributed to the conception and design of the study. GF contributed to the data analysis, and DJR, JT, GF, and TK contributed to the data interpretation. DJR was involved in drafting of the manuscript, and DJR, JT, GF, and TK revised it critically. All authors read and approved the final version of the manuscript.

Ethics approval and consent to participate

This was an observational study using de-identified medical claims data. Because the Japanese Ethical Guidelines for Medical and Health Research Involving Human Subjects (http://www.mhlw.go.jp/file/06-Seisakujouhou-10600000-Daijinkanboukouseikagakuka/0000153339.pdf) do not apply to studies exclusively using de-identified data, we were not obligated to apply for an ethical approval for this study and to obtain informed consent in this study.

Competing interests

DJR, JT, and GF are employed by MSD K.K. TK has no competing interests to declare on this work.

Author details

[1]Medical Affairs, MSD K.K, Kitanomaru Square, 1-13-12 Kudan-kita, Chiyoda-ku, Tokyo 102-8667, Japan. [2]Biostatistics and Research Decision Sciences, MSD K.K, Kitanomaru Square, 1-13-12 Kudan-kita, Chiyoda-ku, Tokyo 102-8667, Japan. [3]The Research Center for Hepatitis and Immunology Department of Liver Disease, National Center for Global Health and Medicine, 1-7-1 Kohnodai, Ichikawa, Chiba 272-8516, Japan.

References

1. Toshikuni N. Therapy with direct-acting antiviral agents for hepatitis C-related liver cirrhosis. Gut Liver. 2016; https://doi.org/10.5009/gnl15458.
2. Schinazi R, Halfon P, Marcellin P, Asselah T. HCV direct-acting antiviral agents: the best interferon-free combinations. Liver Int. 2014;34:69–78.
3. Maasoumy B, Port K, Calle Serrano B, Markova AA, Sollik L, Manns MP, et al. The clinical significance of drug-drug interactions in the era of direct-acting anti-viral agents against chronic hepatitis C. Aliment Pharmacol Ther. 2013;38:1365–72.
4. Zampino R, Marrone A, Restivo L, Guerrera B, Sellitto A, Rinaldi L, et al. Chronic HCV infection and inflammation: clinical impact on hepatic and extra-hepatic manifestations. World J Hepatol. 2013;5:528–40.
5. Tang L, Marcell L, Kottilil S. Systemic manifestations of hepatitis C infection. Infect Agents Cancer. 2016;11:29.
6. Shepard CW, Finelli L, Alter MJ. Global epidemiology of hepatitis C virus infection. Lancet Infect Dis. 2005;5:558–67.
7. Chen SL, Morgan TR. The natural history of hepatitis C virus (HCV) infection. Int J Med Sci. 2006;3:47–52.
8. Lee MH, Yang HI, Lu SN, Jen CL, You SL, Wang LY, et al. Chronic hepatitis C virus infection increases mortality from hepatic and extrahepatic diseases: a community-based long-term prospective study. J Infect Dis. 2012;206:469–77.
9. Lauffenburger JC, Mayer CL, Hawke RL, Brouwer KL, Fried MW, Farley JF. Medication use and medical comorbidity in patients with chronic hepatitis C from a US commercial claims database: high utilization of drugs with interaction potential. Eur J Gastroenterol Hepatol. 2014;26:1073–82.
10. Vespasiani-Gentilucci U, Galati G, Gallo P, De Vincentis A, Riva E, Picardi A. Hepatitis C treatment in the elderly: new possibilities and controversies towards interferon-free regimens. World J Gastroenterol. 2015;21:7412–26.
11. Louie KS, St Laurent S, Forssen UM, Mundy LM, Pimenta JM. The high comorbidity burden of the hepatitis C virus infected population in the United States. BMC Infect Dis. 2012;12:86.
12. Alter MJ. Epidemiology of hepatitis C virus infection. World J Gastroenterol. 2007;13:2436–41.
13. Kamae I, Kumada H, Kobayashi M, Ward T, Webster S, Yuan Y, et al. Epidemiology, treatment and health economics of hepatitis C in Japan (Review). Kanzo. 2014;55:589–603. Japanese
14. Karino Y. Innovation in hepatitis C treatment. J Japan Assoc Rural Med. 2016;65:129–35. Japanese
15. Chung H, Ueda T, Kudo M. Changing trends in hepatitis C infection over the past 50 years in Japan. Intervirology. 2010;53:39–43.
16. International Statistical Classification of Diseases and Related Health Problems 10th Revision. http://apps.who.int/classifications/icd10/browse/2016/en. Accessed 24 May 2017.
17. EphMRA. EphMRA Anatomical Classification Guidelines. https://www.ephmra.org/media/1090/atcguidelines2016final.pdf. Accessed 24 May 2017.
18. Guaraldi G, Orlando G, Zona S, Menozzi M, Carli F, Garlassi E, et al. Premature age-related comorbidities among HIV-infected persons compared with the general population. Clin Infect Dis. 2011;53:1120–6.
19. Schouten J, Wit FW, Stolte IG, Kootstra NA, van der Valk M, Geerlings SE, et al. Cross-sectional comparison of the prevalence of age-associated comorbidities and their risk factors between HIV-infected and uninfected individuals: the AGEhIV cohort study. Clin Infect Dis. 2014;59:1787–97.
20. Höner Zu Siederdissen C, Maasoumy B, Marra F, Deterding K, Port K, Manns MP, et al. Drug-drug interactions with novel all oral interferon-free antiviral agents in a large real-world cohort. Clin Infect Dis. 2016;62:561–7.
21. Kondili LA, Gaeta GB, Ieluzzi D, Zignego AL, Monti M, Gori A, et al. Real-life data on potential drug-drug interactions in patients with chronic hepatitis C viral infection undergoing antiviral therapy with interferon-free DAAs in the PITER Cohort Study. PLoS One. 2017;12:e0172159.
22. Dick TB, Lindberg LS, Ramirez DD, Charlton MR. A clinician's guide to drug-drug interactions with direct-acting antiviral agents for the treatment of hepatitis C viral infection. Hepatology. 2016;63:634–43.
23. Langness JA, Nguyen M, Wieland A, Everson GT, Kiser JJ. Optimizing hepatitis C virus treatment through pharmacist interventions: identification and management of drug-drug interactions. World J Gastroenterol. 2017;23:1618–26.
24. Burger D, Back D, Buggisch P, Buti M, Craxí A, Foster G, et al. Clinical management of drug-drug interactions in HCV therapy: challenges and solutions. J Hepatol. 2013;58:792–800.

21

Co-infection of *Schistosoma mansoni*/hepatitis C virus and their associated factors among adult individuals living in fishing villages, north-western Tanzania

Humphrey D. Mazigo[1*], Stella Kepha[2], Godfrey M. Kaatano[3] and Safari M. Kinung'hi[3]

Abstract

Background: *Schistosoma mansoni* and Hepatitis C virus (HCV) are co-existence in sub-Saharan Africa and co-infection is common among humans population. The immunological responses characterized with Th_2-immune responses for *S. mansoni* and Th_1-immune responses for HCV are responsible for development hepatic morbidities in infected individuals. However, the co-occurrences of *S. mansoni* and HCV infection, their related ultrasound detectable morbidities and associated risk factors at community levels have not been examined in fishing communities, north-western Tanzania. In this context, the present study covers that gap.

Methods: A cross-sectional study was conducted among 1924 asymptomatic individuals aged 15–55 years in four fishing villages (Igombe, Igalagala, Sangabuye and Kayenze) of Northwestern Tanzania. A single stool sample was collected from each study participants and examined for *S. mansoni* eggs using Kato Katz technique. Hepatitis C surface antigen (HCVsAg) was determined from a finger prick blood sample using a rapid test.

Results: Overall, 51.8% (997/1924; 95%CI: 49.6–54.1) of the study participants were infected with *S. mansoni* and had a mean intensity of 223.7epg (95%; 202.4–247.1). Of the study participants, 90 (4.7%) were infected with hepatitis C virus (HCV). Overall, 2. 4% (47/1924) of the study participants were co-infected with *S. mansoni* and hepatitis C virus. Among the co-infected individuals, 42.6%, 70.2% and 19.1% had splenomegaly, hepatomegaly and periportal fibrosis (PPF). Factors associated with *S. mansoni*/HCV co-infection were being aged 26–35 years (aRR = 2. 67, 95%CI: 1.03–6.93, $P < 0.04$), 46–55 years (aRR = 2.89, 95%CI: 1.10–7.57, $P < 0.03$) and having marked hepatomegaly (aRR = 2.32, 95%CI: 1.09–4.9, $P < 0.03$).

Conclusion: In this setting, *S. mansoni* and Hepatitis C are co-endemic and a proportion of individuals were co-infected. Hepatosplenic morbidities characterized with hepatomegaly, splenomegaly, hepatosplenomegaly and PPF were observed in co-infected individuals. These results highlight the need for integrated interventions measures against parasitic and viral diseases.

Keywords: *S. mansoni*, Hepatitis C, Co-infection, Hepatomegaly, Splenomegaly, Periportal fibrosis, Fishing village, Tanzania

* Correspondence: humphreymazigo@gmail.com
[1]Department of Medical Parasitology and Entomology, School of Medicine, Catholic University of Health and Allied Sciences, P.O. Box 1464, Mwanza, Tanzania
Full list of author information is available at the end of the article

Background

Intestinal schistosomiasis caused by *Schistosoma mansoni* infection remains one of the public health concerns in Tanzania [1]. This infection is highly endemic in fishing villages bordering the southern shore and islands within the Lake Victoria [1–3]. One third of the estimated 44 million Tanzanian populations are estimated to be infected with *S. mansoni* [1, 4]. Chronic *S. mansoni* infection is mainly associated with deposition of eggs of the parasites in human body tissues especially the liver [5, 6]. Immunological responses against trapped eggs are responsible for the development of granulomas, chronic exposure to which may end with development of hepatosplenic schistosomiasis [5, 6]. Hepatosplenic morbidities are characterized by hepatic and splenic enlargement, progressive periportal fibrosis (PPF) which can lead to portal hypertension and its associated sequelae such as liver surface irregularities and portal-systemic venous, with the risk of esophageal varices and haemetemesis [5–7].

Conversely, hepatitis C virus (HCV) infection is endemic in sub-Saharan Africa and its prevalence varies from one epidemiological setting to another [8, 9]. Worldwide, 185 million individuals are estimated to be infected with HCV based on antibodies testing, with the highest prevalence observed in Asia and Middle East [10]. In sub-Saharan Africa, the prevalence of HCV infection ranges from 1% in Ethiopia to 50% in Egypt [10, 11]. It is estimated that, 70% of the individuals infected with HCV go on to develop chronic hepatitis and an approximate of 15–20% of them develop cirrhosis [12, 13].

Because of co-endemicity of *S. mansoni* and HCV infection in sub-Saharan Africa, co-infection does occur, especially in areas where intestinal schistosomiasis is highly endemic [9, 14, 15]. The pathogenesis of *S. mansoni* and HCV in co-infected individuals on liver fibrosis is well established [5, 11–13]. However, the pathomechanism of the two infections differs by the fact that *S. mansoni* immunological responses are mainly characterized by Th_2-$CD4^+$ type immune responses [5]; whereas for HCV infection, a type 1 Th_1-$CD8^+$ like responses is thought to play role in hepatic inflammatory responses and viral clearance [16]. Because of the immunological differences, the characteristics of hepatic damage resulting from the two infections also differs [5, 12, 13], with HCV infection causing advanced liver disease, increased incidence of liver cirrhosis and hepatocellular carcinoma [12, 13, 16].

In Tanzania, *S. mansoni* [1] and HCV infections [17–19] are co-endemic. It is estimated that 52% of the Tanzanian population are infected with schistosomiasis (both *S. mansoni* and *S. haematobium*) [4]. In Tanzania, *S. haematobium* is widely distributed, whereas *S. mansoni* is mainly restricted to large water bodies and paddy farming areas [20]. *Schistosoma mansoni* is common in areas surrounding the Lake Victoria shores and islands within the lake [2, 21, 22]. To date, there are no data on the national prevalence of HCV infection and information from the global burden of diseases indicate that, the annual mortality rate per 100,000 people from Hepatitis C in Tanzania has increased by 17.4% since 1990, an average of 0.8% a year [23]. Despite the fact that the two infections are co-endemic in the country, no community study has studied their co-occurrences and their related morbidities, especially in fishing communities. To justify the public health aspects of integrating interventions measures against parasitic and viral diseases at community level, the aim of the present study was to determine the prevalence of *S. mansoni* and hepatitis C co-infections, related hepatosplenic morbidities and associated risk factors among study participants.

Methods

Study area

The current data are from the secondary analysis of the study that was conducted in northwestern Tanzania [7, 24]. Briefly, the study was conducted in fishing villages of Ilemela district, including the villages of Igombe, Igalagala, Sangabuye and Kayenze bordering the Lake Victoria shore on the southern part at Ilemela district, Mwanza region (32-34°E and 2-4^{0}S, north-western Tanzania. The area experiences a temperature range from 18 °C to 28 °C and the mean annual rainfall of 1068 mm. The majority of the inhabitants of these villages are involved in farming and fishing activities. Because of high water contact levels, inhabitants remain at high risk of being infected with *S. mansoni* [2]. The control of *S. mansoni* infection in the study area involves mass chemotherapy using praziquantel drug, which is mainly focused in school children to reduce the long-term morbidities associated with the infection. There is no any program focusing on HCV control, screening and treatment at community.

Study design, inclusion and exclusion criteria

This was an analytical cross-sectional study conducted between September 2012 – December 2012 and the data presented in current work are secondary analysis of the work published elsewhere [7, 24]. The study included participants (i) aged 15–55 years old and (ii) lived in the study villages for more than 2 years (iii) with no history of HCV infection. Study participants with history of treatment against *S. mansoni* infection (praziquantel drug) in the past 6 month, on anti-HCV treatment and clinical diagnosed with HCV infection (advised to seek medical care at the district hospital) were excluded from the study.

Sample size, sampling technique and recruitment

Sample size calculation and sampling procedures have been previously described in details in Mazigo et al.,. [24]. Briefly, a total of 2142 study participants were enrolled into the study of which 1924 were eligible for the final analysis after fulfilling inclusion criteria. A two-step sampling procedures was used to select households and household members to participate in the study. A list of households and household members was obtained and from this, a random sampling procedure was used to select eligible individuals from randomly selected households.

Data collection

Parasitological examination of stool for Schistosoma mansoni and S. haematobium eggs

A single stool and urine samples was collected from all consented study participants using labeled clean containers. From the stool sample, four Kato Katz thick smears were prepared from different sites of each stool sample using a template of 41.7 mg (Vestergaard Frandsen, Lausanne, Switzerland), following a standard protocol [25]. In brief, four Kato-Katz thick smears were prepared on microscope slides and labeled with a participant identification number. After 24 h, the smears were examined for *S. mansoni* eggs independently by two experienced laboratory technician at the laboratory of the National Institute for Medical Research, Mwanza. The number of eggs for *S. mansoni* were counted and recorded separately in the prepared parasitological forms. For quality assurance, a random sample of 10% of the negative and positive Kato Katz thick smears were re-examined by a third technician. For diagnosis of *S. haematobium* infection, collected urine samples were examined grossly for presence of macrohaematuria and using Hemastrix dipstick for presence of microhaematuria. Then, all urine samples were further examined using urine filtration technique with Nuclepore® membrane according to WHO [26].

Examination of hepatitis-C virus infection

For diagnosis of hepatitis- C virus infection, the finger prick blood sample was collected from each study participants and used for screening of hepatitis-C infection using a qualitative rapid test for detection of hepatitis C antigen in whole blood, (ACON Laboratories, Inc., San Diego, CA) according to manufacturer's instructions at the field site laboratory [27]. Briefly, a drop of blood sample was added in the test strip followed by drop of the provided buffer. The results of the test were read after 15–20 min. The test was regarded as positive if the control and test line appeared after the given time. The test was regarded negative if only a single control line appeared.

Screening for human immunodeficiency Virus-1

The Tanzanian National HIV algorithms which recommended (currently has been revised) the use of a rapid test Determine (Alere Determine, Chiba, Japan) and Uni-GOLD (Trinity Biotech PLV, Bray, Ireland) was used for HIV diagnosis. Participants were counseled before and after HIV testing as per recommendation [28].

Ultrasonographical examination of hepatosplenic morbidities

All study participants were examined clinically for presence of any organomegally (enlargement of the liver and spleen) [29]. Two medically personnel trained on Niamey protocol examined study participants using a portable ultrasound machine (Aloka, Tokyo) [30]. Identified pathology was classified as per modified Niamey protocol [30]. The liver texture patterns, peripheral portal branches (PPBs), periportal fibrosis (PPF), thickness of PPB walls, spleen size, splenic vein (SV) diameter and ascites were assessed. Periportal fibrosis (PPF) was defined according to WHO [15] and the degree of PPF was categorized as A, B, C, D, E and F [30]. Periportal fibrosis grade A and B were classified as normal.

Data analysis

A CSPro system was used for double data entry and data analysis was performed using Stata Version 12 (Stata Corp, college station, Texas, USA). Categorical variables were summarized by numbers and percentages. Comparison of proportions/categorical variables was done using chi-square (χ^2)/fisher exact where appropriate. For continuous variables descriptive statistics were reported as means with standard deviation for normally distributed variable and medians with interquartile ranges (IQR) for variables that were not normally distributed. The arithmetic mean of *S. mansoni* egg counts for each participant was calculated from the counts of four Kato Katz thick smears and multiplied by 24 to obtain individual eggs per gram of faeces. *Schistosoma mansoni* egg counts were logarithmically transformed to allow calculation of the geometric mean egg per gram of feaces (GM-epg), which was calculated as an antilog of the mean of the transformed egg counts. Geometric mean egg counts for *S. mansoni* between sex and age were compared using Student-t-test (two groups) or ANOVA (more than two groups). Intensity of infection was categorized according to WHO criteria as: 1–99 epg, 100–399 epg, ≥400 epg defined as low, moderate and heavy intensities of infection respectively [31].

The categorization of the ultrasound measurements was based on the Niamey protocol [30]. To identify factors associated with *S. mansoni*/HCV co-infection, binomial regression model was constructed. At bivariate analysis, factors with *P*-values of 0.2 were considered for multiple binomial regression analysis. Because PPF grades, splenomegaly and left liver lobe hepatomegaly were related, only left liver lobe hepatomegaly was considered for multiple binomial regressions. A *P*-value of <0.05 was considered significant.

Ethical consideration

Ethical approval was sought from the Research and Ethics Committees of Bugando University College of Health Sciences and Allied Sciences-Institutional Review Board, (BREC/001/32/2011). Ethical clearance was granted by the National Ethical Review Committee, National Institute for Medical Research, Tanzania. Swahili translated informed assent and consent forms were used to obtain children and adult participants' consent respectively. For illiterate individuals, a thumb print was used to sign the assent and consent forms after a clear description of the study objective was explained to them and accepted to participate.

Results

Demographic characteristics of the study participants

A total of 1924 study participants aged 15–55 years were enrolled into the present study (Fig. 1). Of these participants, 46.7% ($n = 899/1924$) and 53.3% ($n = 1025$) were male and female respectively. The mean age of the study participants was 32.75 ± 11.15 years. The main economic activities of the study participants were farming (72.5%, $n = 1396$), fishing (13.9%, $n = 268$) and small-scale business (13.5%, $n = 260$). Overall, 33.3% ($n = 638$) and 66.7% ($n = 1284$) of the study participants were illiterate and literate respectively. Table 1 shows demographic characteristics of the study participants.

Prevalence and intensity of *Schistosoma mansoni* infection

The overall prevalence of *S. mansoni* was 51.8% (997/1924, 95%CI: 49.6–54.1) with male in individuals having the highest prevalence compared to female individuals (44.1% versus 60.6%, $P < 0.001$) (Table 2). Similarly, the youngest age group (15–25 years) having the highest prevalence compared to older age groups ($\chi^2 = 77.0276$, $P < 0.001$). In relation to village of residence, study participants from Igalagala and Kayenze villages had the highest prevalence of *S. mansoni* infection than participants from other participating villages ($\chi^2 = 42.4633$, $P < 0.001$). Similarly, in relation to occupation, participants reported to be involved in fishing activities had the highest prevalence compared to study participants involved in farming and small scale business ($\chi^2 = 30.8409$, $P < 0.001$) (Table 2).

The overall, Geometrical mean egg per gram of feaces (GMepg) was 223.7(95%CI: 202.4–247.1, range: 24-30192epg), with male individuals having the highest infection intensity ($t = -4.7597$, $P < 0.001$). Similarly, the youngest age group had the highest infection intensity (F = 1.62, $P < 0.001$).

Seroprevalence of hepatitis C virus infection

The overall prevalence of Hepatitis C virus (HCV) infection was 4.7% (90/1924, 95%CI: 3.7–5.7). There was no sex difference in prevalence of HCV ($\chi^2 = 0.0001$, $P = 0.99$) (Table 3). Age difference in prevalence of HCV infection was observed with the oldest age group having the highest prevalence ($\chi^2 = 25.0304$, $P < 0.001$). Similarly, study participants from Kayenze village recorded the highest prevalence of HCV infection compared to participants from other participating villages ($\chi^2 = 11.9520$, $P < 0.01$).

Co-infection of *Schistosoma mansoni* and hepatitis C virus

The overall prevalence of co-infection of *S. mansoni* and hepatitis C was 2.4% (47/1924). The overall GMepg of the study participants who were co-infected with *S. mansoni*/HCV infection was 206.95GMepg (95%CI: 128.4–333.6). Among the co-infected, a sex difference was observed with male individual's having the GMepg of 225.9epg (95%CI; 106.9–477.1) and for female individuals had GMepg of 188.9epg (95%CI: 98.9–360.6).

Hepatosplenic morbidities in *S. mansoni* and hepatitis C virus co-infected individuals

Among the study participants who were infected with hepatitis C virus ($n = 90$), 45.6% ($n = 41$) and 20% ($n = 18$) had enlarged and marked enlarged left liver lobe (left liver lobe hepatomegaly). For splenomegaly, 23.3%(21/90) and 10%(9/90) of the study participants had moderate and severely enlarged spleen. In relation to co-infection, study participants who were co-infected with *S. mansoni* and HCV ($n = 47$), 44.7% (21/47) and 25.5% (12/47) had moderate and marked enlarged left liver lobe. For the splenomegaly, 27.7% (13/47) and 14.9% (7/47) of the co-infected study participants had moderate and severely enlarged spleen. Similarly, 36.2% ($n = 17/47$) of the co-infected individuals had hepatosplenomegaly (enlarged both left liver lobe and spleen).

Overall, the prevalence of periportal fibrosis (PPF) among study participants infected with HCV was 15.6% (14/90) (PPF grades, C = 2, D = 11 and E-F = 1). For co-infected study participants (n = 47), 19.1% (9/47) had PPF (PPF grades, C = 1, D = 7 and E-F = 1).

Factors associated with *Schistosoma mansoni* and Hepatitis C virus co-infections

At bivariate analysis, age groups 26–35 years and 46–55 years, living at Kayenze village, having marked left liver lobe hepatomegaly, having splenomegaly and PPF grade D were associated with *S. mansoni*

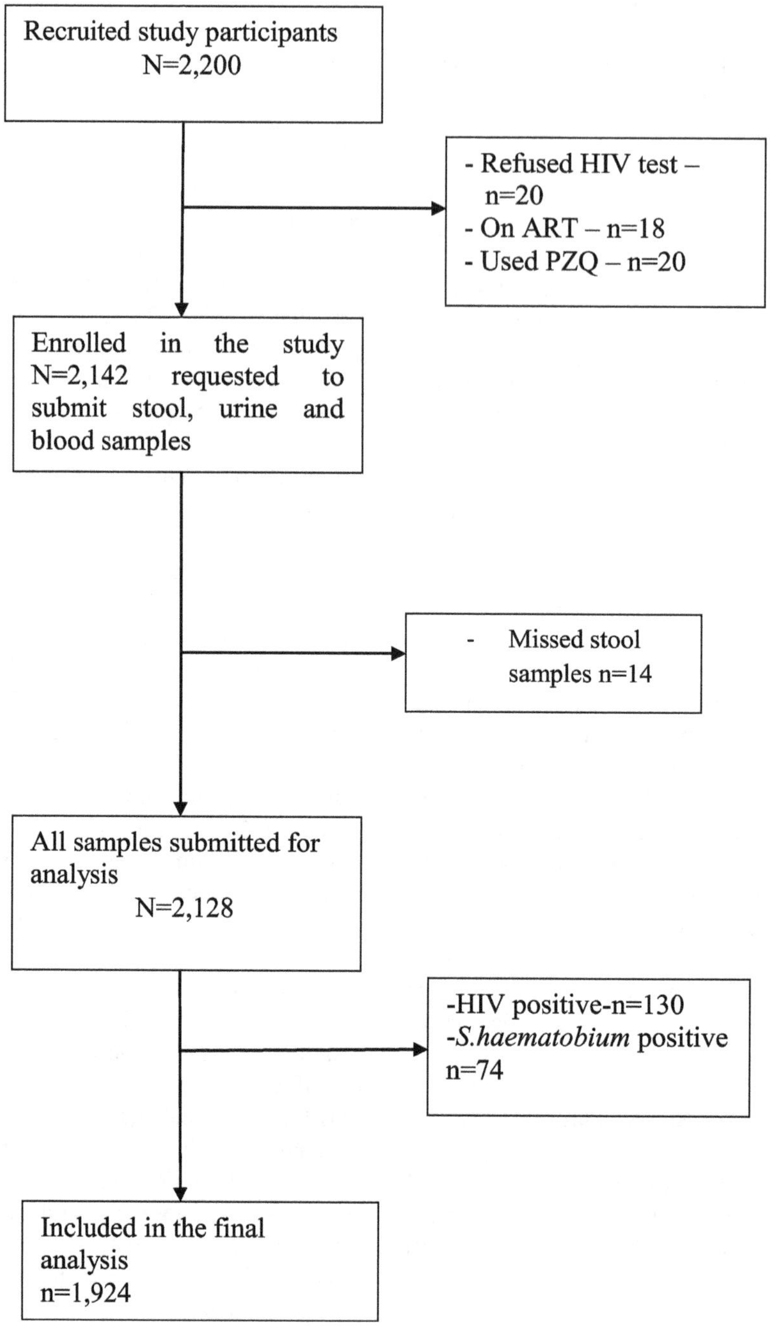

Fig. 1 Flow chart detailing participation and adherence of study participants in the study

and hepatitis C virus co-infection (Table 4). At multiple binomial regression analysis, belong to the age group 26–35 years (aRR = 2.67, 95%CI: 1.03–6.93, $P < 0.04$) and 46–55 years (aRR = 2.89, 95%CI: 1.10–7.57, $P < 0.03$), living at Kayenze village (aRR = 3.67,95%CI: 1.62–8.31, $P < 0.002$) and having marked hepatomegaly (aRR = 2.32,95%CI: 1.09–4.91, $P < 0.03$) remained independently associated with co-infection of *S. mansoni* and hepatitis C virus infections (Table 4).

Discussion

The findings of the present study on *S. mansoni* infection confirms the report of the previous reports in northwestern Tanzania [2, 3, 32], which demonstrated high prevalence of *S. mansoni* and infection intensity among adult population [2, 3]. Furthermore, our findings confirm high infection intensity among male individuals and young age groups [2, 3]. The variation in exposure to risk areas such as the lake and time spent in water

Table 1 Demographic characteristics of the study participants

Characteristics	N	Sex		χ^2	P-value
		Female n(%)	Male n(%)		
Age groups (in years)					
15–25	584	330(57.2)	250(43.1)	6.9748	0.01
26–35	553	272(49.2)	281(50.8)		
36–45	385	209(54.3)	176(45.7)		
46–55	402	212(52.7)	190(47.3)		
Village of residence					
Sangabuye	482	259(53.7)	223(46.3)	10.3077	0.02
Kayenze	708	378(53.4)	330(46.6)		
Igombe	456	262(57.5)	194(42.5)		
Igalagala	278	126(45.3)	152(54.7)		
Education level					
Literate	1284	614(47.8)	670(52.2)	52.4112	0.001
Illiterate	638	418(65.5)	220(34.5)		
Occupation					
Small scale business	260	187(71.9)	73(28.1)	291.1728	0.001
Farming	1396	827(59.2)	569(40.8)		
Fishing	268	22(8.0)	247(92.1)		

Table 2 Prevalence of *Schistosoma mansoni* in relation to demographic characteristics of the study participants

Characteristics	N	*Schistosoma mansoni*		χ^2	P-values
		Negative	Positive		
Sex					
Male	899	354(39.4)	545(60.6)	52.3860	0.001
Female	1025	573(55.9)	452(44.1)		
Age groups (in years)					
15–25	584	211(36.1)	373(63.9)	77.0276	0.001
26–35	553	253(45.7)	300(54.3)		
36–45	385	225(58.4)	260(41.6)		
46–55	402	242(60.2)	160(39.8)		
Village of residence					
Sangabuye	482	264(54.8)	218(45.2)	42.4633	0.001
Kayenze	708	290(40.9)	418(59.1)		
Igombe	456	259(56.8)	197(43.2)		
Igalagala	278	114(41.0)	164(58.9)		
Occupation					
Small scale business	260	142(54.6)	118(45.4)	30.8409	0.001
Farming	1396	712(51.0)	684(48.9)		
Fishing	268	196(35.8)	172(64.2)		

Table 3 Prevalence of hepatitis C virus in relation to demographic characteristics of the study participants

Characteristics	N	Hepatitis C virus infection		χ^2	P-value
		Negative	Positive		
Sex					
Male	1025	977(95.3)	48(4.7)	0.0001	0.99
Female	899	857(95.3)	42(4.7)		
Age groups (in years)					
15–25	584	575(98.5)	9(1.5)	25.0304	0.001
26–35	553	522(94.4)	31(5.6)		
36–45	385	368(95.6)	17(4.4)		
46–55	402	369(91.8)	33(8.2)		
Village of residence					
Sangabuye	482	462(95.9)	20(4.2)	11.9520	0.01
Kayenze	708	662(93.5)	46(6.5)		
Igombe	456	446(97.8)	10(2.2)		
Igalagala	278	264(94.9)	14(5.0)		

sources (lake) partly explain the observed differences in prevalence and infection intensity between sex and between age groups [33–35]. In addition, a noted difference in prevalence of *S. mansoni* infection between villages was observed. Partly, this observation is explained by geographical location of the villages from the Lake Victoria shores, with Kayenze and Igalagala villages are located at the shoreline of the lake [2]. The geographical variations of *S. mansoni* infection even in villages located in the same area have been noted elsewhere in Africa [6, 33, 35].

Our findings noted a low prevalence of HCV infection among adult population in fishing communities. Population based studies in health adult individuals have reported a prevalence of 0.7% of HCV infection in Dar Es Salaam [36] and 1.2% in Northwestern Tanzania based on antibodies detection using ELISA technique [18]. In special groups such as blood donors, lower prevalence of HCV infection (1.5%) was reported in Dar Es Salaam, Tanzania [19]. Similarly, a lower prevalence of HCV antibodies (1.2%) was reported among health workers [37]. In contrast, a high seroprevalence of HCV infection (57% based on HCV antibody) was reported among a cohort of opioid treatment patients in Dar Es Salaam, Tanzania [38]. Compared to findings from other African countries, a prevalence of 8.1% [39], 12.8% [40] and 13.7% [41] of anti-HCV infection has been reported in Angola Nigeria and Democratic Republic of Congo. The observed variation in prevalence among different groups mainly reflects different levels of exposure to risk factors [38]. Hepatitis C virus infection is transmitted predominantly through exposure to contaminated blood and body fluids, thus, groups of individuals with high

Table 4 Risk factors associated with *S. mansoni* and Hepatitis C virus infections among individuals living in fishing villages of northwestern Tanzania

Variable	cRR	95%CI	*P*-value	aRR	95%CI	*P*-value
Sex						
Female	1			1		
Male	1.66	0.9–2.9	0.1	1.45	0.8–2.7	0.24
Age groups (in years)						
15–25	1			1		
26–35	3.18	1.2–8.3	0.02	2.67	1.0–6.9	0.04
36–45	0.77	0.2–2.8	0.69	0.83	0.2–3.1	0.79
46–55	3.06	1.2–8.1	0.02	2.89	1.1–7.6	0.03[a]
Occupation						
Small scale business	1			1		
Farming	1.58	0.6–4.4	0.9	1.31	0.5–3.6	0.6
Fishing	2.93	0.9–9.4	0.1	1.89	0.6–6.3	0.3
Village of residence						
Sangabuye	1			1		
Kayenze	3.53	1.6–7.9	0.002	3.67	1.6–8.3	0.02[a]
Igombe	0.57	0.16 – 1.9	0.37	0.66	0.2–2.3	0.51
Igalagala	2.26	0.8–6.3	0.12	2.14	0.8–5.9	0.14
Education level						
Literate	1			–	–	–
Illiterate	1.18	0.66–2.0	0.58	–	–	–
Left liver lobe hepatomegaly						
Normal	1			1		
Moderate	1.60	0.8–3.1	0.16	1.79	0.9–3.5	0.1
Marked	2.26	1.1–4.8	0.03	2.32	1.1–4.9	0.03[a]
Splenomegaly						
Normal	1			–	–	–
Moderate	1.86	0.9–3.5	0.05	–	–	–
Marked	2.97	1.4–6.5	0.01	–	–	–
Periportal fibrosis (PPF) grades						
Normal	1					
Grade C	0.54	0.1–3.8	0.54	–	–	–
Grade D	2.39	1.1–5.1	0.03	–	–	–
Grade E & F	1.02	0.1–7.1	0.98	–	–	–

[a]Significant factors, *cRR* Crude Risk Ration, *aRR* Adjusted Risk Ratio

exposure to body fluids such as health workers and drug abusers always present with high prevalence of HCV infection [12, 38].

Our analysis on prevalence of HCV infection noted age difference in the prevalence of this viral infection. The older age groups (≥36 years) had the highest prevalence of HCV infection. The report of global burden of diseases indicates that hepatitis C virus infection is more common in the older age groups (75–79 years) in Tanzania [23]. This observation depicts the chronicity of the viral infection [12, 13]. Perhaps, the infection starts at young ages and its related morbidities and mortality are observed at older age groups [12].

In the present study a proportion of study participants were co-infected and had different patterns of hepatosplenic morbidities related to *S. mansoni* and Hepatitis C virus infection. Similar findings have been observed in endemic areas of sub-Saharan Africa, where both *S. mansoni* and HCV are co-endemic [8–10, 14]. However, the prevalence of co-infection of *S. mansoni* and HCV observed in the present study was comparable to findings of similar study in Ethiopia (4%) [15] and lower than what was observed in Egypt (33% and 40.2%) [42, 43]. Specifically, in Egypt, the prevalence of HCV is very high compared to many of the sub-Saharan African countries [8, 10], thus, co-infection of *S. mansoni* and HCV is also very high [8, 10]. It is worthwhile noting that, the present study used rapid diagnostic test to detected hepatitis C surface antigens (HCVsAg) which may have lower sensitivity than HCV antibodies detection methods used in previous studies [44]. Perhaps in these setting, the prevalence could be very high if HCV antibodies detection method could have been used. This is an open area calling for further studies using the more reliable diagnostic technique with improved sensitivity and preferably with a large sample size to establish the associated effects.

In the present study, study participants had hepatosplenic morbidities characterized by hepatic and splenic enlargements and periportal fibrosis characterized with different grades. Similar observations with different PPF grades and hepatosplenomegaly have been reported by previous studies [2, 3]. In co-infected individuals studies have shown that, *S. mansoni* infections increases HCV morbidities and chronicity of the liver pathology [45], increases HCV RNA titres, incidence of cirrhosis/hepatocellular carcinoma and higher mortality rates [45]. The effects of *S. mansoni* infection in HCV infected patients have been reviewed in details elsewhere [8]. However, the role of *S. mansoni* infection in exacerbating hepatic morbidities related to HCV infection remain a topic of debate, with other studies reporting no evidence that *S. mansoni* infection affect the outcome of HCV in infected individuals [46]. Given the low prevalence of HCV infection observed in the present study population, this HCV infection is likely to account for only a small proportion of chronic liver disease in the studied population. In addition, it is difficult to draw a solid conclusion on the role of *S. mansoni* infection in HCV co-infected patients in a study which had only 17 study participants who were co-infected and had hepatosplenic morbidities [45]. Large sample sizes will be needed in further studies to add more evidence.

The main risk factors associated with *S. mansoni*/ HCV infection were mainly being of older age group (46–55 years), village of residence and having left liver lobe hepatomegaly. The association of these infections with older ages indicates that, these are chronic infections, which needs time for their obvious related morbidities such as hepatomegaly and fibrosis/ liver cirrhosis to manifest [6, 12, 13]. The association with village of residence mainly defines the presence of exposure factors in these villages [7, 15]. Individually, epidemiological studies have shown that, *S. mansoni* infection is associated with village of residence, age, occupation, specifically fishing, being male and hepatosplenic morbidities [1, 6, 7, 47]. Older age groups, being male and residing in rural areas have been demonstrated to be associated with HCV infection [11].

The present study was subject to limitation, being a cross-sectional study in nature, partly may contribute to lack of temporal association between the *S. mansoni*/ HCV as the main outcomes with some of the study variables. Also, the use of only one diagnostic technique to diagnosed HCV infection (HCVsAg), partly, may have underestimated the prevalence of HCV infection in the study population. In addition, the use of a single stool sample to examine for *S. mansoni* infection owing the day to day variability of parasite eggs output and low sensitivity of the Kato Katz technique in detecting individuals with light infection intensity may have under estimated the prevalence of *S. mansoni* infection in the studied population.

Conclusion

The present study setting is endemic to *S. mansoni* and Hepatitis C virus infections and a small proportional of individuals are co-infected. *Schistosoma mansoni* related PPF grades, hepatomegaly, splenomegaly and hepatosplenomegaly were also present in co-infected individuals. Co-infection of *S. mansoni*/HCV was mainly associated with older age, village of residence and having hepatomegaly. Further studies are recommended in these areas to understanding the impact of *S. mansoni*/HCV co-infection before implementation of integrated interventions measures can be thought.

Abbreviations

ARR: Adjusted Risk Ratios; cRR: Crude Odd Ratio; Epg: Egg per Gram of Feaces; GMepg: Geometrical Mean egg per gram of feaces; HCV: Hepatitis C Virus; HCVsAg: Hepatitis C Virus surface antigen; Mg: Milligram; PPF: Periportal fibrosis; Th: Lymphocytes type T- helper

Acknowledgements

We thank the study participants from the study villages of Igombe, Igalagala, Sangabuye and Kayenze for their participation in the study, as well as school teachers and school children for their cooperation. We are grateful to the National Institute for Medical Research and Catholic University of Health Sciences for logistical support.

Funding

This work was supported by Training Health Researchers into Vocational Excellence in East Africa (THRiVE), grant number 087540 funded by the Wellcome Trust to HDM. Its contents are solely the responsibility of the authors and do not necessarily represent the official views of the supporting offices.

Authors' contributions

HDM and GMK designed the study, participated in data collection and analysis, and drafted the first version of the manuscript. HDM, SMK and SK participated in data analysis. All authors read and approved the final manuscript, contributed to the critical review and made substantial contribution to its content.

Ethics approval and consent to participate

Ethical approval was sought from the Research and Ethics Committees of Bugando University College of Health Sciences and Allied Sciences-Institutional Review Board, (BREC/001/32/2011). Ethical clearance was granted by the National Ethical Review Committee, National Institute for Medical Research, Tanzania. Swahili translated informed assent and consent forms were used to obtain children and adult participants' consent respectively. For illiterate individuals, a thumb print was used to sign the assent and consent forms after a clear description of the study objective was explained to them and accepted to participate.

Consent for publication

Not applicable.

Competing interests

The authors declare that they have no competing interests.

Author details

[1]Department of Medical Parasitology and Entomology, School of Medicine, Catholic University of Health and Allied Sciences, P.O. Box 1464, Mwanza, Tanzania. [2]Pwani University, Kilifi 195-80108, Kenya. [3]National Institute for Medical Research, Mwanza Research Centre, Mwanza, Tanzania.

References

1. Mazigo HD, Nuwaha F, Kinung'hi SM, Morona D, Pinot de Moira A, Wilson S, Heukelbach J, Dunne DW. Epidemiology and control of human schistosomiasis in Tanzania. Par Vect. 2012;5:274.
2. Malenganisho WL, Magnussen P, Friis H, Siza J, Kaatano G, Temu M, Vennervald BJ. Schistosoma mansoni morbidity among adults in two villages along Lake Victoria shores in Mwanza District, Tanzania. Trans R Soc Trop Med Hyg. 2008;102(6):532–41.
3. Kardorff R, Gabone RM, Mugashe C, Obiga D, Ramarokoto CE, Mahlert C, Spannbrucker N, Lang A, Gunzler V, Gryseels B, et al. Schistosoma mansoni-related morbidity on Ukerewe Island, Tanzania: clinical, ultrasonographical and biochemical parameters. Trop Med Int Health. 1997;2(3):230–9.
4. Rollinson D, Knopp S, Levitz S, Stothard JR, Tchuem Tchuente LA, Garba A, Mohammed KA, Schur N, Person B, Colley DG, et al. Time to set the agenda for schistosomiasis elimination. Acta Trop. 2013;128(2):423–40.
5. Dunne DW, Pearce EJ. Immunology of hepatosplenic schistosomiasis mansoni: a human perspective. Microbes Infect. 1999;1(7):553–60.
6. Booth M, Vennervald BJ, Kabatereine NB, Kazibwe F, Ouma JH, Kariuki CH, Muchiri E, Kadzo H, Ireri E, Kimani G, et al. Hepatosplenic morbidity in two neighbouring communities in Uganda with high levels of Schistosoma

mansoni infection but very different durations of residence. Trans R Soc Trop Med Hyg. 2004;98(2):125–36.
7. Mazigo HD, Dunne DW, Morona D, Lutufyo TE, Kinung'hi SM, Kaatano G, Nuwaha F. Periportal fibrosis, liver and spleen sizes among S. mansoni mono or co-infected individuals with human immunodeficiency virus-1 in fishing villages along Lake Victoria shores, North-Western, Tanzania. Parasit Vectors. 2015;8:260.
8. Gasim GI, Bella A, Adam I. Schistosomiasis, hepatitis B and hepatitis C co-infection. Virol J. 2015;12:19.
9. Kamal S. Progression of hepatitis C virus infection with and without schistosomiasis. National Academy of Sciences. 2004;
10. Hanafiah M, Groeger J, Flaxman AD, Wiersma ST. Global epidemiology of hepatitis C virus infection: new estimates of age-specific antibody to HCV seroprevalence. Hepatology. 2013;57:1333–42.
11. Van-Lume DS, Albuquerque Mde F, Souza AI, Domingues AL, Lopes EP, Morais CN, Montenegro SM. Association between Schistosomiasis mansoni and hepatitis C: systematic review. Rev Saude Publica. 2013;47(2):414–24.
12. Seeff LB. Natural history of hepatitis C. Hepatology. 1997;26(3 Suppl 1): 21S–8S.
13. Seeff LB. The natural history of chronic hepatitis C virus infection. Clin Liver Dis. 1997;1(3):587–602.
14. Blanton RE, Salam EA, Kariuki HC, Magak P, Silva LK, Muchiri EM, Thiongo F, Abdel-Meghid IE, Butterworth AE, Reis MG, et al. Population-based differences in Schistosoma mansoni- and hepatitis C-induced disease. J Infect Dis. 2002;185(11):1644–9.
15. Berhe N, Myrvang B, Gundersen SG. Intensity of Schistosoma mansoni, hepatitis B, age, and sex predict levels of hepatic periportal thickening/ fibrosis (PPT/F): a large-scale community-based study in Ethiopia. Am J Trop Med Hyg. 2007;77(6):1079–86.
16. Sobue S, Nomura T, Ishikawa T, Ito S, Saso K, Ohara H, Joh T, Itoh M, Kakumu S. Th1/Th2 cytokine profiles and their relationship to clinical features in patients with chronic hepatitis C virus infection. J Gastroenterol. 2001;36(8):544–51.
17. Miller WC, Shao JF, Weaver DJ, Shimokura GH, Paul DA, Lallinger GJ. Seroprevalence of viral hepatitis in Tanzanian adults. Tropical Medicine and Internationa Health. 1998;3(9):757–63.
18. Tess BH, Levin A, Brubaker G, Shao J, Drummond JE, Alter HJ, O'Brien TR. Seroprevalence of hepatitis C virus in the general population of northwest Tanzania. Am J Trop Med Hyg. 2000;62(1):138–41.
19. Matee MI, Magesa PM, Lyamuya EF. Seroprevalence of human immunodeficiency virus, hepatitis B and C viruses and syphilis infections among blood donors at the Muhimbili National Hospital in Dar es Salaam, Tanzania. BMC Public Health. 2006;6:21.
20. Lwambo NJ, Siza JE, Brooker S, Bundy DA, Guyatt H. Patterns of concurrent hookworm infection and schistosomiasis in schoolchildren in Tanzania. Trans R Soc Trop Med Hyg. 1999;93(5):497–502.
21. Mugono M, Konje E, Kuhn S, Mpogoro FJ, Morona D, Mazigo HD. Intestinal schistosomiasis and geohelminths of Ukara Island, North-Western Tanzania: prevalence, intensity of infection and associated risk factors among school children. Parasit Vectors. 2014;7:612.
22. Kardorff R, Stelma FF, Vocke AK, Yazdanpanah Y, Thomas AK, Mbaye A, Talla I, Niang M, Ehrich JH, Doehring E, et al. Ultrasonography in a Senegalese community recently exposed to Schistosoma mansoni infection. Am J Trop Med Hyg. 1996;54(6):586–90.
23. Wiktor SZ, Hutin YJ. The global burden of viral hepatitis: better estimates to guide hepatitis elimination efforts. Lancet. 2016;388(10049):1030–1.
24. Mazigo HD, Dunne DW, Wilson S, Kinung'hi SM. Pinot de Moira A, Jones FM, Morona D, Nuwaha F: Co-infection with Schistosoma mansoni and Human Immunodeficiency Virus-1 (HIV-1) among residents of fishing villages of north-western Tanzania. Parasit Vectors. 2014;7:587.
25. Katz N, Chaves A, Pellegrino J. A simple device for quantitative stool thick-smear technique in Schistosomiasis mansoni. Rev Inst Med Trop Sao Paulo. 1972;14(6):397–400.
26. World Health Organization.: Basic laboratory methods in medical parasitology. 1991.
27. Ghany MG, Strader DB, Thomas DL, Seeff LB. Diagnosis, management, and treatment of hepatitis C: an update. Hepatology. 2009;49(4):1335–74.
28. Lyamuya EF, Aboud S, Urassa WK, Sufi J, Mbwana J, Ndugulile F, Massambu C. Evaluation of simple rapid HIV assays and development of national rapid HIV test algorithms in Dar es Salaam, Tanzania. BMC Infectious Diseases. 2009;9:19.
29. Vennervald BJ, Kenty L, Butterworth AE, Kariuki CH, Kadzo H, Ireri E, Amaganga C, Kimani G, Mwatha J, Otedo A, et al. Detailed clinical and ultrasound examination of children and adolescents in a Schistosoma mansoni endemic area in Kenya: hepatosplenic disease in the absence of portal fibrosis. Trop Med Int Health. 2004;9(4):461–70.
30. Richter J, Hatz C, Campagne G, Bergquist N, Jenkins JM: Ultrasound in schistosomiasis: a practical guide to the standard use of ultrasonography for assessment of schistosomiasis-related morbidity: Second international workshop, October 22–26 1996, Niamey, Niger. Tropical Diseases Research, World Health Organization, Geneva 2000.
31. World Health Organization.: Prevention and control of schistosomiasis and soil-transmitted helminthiasis. *World Health Organization technical report series* 2002, 912:i.
32. Mazigo HD, Nuwaha F, Kinung'hi SM, Morona D, Pinot de Moira A, Wilson S, Heukelbach J, Dunne DW. Epidemiology and control of human schistosomiasis in Tanzania. *Parasit Vect.* 2012;5:274.
33. Boisier P, Ramarokoto CE, Ravoniarimbinina P, Rabarijaona L, Ravaoalimalala V. Geographic differences in hepatosplenic complications of schistosomiasis mansoni and explanatory factors of morbidity. Tropical Med Int Health. 2001;6(9):699–706.
34. Barreto ML. Geographical and socioeconomic factors relating to the distribution of Schistosoma mansoni infection in an urban area of north-east Brazil. Bull World Health Organ. 1991;69(1):93–102.
35. Barakat R, Farghaly A, El Masry AG, El-Sayed MK, Hussein MH. The epidemiology of schistosomiasis in Egypt: patterns of Schistosoma mansoni infection and morbidity in Kafer El-Sheikh. Ame J Trop Med Hyg. 2000;62(2 Suppl):21–7.
36. Miller WC, Shao JF, Weaver DJ, Shimokura GH, Paul DA, Lallinger GJ. Seroprevalence of viral hepatitis in Tanzanian adults. Tropical Med Int Health. 1998;3(9):757–63.
37. Muller A, Stoetter L, Kallluvya S, Stich A, Majinge C, Weissbrich B, Kasang C: Prevalence of heaptitis B virus infection among health care workers in a tertiary hopsital in Tanzania. BMC Infectious Diseases 2015, 15(386).
38. Lambdin BH, Lorvick J, Mbwambo JK, Rwegasha J, Hassan S, Lum P, Kral AH. Prevalence and predictors of HCV among a cohort of opioid treatment patients in Dar es Salaam, Tanzania. Int J Drug Policy. 2017;45:64–9.
39. Guimaraes Nebenzahl H, Lopes A, Castro R, Pereira F. Prevalence of human immunodeficiency virus, hepatitis C virus,hepatitis B virus and syphillis among individuals attending anonymous testing for HIV in Luanda, Angola. S Afr Med J. 2013;103:186–8.
40. Oje OJ, Sule WF, Famurewa D. Dual positivity of hepatitis B surface antigen and anti-hepatitis C virus antibody and associated factors among apparently healthy patients of Ekiti State, Nigeria. Viral Immunol. 2012;25(6):448–55.
41. Iles JC, Abby Harrison GL, Lyons S, Djoko CF, Tamoufe U, Lebreton M, Schneider BS, Fair JN, Tshala FM, Kayembe PK, et al. Hepatitis C virus infections in the Democratic Republic of Congo exhibit a cohort effect. Infect Genet Evol. 2013;19:386–94.
42. Angelico M, Renganathan E, Gandin C, Fathy M, Profili MC, Refai W, De Santis A, Nagi A, Amin G, Capocaccia L, et al. Chronic liver disease in the Alexandria governorate, Egypt: contribution of schistosomiasis and hepatitis virus infections. J Hepatol. 1997;26(2):236–43.
43. el-Esnawy NA, Al-Herrawy AZ. Seroprevalence of certain hepatitis viruses among Egyptian workers infected with schistosomiasis. J Egypt Public Health Assoc. 2000;75(3–4):357–66.
44. Tsega E, Nordenfelt E, Hansson BG. Hepatitis C virus infection and chronic liver disease in Ethiopia where hepatitis B infection is hyperendemic. Trans R Soc Trop Med Hyg. 1995;89(2):171–4.
45. Kamal SM, Rasenack JW, Bianchi L, Al Tawil A, El Sayed KK, Peter T, Mansour H, Ezzat W, Koziel M. Acute hepatitis C without and with schistosomiasis: correlation with hepatitis C-specific CD4(+) T-cell and cytokine response. Gastroenterology. 2001;121(3):646–56.
46. Allam WR, Barakat A, Zakaria Z, Galal G, Abdel-Ghafar TS, El-Tabbakh M, Mikhail N, Waked I, Abdelwahab SF. Schistosomiasis does not affect the outcome of HCV infection in genotype 4-infected patients. Am J Trop Med Hyg. 2014;90(5):823–9.
47. Mazigo HD, Dunne DW, Wilson S, Kinung Hi SM, de Moira A, Jones FM, Morona D, Nuwaha F. Co-infection with Schistosoma mansoni and Human Immunodeficiency Virus-1 (HIV-1) among residents of fishing villages of north-western Tanzania. Parasites Vectors. 2014;7(1):587.

Permissions

All chapters in this book were first published in ID, by BioMed Central; hereby published with permission under the Creative Commons Attribution License or equivalent. Every chapter published in this book has been scrutinized by our experts. Their significance has been extensively debated. The topics covered herein carry significant findings which will fuel the growth of the discipline. They may even be implemented as practical applications or may be referred to as a beginning point for another development.

The contributors of this book come from diverse backgrounds, making this book a truly international effort. This book will bring forth new frontiers with its revolutionizing research information and detailed analysis of the nascent developments around the world.

We would like to thank all the contributing authors for lending their expertise to make the book truly unique. They have played a crucial role in the development of this book. Without their invaluable contributions this book wouldn't have been possible. They have made vital efforts to compile up to date information on the varied aspects of this subject to make this book a valuable addition to the collection of many professionals and students.

This book was conceptualized with the vision of imparting up-to-date information and advanced data in this field. To ensure the same, a matchless editorial board was set up. Every individual on the board went through rigorous rounds of assessment to prove their worth. After which they invested a large part of their time researching and compiling the most relevant data for our readers.

The editorial board has been involved in producing this book since its inception. They have spent rigorous hours researching and exploring the diverse topics which have resulted in the successful publishing of this book. They have passed on their knowledge of decades through this book. To expedite this challenging task, the publisher supported the team at every step. A small team of assistant editors was also appointed to further simplify the editing procedure and attain best results for the readers.

Apart from the editorial board, the designing team has also invested a significant amount of their time in understanding the subject and creating the most relevant covers. They scrutinized every image to scout for the most suitable representation of the subject and create an appropriate cover for the book.

The publishing team has been an ardent support to the editorial, designing and production team. Their endless efforts to recruit the best for this project, has resulted in the accomplishment of this book. They are a veteran in the field of academics and their pool of knowledge is as vast as their experience in printing. Their expertise and guidance has proved useful at every step. Their uncompromising quality standards have made this book an exceptional effort. Their encouragement from time to time has been an inspiration for everyone.

The publisher and the editorial board hope that this book will prove to be a valuable piece of knowledge for researchers, students, practitioners and scholars across the globe.

List of Contributors

Christina Greenaway
Division of Infectious Diseases, Jewish General Hospital, McGill University, 3755 Côte St. Catherine Road, Room E-0057, Montreal PQ H3T 1E2, Canada
Centre for Clinical Epidemiology, Lady Davis Research Institute for Medical Research, Jewish General Hospital, McGill University, Montreal, Canada

Viet Anh Tran and Claire Nour Abou Chakra
Centre for Clinical Epidemiology, Lady Davis Research Institute for Medical Research, Jewish General Hospital, McGill University, Montreal, Canada

Laurent Azoulay
Centre for Clinical Epidemiology, Lady Davis Research Institute for Medical Research, Jewish General Hospital, McGill University, Montreal, Canada
Department of Oncology, McGill University, Montreal, Canada

Robert Allard
Department of Oncology, McGill University, Montreal, Canada
Montreal Public Health Department, Montreal, Canada

Joseph Cox
Sexually Transmitted Infections Division, Montreal Public Health Department, Montreal, Canada

Russ Steele
Centre for Clinical Epidemiology, Lady Davis Research Institute for Medical Research, Jewish General Hospital, McGill University, Montreal, Canada
Department of Mathematics and Statistics, McGill University, Montreal, Canada

Marina Klein
Division of Infectious Diseases, McGill University Health Center, McGill University, Montreal, Canada

Elena Ivanova Reipold, Alessandra Trianni, Stefano Ongarello and Teri Roberts
FIND, MSF Access Campaign, Geneva, Switzerland

Claudia Denkinger
FIND, MSF Access Campaign, Geneva, Switzerland
Beth Israel Deaconess Medical Center, Harvard Medical School, Boston, MA, USA

Nivedha Panneer and Veronica Miller
Forum for Collaborative HIV Research, Washington D.C, USA

Douglas Krakower
Beth Israel Deaconess Medical Center, Harvard Medical School, Boston, MA, USA

Philippa Easterbrook
Global Hepatitis Programme, HIV Department, World Health Organization, Geneva, Switzerland

David C. Boettiger, Matthew G. Law, Gregory J. Dore, Rebecca Guy, Denton Callander and Gail Matthews
The Kirby Institute, UNSW Sydney, Sydney, NSW, Australia

Basil Donovan
The Kirby Institute, UNSW Sydney, Sydney, NSW, Australia
Sydney Sexual Health Centre, Sydney, NSW, Australia

Catherine C. O'Connor
The Kirby Institute, UNSW Sydney and Sexual Health Service, Sydney Local Health District, Sydney, NSW, Australia
Central Clinical School, Sydney University, Sydney, NSW, Australia

Christopher K. Fairley
Melbourne Sexual Health Centre, Alfred Health and Monash University, Melbourne, Victoria, Australia

Margaret Hellard
Viral Hepatitis Elimination Program, Burnet Institute, Melbourne, Victoria, Australia

A. M. Falla
Department of Public Health, Erasmus MC, University Medical Center Rotterdam, Rotterdam, the Netherlands
Division of Infectious Disease Control, Municipal Public Health Service Rotterdam-Rijnmond, 3000, LP, Rotterdam, The Netherlands

A. A. Ahmad
Department of Health Sciences, Hamburg University of Applied Sciences, Faculty Life Sciences / Public Health Research, Ulmenliet 20, 21033 Hamburg, Germany
Department of Internal Medicine, University Medical Center Hamburg-Eppendorf, Martinistr 52, 20246 Hamburg, Germany

E. Duffell and T. Noori
European Centre for Disease Prevention and Control, Granits väg 8, 171 65 Solna, Sweden

I. K. Veldhuijzen
Division of Infectious Disease Control, Municipal Public Health Service Rotterdam-Rijnmond, 3000, LP, Rotterdam, The Netherlands
Center for Infectious Disease Control, National Institute for Public Health and the Environment, Bilthoven, the Netherlands

Maria Pokorska-Śpiewak, Barbara Kowalik-Mikołajewska, Małgorzata Aniszewska, Magdalena Pluta and Magdalena Marczyńska
Department of Children's Infectious Diseases, Medical University of Warsaw, ul. Wolska 37, 01-201 Warsaw, Poland
Hospital of Infectious Diseases, ul.Wolska 37, 01-201 Warsaw, Poland

Kristel Kivimets
National Institute for Health Development, 42, 11619 Tallinn, Hiiu, Estonia

Anneli Uusküla
Department of Family Medicine and Public Health, University of Tartu, Ravila 19, 50411 Tartu, Estonia

Jeffrey V. Lazarus
Barcelona Institute for Global Health (ISGlobal), Hospital Clínic, University of Barcelona, Carrer de Casanova, 143, 08036 Barcelona, Spain
CHIP, Rigshospitalet, University of Copenhagen, Blegdamsvej 9, DK-2100 Copenhagen, Denmark

Kristi Ott
West Tallinn Central Hospital, Infectious Diseases Clinic, Paldiski maantee 68, 10617 Tallinn, Estonia

Caroline Manchiero, Arielle Karen da Silva Nunes, Mariana Carvalheiro Magri and Bianca Peixoto Dantas
Medical Research Laboratory for Virus (Laboratório de Investigação Médica por Vírus - LIM47) of the Clinics Hospital, School of Medicine, University of São Paulo (Universidade de São Paulo - USP), São Paulo, Brazil

Antonio Alci Barone and Fátima Mitiko Tengan
Medical Research Laboratory for Virus (Laboratório de Investigação Médica por Vírus - LIM47) of the Clinics Hospital, School of Medicine, University of São Paulo (Universidade de São Paulo - USP), São Paulo, Brazil
Department of Infectious and Parasitic Diseases, School of Medicine, University of São Paulo, São Paulo, Brazil

Celso Carmo Mazza
Department of Infectious and Parasitic Diseases, School of Medicine, University of São Paulo, São Paulo, Brazil

Cristina Aurora São Pedro Soeiro, Celina Andreia Melo Gonçalves, Marta Sofia Correia Marques, Maria Josefina Vazquez Méndez, Ana Paula Ribeiro Almeida Tavares, Ana Maria Lacerda Morgado Fernandes de Carvalho de Aboim Horta and Rui Manuel do Rosário Sarmento-Castro
Infectious Diseases Department, Centro Hospitalar do Porto, Largo do Prof. Abel Salazar, 4099-001 Porto, Portugal

Weiming Tang
University of North Carolina Project-China, No. 2 Lujing Road, Guangzhou 510095, China
Guangdong Provincial Dermatology Hospital (Dermatology Hospital, Southern Medical University), Guangzhou, China
SESH Global, Guangzhou, China
School of Medicine, University of North Carolina at Chapel Hill, Chapel Hill, NC, USA

Joseph D. Tucker
University of North Carolina Project-China, No. 2 Lujing Road, Guangzhou 510095, China
SESH Global, Guangzhou, China
School of Medicine, University of North Carolina at Chapel Hill, Chapel Hill, NC, USA
London School of Hygiene and Tropical Medicine, Keppel St, London, UK

Wen Chen
School of Public Health, Sun Yat-sen University, Guangzhou, China
Center for Migrant Health Policy, Sun Yat-sen University, Guangzhou, China

Ali Amini, Debi Boeras, Jane Falconer, Helen Kelly, Rosanna Peeling and Olivia Varsaneux
London School of Hygiene and Tropical Medicine, Keppel St, London, UK

Philippa Easterbrook
Global Hepatitis Programme, HIV Department, World Health Organization, Geneva, Switzerland

Ngoc Nghiem My
Oxford University Clinical Research Unit, Vietnam Wellcome Trust Major Overseas Programme, 764 Vo Van Kiet, District 5, Ho Chi Minh City, Vietnam

Alessandra Berto, Jeremy Day and Guy E. Thwaites
Oxford University Clinical Research Unit, Vietnam Wellcome Trust Major Overseas Programme, 764 Vo Van Kiet, District 5, Ho Chi Minh City, Vietnam
Centre for Tropical Medicine and Global Health, Nuffield Department of Clinical Medicine, University of Oxford, Oxford, UK

Nguyen Van Vinh Chau
Hospital for Tropical Diseases, Ho Chi Minh City, Vietnam

Stephen Baker
Oxford University Clinical Research Unit, Vietnam Wellcome Trust Major Overseas Programme, 764 Vo Van Kiet, District 5, Ho Chi Minh City, Vietnam
Centre for Tropical Medicine and Global Health, Nuffield Department of Clinical Medicine, University of Oxford, Oxford, UK
The London School of Hygiene and Tropical Medicine, London, UK

Thomas C. Darton
Oxford University Clinical Research Unit, Vietnam Wellcome Trust Major Overseas Programme, 764 Vo Van Kiet, District 5, Ho Chi Minh City, Vietnam
Department of Infection, Immunity and Cardiovascular Disease, University of Sheffield, Sheffield, UK

Emily Adland
Department of Paediatrics, Peter Medawar Building for Pathogen Research, South Parks Road, Oxford OX1 3SY, UK

Gerald Jesuthasan, Louise Downs, Monique Andersson and Katie Jeffery
Department of Infectious Diseases and Microbiology, John Radcliffe Hospital, Headley Way, Headington, Oxford OX3 9DU, UK

Philippa C. Matthews
Department of Infectious Diseases and Microbiology, John Radcliffe Hospital, Headley Way, Headington, Oxford OX3 9DU, UK
Nuffield Department of Medicine, Peter Medawar Building for Pathogen Research, South Parks Road, Oxford OX1 3SY, UK

Paul Klenerman
Department of Infectious Diseases and Microbiology, John Radcliffe Hospital, Headley Way, Headington, Oxford OX3 9DU, UK
Department of Hepatology, John Radcliffe Hospital, Headley Way, Headington, Oxford OX3 9DU, UK
Nuffield Department of Medicine, Peter Medawar Building for Pathogen Research, South Parks Road, Oxford OX1 3SY, UK
Oxford NIHR Biomedical Research Centre, John Radcliffe Hospital, Headley Way, Headington, Oxford OX3 9DU, UK

Victoria Wharton, Gemma Wilde and Jane Collier
Department of Hepatology, John Radcliffe Hospital, Headley Way, Headington, Oxford OX3 9DU, UK

Anna L. McNaughton
Nuffield Department of Medicine, Peter Medawar Building for Pathogen Research, South Parks Road, Oxford OX1 3SY, UK

Eleanor Barnes
Department of Hepatology, John Radcliffe Hospital, Headley Way, Headington, Oxford OX3 9DU, UK
Nuffield Department of Medicine, Peter Medawar Building for Pathogen Research, South Parks Road, Oxford OX1 3SY, UK
Oxford NIHR Biomedical Research Centre, John Radcliffe Hospital, Headley Way, Headington, Oxford OX3 9DU, UK

Evan B. Cunningham, Behzad Hajarizadeh, Janaki Amin, Philippa S. Marks, Sophie Quiene, Tanya L Applegate, Gregory J Dore and Jason Grebely
The Kirby Institute, UNSW Sydney, Sydney, NSW, Australia

Olav Dalgard and Håvard Midgard
Akershus University Hospital, Oslo, Norway

Graham R Foster
The Liver Unit, Queen Mary University of London, London, UK

Philip Bruggmann
Arud Centres for Addiction Medicine, Zurich, Switzerland

Brian Conway
Vancouver Infectious Diseases Center, Vancouver, BC, Canada,

Markus Backmund
Ludwig Maximilians-University Munich, Munich, Germany

Geert Robaeys
Department of Gastroenterology and Hepatology, Ziekenhuis Oost Limburg, Genk, Belgium
Department of Hepatology, UZ Leuven, Leuven, Belgium
UHasselt, Hasselt, Belgium

David Shaw
Royal Adelaide Hospital, Adelaide, South Australia, Australia

Adrian Dunlop
School of Medicine and Public Health, University of Newcastle, Newcastle, NSW, Australia

Margaret Hellard
Burnet Institute, Melbourne, VIC, Australia

Julie Bruneau
Research Center, Centre Hospitalier de l'Universite de Montreal (CRCHUM), Montreal, Quebec, Canada

Stefan Bourgeois
Stuivenberg ZNA, Antwerp, Belgium

Maria Christine Thurnheer
Department of Infectious Diseases, Bern University Hospital, University of Bern, Bern, Switzerland

Eric W. Hall and Patrick S. Sullivan
Department of Epidemiology, Emory University Rollins School of Public Health, 1518 Clifton Road, GCR 432, Atlanta, GA 30322, USA

Eli S. Rosenberg
Department of Epidemiology and Biostatistics, University at Albany School of Public Health, 1 University Place, rm 123, Rensselaer, NY 12144, USA

O. S. Moen
Gastroenterology and Nutrition Research Group, Department of Clinical Medicine, UiT The Arctic University of Norway, Tromsø, Norway

L. Bernfort
Department of Medical and Health Sciences, University of Linköping, Linköping, Sweden

H. Kileng, E. J. Paulssen, J. Florholmen and R. Goll
Gastroenterology and Nutrition Research Group, Department of Clinical Medicine, UiT The Arctic University of Norway, Tromsø, Norway
Department of Internal Medicine, Section of Gastroenterology, University Hospital of North Norway, Tromsø, Norway

T. Gutteberg
Research Group for Host-Microbe Interactions, Department of Medical Biology, UiT The Arctic University of Norway, Tromsø, Norway
Department of Microbiology, University Hospital of North Norway, Tromsø, Norway

M. G. Kristiansen
Department of Medicine, Nordland Hospital, Bodø, Norway

L. K. Berg
Department of Medicine, Helgeland Hospital, Mo i Rana, Norway

Mohamed A. Daw and Nadia E. M. Sifennasr
Department of Medical Microbiology &Immunology, Faculty of Medicine, University of Tripoli, CC 82668 Tripoli, Libya

Lutfi A. Buktir Ali
Department of Infectious Disease, Tripoli Medical Centre, Tripoli, CC 82668 Tripoli, Libya

Amina M. Daw
Department of General Medicine, Faculty of Medicine, University of Tripoli, CC 82668 Tripoli, Libya

Aghnyia A. Dau
Department of Surgery, Tripoli Medical Centre, Faculty of Medicine, University of Tripoli, CC 82668 Tripoli, Libya

Mohamed M. Agnan
Department of Toxicology, Faculty of Medical Technology, AlgabalAl-garbi University, Nalut, Libya

Abdallah El-Bouzedi
Department of Laboratory Medicine, Faculty of Biotechnology, Tripoli University, CC 82668 Tripoli, Libya

Vincent Alcazer
Département d'hématologie clinique, Hospices Civils de Lyon, Centre Hospitalier Lyon Sud, 69495 Pierre-Bénite, France
Inserm U1052, Centre de Recherche en Cancérologie de Lyon, 69008 Lyon, France

Patrick Miailhes and Laurent Cotte
Service des maladies infectieuses et tropicales, Hospices Civils de Lyon, Hôpital de la Croix Rousse, 69004 Lyon, France

Christophe Ramière and Caroline Charre
Inserm U1052, Centre de Recherche en Cancérologie de Lyon, 69008 Lyon, France
Laboratoire de virologie, Hospices civils de Lyon, Hôpital de la Croix Rousse, 69004 Lyon, France
INSERM U1111, Centre International de Recherche en Infectiologie, Lyon, France

Truong Tam Nguyen
University of Medicine Pham Ngoc Thach, Ho Chi Minh City, Vietnam
Pathogenesis and Control of Chronic Infections, INSERM, Université de Montpellier, CHU Montpellier, Montpellier, France

Karine Bollore and Edouard Tuaillon
Pathogenesis and Control of Chronic Infections, INSERM, Université de Montpellier, CHU Montpellier, Montpellier, France

Véronique Lemee, Charline Dubos and Jean-Christophe Plantier
Normandie Univ., CHU Rouen, Laboratoire de Virologie, Rouen, France

Hai Vinh Vu
Department of Infectious and Tropical Diseases, Viet Tiep Hospital, Hai Phong, Vietnam

Karine Lacombe
Department of Infectious and Tropical Diseases, Saint-Antoine Hospital, AP-HP, Sorbonne Universités, Université Paris 06, INSERM S 1136, iPLESP, Paris, France

Xuan Lien Truong Thi and Que Anh Luong
Pasteur Institute, Ho Chi Minh City, Vietnam

Huong Duong Thi
Department of Public Health, University of Medicine and Pharmacy, Hai Phong, Vietnam

Didier Laureillard
Pathogenesis and Control of Chronic Infections, INSERM, Université de Montpellier, CHU Nîmes, Montpellier, France

Maud Lemoine
Department of Hepatology, St Mary's Hospital, Imperial College, London, UK

Robin Nesbitt, Nang Thu Thu Kyaw, Elkin Bermudez, Kyi Pyar Soe, Rey Anicete, Phyu Ei Mon, Win Le Shwe Sin Ei, Susannah Christofani and Marcelo Fernandez
MSF-Switzerland, Myanmar Project, #101 Dhama Zedi Road, Kamayut Tsp, Yangon, Myanmar

Iza Ciglenecki
MSF, Geneva, Switzerland

Janet Ousley
MSF-Switzerland, Myanmar Project, #101 Dhama Zedi Road, Kamayut Tsp, Yangon, Myanmar
Medecins Sans Frontiers, 333 7th Avenue, 2nd Floor, New York, NY 10001, USA

Femke Lambers, Wendy van der Veldt and Udi Davidovich
Department of Infectious Diseases, Research and Prevention, Public Health Service of Amsterdam, Amsterdam, the Netherlands

Maria Prins
Department of Infectious Diseases, Research and Prevention, Public Health Service of Amsterdam, Amsterdam, the Netherlands
Department of Infectious Diseases (Centre for Infection and Immunology Amsterdam (CINIMA), Academic Medical Centre (University of Amsterdam), Amsterdam, the Netherlands

Daniel J. Ruzicka and Jumpei Tetsuka
Medical Affairs, MSD K.K, Kitanomaru Square, 1-13-12 Kudan-kita, Chiyoda-ku, Tokyo 102-8667, Japan

Go Fujimoto
Biostatistics and Research Decision Sciences, MSD K.K, Kitanomaru Square, 1-13-12 Kudan-kita, Chiyoda-ku, Tokyo 102-8667, Japan

Tatsuya Kanto
The Research Center for Hepatitis and Immunology Department of Liver Disease, National Center for Global Health and Medicine, 1-7-1 Kohnodai, Ichikawa, Chiba 272-8516, Japan

Humphrey D. Mazigo
Department of Medical Parasitology and Entomology, School of Medicine, Catholic University of Health and Allied Sciences, Mwanza, Tanzania

Stella Kepha
Pwani University, Kilifi 195-80108, Kenya

Godfrey M. Kaatano and Safari M. Kinung'hi
National Institute for Medical Research, Mwanza Research Centre, Mwanza, Tanzania

Index